Clinical Cases in Avian and Exotic Animal Hematology and Cytology

Clinical Cases in Avian and Exotic Animal Hematology and Cytology

TERRY W. CAMPBELL
and
KRYSTAN R. GRANT

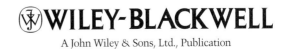

WILEY-BLACKWELL

A John Wiley & Sons, Ltd., Publication

Edition first published 2010
© 2010 Terry W. Campbell and Krystan R. Grant

Blackwell Publishing was acquired by John Wiley & Sons in February 2007.
Blackwell's publishing program has been merged with Wiley's global Scientific,
Technical, and Medical business to form Wiley-Blackwell.

Editorial office
2121 State Avenue, Ames, Iowa 50014-8300, USA

For details of our global editorial offices, for customer services, and for
information about how to apply for permission to reuse the copyright material in
this book, please see our website at www.wiley.com/wiley-blackwell.

Library of Congress Cataloging-in-Publication Data

Campbell, Terry W., 1949-
   Clinical cases in avian and exotic animal hematology and cytology /
Terry W. Campbell and Krystan R. Grant.
      p. ; cm.
   Includes bibliographical references and index.
   Summary: "Clinical Cases in Avian and Exotic Animal Hematology and
Cytology demonstrates how to use hemic cytology and cytodiagnosis as part of
the assessment of an exotic animal patient. The clinical case presentation uses a
hands-on, practical approach to facilitate learning, teaching, and
comprehension. Well-illustrated throughout, each case presents the signalment,
history, and physical exam findings. It then moves on to interpretive discussion
and summarizes how to use the techniques in clinical practice. This book serves
as a helpful guide for exotics veterinarians, zoo and aquarium veterinarians, and
veterinary hematologists"–Provided by publisher.
   ISBN 978-0-8138-1661-6 (hardback : alk. paper)   1. Veterinary
hematology–Case studies.   2. Veterinary cytology–Case studies.
3. Birds–Diseases–Diagnosis–Case studies.   4. Exotic
animals–Diseases–Diagnosis–Case studies.   I. Grant, Krystan R.   II. Title.
   [DNLM: 1. Animal Diseases–diagnosis–Case Reports.   2. Animal
Diseases–therapy–Case Reports.   3. Cytodiagnosis–veterinary–Case Reports.
4. Hematologic Tests–veterinary–Case Reports. SF 771 C174c 2010]
   SF769.5.C36 2010
   636.089'615–dc22   2009045135

A catalog record for this book is available from the U.S. Library of Congress.

Set in 11/12 pt Times by Aptara® Inc., New Delhi, India
Printed in Singapore

Disclaimer

1   2010

CONTENTS

Section 6: Avian Cytology Case Studies

Section 7: Herptile Cytology Case Studies

Section 8: Fish Cytology Case Studies

PREFACE

This book provides representative examples of hematology and cytology cases encountered in exotic animal practice. Cases in the book were selected based on the important role of cytodiagnosis or hematology in the medical management of the exotic animal patient. The cases in the book offer a variety of hematologic and cytodiagnostic interpretations.

Cases representing animals with anemia include blood loss, hemolytic, iron deficiency, Heinz body, and nonregenerative anemia. An example of polycythemia as well as the effects of lead toxicosis on the hemogram is provided. A variety of abnormal leukograms, such as leukocytosis, leukopenia, leukemia, and stress responses, are represented in the text. Representations of normal and abnormal hemic cytologies are provided. These include normal hemic cells, toxic neutrophils and heterophils, left shifts, and leukemia. Blood parasites, such as *Leukocytozoon, Hemoproteus, Plasmodium,* and *Hemogregarine,* and bacteremia are also represented.

Example cases of the basic cytodiagnosis interpretations are also represented. These include normal cytology, inflammation, hyperplasia or benign neoplasia, and malignant neoplasia. Inflammatory lesions are represented by neutrophilic or heterophilic, mixed cell, macrophagic, and eosinophilic inflammation. Along with these inflammatory lesions, a specific etiologic agent, such as bacterial, mycobacterial, fungal, viral, parasitic, or foreign body, is represented. Tissue hyperplasia or benign neoplasia is represented by epithelial hyperplasia, papilloma, adenoma, lipoma, mast cell tumor, and chondroma. Representations of malignant neoplasia include carcinomas, such as undifferentiated carcinoma, adenocarcinoma, and squamous cell carcinoma; sarcomas, such as undifferentiated soft tissue sarcoma, liposarcoma, hemangiosarcoma, and malignant melanoma; and discrete cell neoplasms, such lymphoma, histiocytoma, and mast cell tumor.

Effusions are also represented. These include transudate, modified transudate, exudate, and hemorrhagic effusion. Examples of specific fluid analysis include synovial fluid, such as articular gout and synovial cysts, and a salivary mucocele.

Guideline for Using the Clinical Cases Presented in this Book

This book is offered as a companion to TW Campbell and CK Ellis, *Avian and Exotic Animal Hematology and Cytology,* Ames, Iowa, Blackwell Publishing, 2007, and is designed to assess one's level of knowledge in the use of hematology and cytology in the diagnosis of health disorders involving exotic animal patients. The clinical cases presented were obtained from animal medical records, and each was chosen for its relevant hematology or cytology data. Although not a focus of the book, other clinical data, such as serum or plasma biochemistry profiles (presented in conventional units), imaging, and histology, are also presented with some case studies. Veterinarians, veterinary students, and veterinary technicians in clinical practice will find this additional information useful as an example of how each case was managed medically or surgically. Veterinary clinical pathologists and laboratory technicians will also find this added information beneficial in providing a complete overview of each case. Often the pathologist and laboratory technicians are exposed to only a small part of the clinical cases that they help to manage. Overall, this book is designed to test one's skills in the interpretation of laboratory data and cytology with the added benefit of providing self-assessment material for all aspects in the management of the exotic animal patient.

Results of the serum or plasma biochemistry profiles presented in these case studies were obtained using the Roche Hitachi 911 chemistry analyzer (Roche Diagnostics Corporation, Indianapolis, IN). Study cases that include mammalian blood cell counts were obtained using the Advia® 120 Hematology System (Siemens Medical

Solutions Diagnostics, Tarrytown, NY). Total leukocyte counts from lower vertebrates (birds, reptiles, and fish) in the case studies were obtained by manual methods using either the direct (Natt and Herrick's method) or semidirect (phloxine B method) manual method (Campbell and Ellis, 2007).

The cases are presented in a manner that allows the reader to learn by making his or her own description of microscopic images and interpretation of the data. Following each data set, an interpretive discussion and case summaries are provided to be used by the reader for self-assessment of proficiency in interpretation of the data.

It is possible that one may have managed a case differently from what was described in the text. Each case presented in this book follows the case management as it was described in the medical records including the outcome, when known. Any differences of opinion can be used as a comparison of clinical management styles.

The clinical case studies are organized according to the animal type and diagnostic focus (either hematology or cytology):

Section 1: Mammalian Hematology Case Studies
Section 2: Avian Hematology Case Studies
Section 3: Herptile Hematology Case Studies
Section 4: Fish Hematology Case Studies
Section 5: Mammalian Cytology Case Studies
Section 6: Avian Cytology Case Studies
Section 7: Herptile Cytology Case Studies
Section 8: Fish Cytology Case Studies

The reader should note that the term "herptile" used in the title for Sections 3 and 7 is an arcane lexicon, in this case, a word used only by those who deal with reptiles and amphibians. Thus, reptiles and amphibians are collectively known as herptiles. The term likely comes from the word herpetology, the study of reptiles and amphibians. The term "herp," another arcane lexicon used by this group, refers to an animal that is either a reptile or an amphibian.

The following questions are to be answered by the reader while navigating through the clinical cases and are designed to guide the reader in the management of real-life cases. Many quality reference texts on avian and exotic animal medicine are available to provide the reader with in-depth information on specific aspects in the management of real-life clinical cases and aid the reader in answering these questions:

1. What is the significant historical information needed in order to assess the husbandry provided to the patient? What husbandry advice would you give to the owner of this patient?
2. What historical information is needed in order to assess the cause of the primary complaint?
3. How would one perform a physical examination on this patient?
4. How does one determine the gender in this species?
5. On the basis of the historical information and physical examination findings, what are the likely rule-outs concerning this case?
6. What, if any, diagnostic tests are needed in order to evaluate the patient and arrive at a more definitive rule-out?
7. How would one obtain a blood sample from this patient and how much blood could one safely take? What is the best restraint method in order to do this?
8. What is the best way to handle the blood once it was obtained in order to perform a complete blood cell count and serum/plasma chemistry profile?
9. How would you interpret the complete blood count?
10. How would you interpret the plasma chemistry panel?
11. If needed, how would one obtain the cytologic sample for the assessment of this patient? How would you prepare this sample for cytological evaluation? What stain would you use?
12. How would you interpret the cytologic specimen?
13. How would you restrain and position the patient for a radiographic evaluation?
14. How would you interpret the radiographs, if available?
15. On the basis of the history, physical examination, blood profile, and radiographic evaluation, what is the most likely diagnosis?
16. What would you do next in the management of this case?
17. If needed, how would you anesthetize this patient?
18. If needed, how would you surgically manage this patient? How would you perform a surgical closure in this patient? When should one remove the skin sutures?
19. What instructions would you provide to the client?
20. What is the prognosis for this patient?

ACRONYMS AND ABBREVIATIONS

A/G	Albumin/globulin		MCHC	Mean cell hemoglobin concentration
ALT	Alanine aminotransferase		mCi	Millicuries
AP or ALP	Alkaline phosphatase		MCV	Mean cell volume
AST	Aspartate aminotransferase		M:E	Myeloid–erythroid
BCS	Body condition score		mEq	Milliequivalents
BID	Twice daily		mg	Milligram
BUN	Blood urea nitrogen		Min	Minimum
CBC	Complete blood count		mL	Milliliters
cc	Cubic centimeter		mm	Millimeters
CK	Creatine kinase		MPV	Mean platelet volume
cm	Centimeters		MRI	Magnetic resonance imaging
CNS	Central nervous system		N:C	Nucleus–cytoplasm
CR	Computed radiography		N/L	Neutrophils/lymphocytes
CT	Computed tomography		nmol	Nanomole
dL	Deciliter		Oz	Ounce
DV	Dorsoventral		PCV	Packed cell volume
E-collar	Elizabethan collar		PE	Physical examination
EDTA	Ethylenediaminetetraacetic acid		pmol	Picomole
F	Fahrenheit		PO	Per os
fL	Femtoliters		ppm	Parts per million
FNA	Fine-needle aspirate		ppt	Parts per thousand
Ft	Feet		QID	Four times daily
g	Gram		q 24 hours	Every 24 hours
GFR	Glomerular filtration rate		q 72 hours	Every 72 hours
GGT	γ-Glutamyltransferase		RBC	Red blood cell
GI	Gastrointestinal		RDW	Red cell distribution width
GMS	Gomori methenanime silver		SC	Subcutaneously
Gy	Gray		sp. or spp.	Species
Hb	Hemoglobin		Tc	Technetium
HCO_3	Bicarbonate		Tc-99m HDP	Technetium 99 high-density plasma
IM	Intramuscularly		TIBC	Total iron-binding capacity
IO	Intraosseous		TID	Three times daily
ISIS	International Species Information System		μm	Micron
IU	International units		UIBC	Unsaturated iron-binding capacity
IV	Intravenously		μL	Microliter
kg	kilogram		UV	Ultraviolet
LRS	Lactated Ringer's solution		VD	Ventral–dorsal
Max	Maximum		WBC	White blood cell

Clinical Cases in Avian and Exotic Animal Hematology and Cytology

Section 1
Mammalian Hematology Case Studies

A 6-Year-Old Otter Undergoing a Routine Physical Examination

Signalment

A 6-year-old intact North American male river otter (*Lontra canadensis*) was examined as part of a routine physical examination.

History

The patient was housed with two other male otters of the same age. No significant health problems had been observed in any of the otters. The otters were weighed weekly, and there had been no change in the appetite, behavior, or weight.

Physical Examination Findings

The 10 kg otter appeared healthy on physical examination (Figs. 1.1–1.4 and Tables 1.1 and 1.2).

Other Diagnostic Information

A fecal occult blood was positive; however, no red blood cells or other abnormalities were seen on a fecal cytology.

Whole body ventral–dorsal and lateral radiographs revealed no abnormalities in the abdominal organs. The T14-L1 intervertebral disk space was narrowed with sclerotic end plates and was indicative of spondylosis deformans.

Endoscopic examination revealed evidence of fresh blood in the stomach and small punctate ulcers. Some shrimp tails remained in the stomach several hours after the last meal. The gastric mucosa was irregular, suggesting a possible infection associated with *Helicobacter* sp. The duodenum appeared normal. The esophagus was very long and the pylorus was open and easy to enter. Histopathologic examination of biopsies

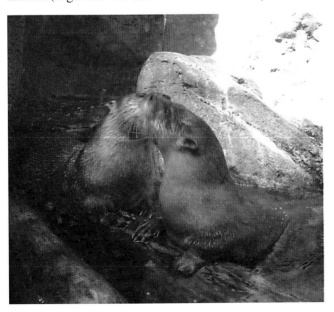

Fig. 1.1. The North American river otter in an exhibit with his cage mate.

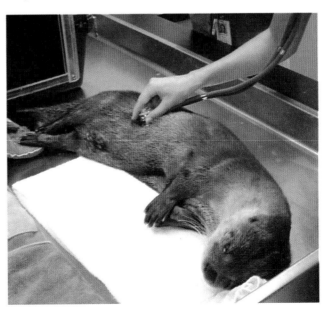

Fig. 1.2. The otter under anesthesia for physical examination and blood collection.

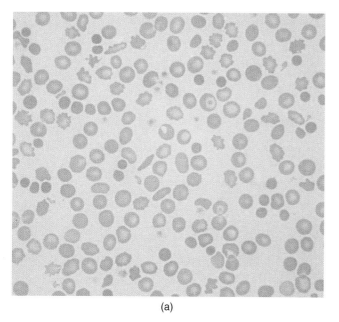

(a)

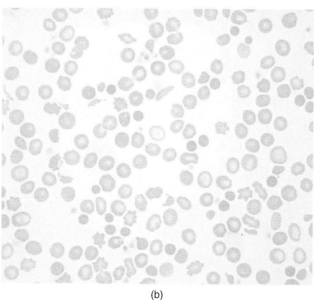

(b)

Fig. 1.3. (a and b) Blood films from an otter (Wright–Giemsa stain, 50×).

taken during the endoscopic examination revealed no abnormalities.

Interpretive Discussion

Figures 1.3 and 1.4 reveal erythrocyte abnormalities. Many of the erythrocytes are hypochromatic as indicated by extended central pallor and thin rim of hemoglobin. There are many keratocytes and schistocytes present. The erythrocytes (blister cells) appear to be developing vacuoles or blisters that enlarge. These blisters eventually break open to form "apple stem cells" and keratocytes. Spiculated erythrocytes (those

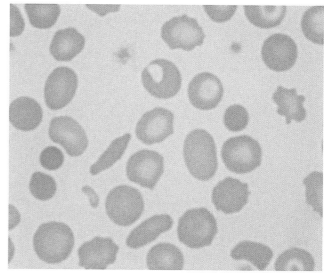

Fig. 1.4. A blood film from an otter (Wright–Giemsa stain, 100×).

with more than two pointed projections) are also seen. The projections fragment from the cells to form the schistocytes.

The packed cell volume (PCV), hemoglobin concentration (Hb), mean cell volume (MCV), and

Table 1.1. Hematology results.

	Day 1	Ranges for otters at aquarium
WBC (10^3/μL)	7.1	2.7–5.3 (3.8)
Neutrophils (10^3/μL)	4.4	1.6–3.9 (2.4)
Neutrophils (%)	62	38–73 (61)
Lymphocytes (10^3/μL)	2.4	0.7–1.6 (1.1)
Lymphocytes (%)	34	16–48 (31)
Monocytes (10^3/μL)	0.2	0–0.2 (0.1)
Monocytes (%)	3	1–5 (2)
Eosinophils (10^3/μL)	0.1	0–0.4 (0.2)
Eosinophils (%)	1	1–8 (4)
Basophils (10^3/μL)	0	0
Basophils (%)	0	0
Plasma protein (g/dL)	7.4	7.4–8.1 (7.7)
RBC (10^6/μL)	11.5	10.9–14.6 (12.3)
Hb (g/dL)	9.9	16.0–19.6 (17.0)
PCV (%)	38	48–60 (52)
MCV (fL)	33.0	39–45 (42)
MCHC (g/dL)	26.0	32–34 (33)
Reticulocytes per microliter		10,910–14,620 (12,673)
Reticulocytes (%)		0.1
RDW	8.8	13.6–18.0 (15.1)
Platelets (10^3/μL)	762	311–474 (371)
MPV (fL)	5.9	6.0–6.9 (6.6)
Clumped platelets	0	0
Keratocytes	Moderate	0
Echinocytes	Few	0 to few
Hypochromasia	Slight	0
Reactive lymphs	Few	0

Table 1.2. Plasma biochemical results.

	Day 1	Ranges for otters at aquarium
Glucose (g/dL)	109	91–136 (114)
BUN (mg/dL)	38	27–43 (36)
Creatinine (mg/dL)	0.4	0.4–0.7 (0.5)
Phosphorus (mg/dL)	4.6	2.2–4.8 (3.6)
Calcium (mg/dL)	8.9	8.5–9.4 (9.0)
Total protein (g/dL)	7.0	6.6–7.4 (7.0)
Albumin (g/dL)	2.9	2.6–3.2 (3.0)
Globulin (g/dL)	4.1	3.6–4.2 (4.0)
A/G ratio	0.7	0.7–0.9 (0.8)
Cholesterol (mg/dL)	177	88–235 (175)
Total bilirubin (mg/dL)	0.1	0.1–0.2 (0.2)
CK (IU/L)	149	148–588 (375)
ALP (IU/L)	61	60–118 (82)
ALT (IU/L)	104	91–127 (112)
AST (IU/L)	122	88–174 (125)
GGT (IU/L)	9	7–14 (10)
Sodium (mg/dL)	147	143–149 (146)
Potassium (mg/dL)	3.7	3.7–4.0 (3.9)
Chloride (mg/dL)	114	107–115 (112)
Bicarbonate (mg/dL)	20.8	17–25 (21)
Anion gap	15	10–20 (16)
Calculated osmolality	300	291–303 (297)
Lipemia (mg/dL)	9	—
Hemolysis (mg/dL)	9	—
Icterus (mg/dL)	0	—

Table 1.3. Plasma iron profile results.

	Day 1	Ranges for otters at aquarium
Iron (µg/dL)	35	112–160 (135)
TIBC (µg/dL)	434	286–409 (320)
Saturation (%)	8	27–58 (44)
UIBC (µg/dL)	399	116–297 (186)

mean cell hemoglobin concentration (MCHC) on the hemogram are decreased, which is indicative of an iron-deficiency anemia. The appearance of microcytic, hypochromic erythrocytes on the blood film is also indicative of an iron-deficiency anemia, a condition that is nearly always caused by chronic blood loss in an adult animal. The positive fecal occult blood is suggestive of gastrointestinal blood loss in this patient; however, the two healthy otters that share his habitat also exhibited positive fecal occult blood tests. Thus, it is likely that the results of the fecal occult blood testing are false-positive owing to the meat diet of the otters. The endoscopic examination suggested the possibility of blood being lost from the upper gastrointestinal tract as would be seen with *Helicobacter* involvement; however, histologic examination of biopsy samples failed to confirm pathology associated with that area (Table 1.3).

Variability in the normal serum iron, total iron-binding capacity (TIBC), and percent saturation of transferrin occurs among mammalian species; however, in general, healthy animals have an average serum iron concentration of 100 µg/dL, a TIBC of 300 µg/dL, and transferrin saturation of 33%. Using these values, this otter patient has a confirmed iron deficiency based on reduced serum iron concentration and transferrin saturation with an increased TIBC.

The platelet count is greater than expected. This is a common finding associated with iron-deficiency anemia in other mammalian species. The exact cause of this is unknown.

The otter had a mild leukocytosis, mature neutrophilia, and lymphocytosis, which are suggestive of a physiological leukocytosis. This is not surprising owing to the nature of capture and delivery of a chemical restraint needed in order to obtain the blood sample.

Summary

The otter underwent a 4-month treatment for a presumed chronic blood loss anemia resulting in the loss of iron from the gastrointestinal tract in association with a *Helicobacter* sp. infection. He was also treated with injectable supplemental iron. Because the otter never appeared weak or ill from his anemia, a reevaluation examination was performed 4 months following the initial examination. The erythrocyte parameters had returned to normal by that time.

A 10-Year-Old Ferret with Lethargy and Anorexia

Signalment

A 10-year-old castrated male Fitch ferret (*Mustela putorius furo*) was presented for anorexia and lethargy (Fig. 2.1).

History

The ferret recently exhibited bouts of intermittent melena. The ferret is housed with two other ferrets that appear healthy. Other pets in the household include two dogs and two cats. The client lives on a small farm where a small number of livestock (cattle and chickens) are kept. The ferrets are fed a commercial kibbled diet.

Physical Examination Findings

A geriatric ferret was 10% dehydrated and was moderately lethargic. A small amount of watery discharge was noted from his left eye. There was also a significant amount of debris in both ears that contained a mixed yeast and bacterial infection based on cytological examination. See Figures 2.2–2.5 and Tables 2.1 and 2.2.

Interpretive Discussion

In Fig. 2.2, the dark tarry stool is representative of melena. Figure 2.3 represents ear mites (*Otodectes*). Figure 2.4 shows the Wright–Giemsa stained blood film, which reveals numerous echinocytes and a schistocyte. An erythrocyte in the center as well as a few others appears to contain a pale structure, suggestive of Heinz bodies. Figure 2.5 shows staining of the blood with a stain used to detect reticulocytes and reveals blue structures within the erythrocytes, indicative of Heinz bodies.

On day 1, the ferret appears to be exhibiting a stress leukogram; however, considering the geriatric status of the ferret, it is also likely that the neutrophils/lymphocytes ratio has changed with age, resulting in decreased lymphocytes and increased neutrophils compared to younger ferrets. The ferret has a significant anemia based on the low PCV, RBC, and hemoglobin concentration. The cause of the anemia is likely in part related to blood loss in the gastrointestinal tract as indicated by melena. The refractometric plasma protein is low, which supports blood loss; however, this finding is not supported by the normal protein or perhaps elevated value found in the biochemical profile. Because the ferret appears clinically dehydrated, the anemia may actually be worse than it appears and the red cell indices and total protein values would expect to decrease with fluid replacement therapy. The anemia may also be related in part to a hemolytic anemia associated with Heinz body formation in the erythrocytes in which a moderate number of large Heinz bodies and a few small Heinz bodies were reported on the hemogram. At this time, the anemia appears to be poorly regenerative as indicated by the lack of a significant polychromasia and reticulocyte count. The platelet count is low owing to either excessive peripheral utilization of platelets associated with gastrointestinal hemorrhage or perhaps as an analytic artifact associated with clumping of platelets as indicated by the interpretation of the blood film. The presence of echinocytes is typically an artifactual finding.

The plasma biochemical profile on day 1 indicates a possible hyperproteinemia with a hyperglobulinemia suggestive of an immune response based on the first set of reference values but not supported by the second set of reference values.

The hemogram on day 6 indicates no significant change in the leukogram; however, there is a marked improvement to the erythrocyte parameters. The ferret is exhibiting a significant regenerative response to his erythrocytes, platelets, and refractometric total protein. He is no longer anemic and appears to be recovering from a blood loss anemia. The unexplained presence of

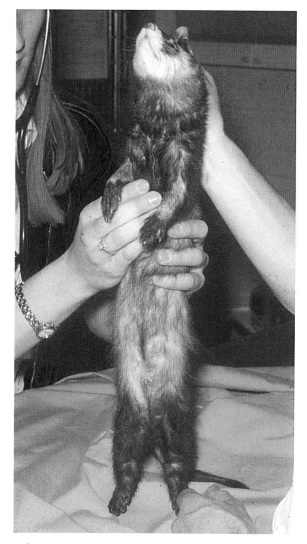

Fig. 2.1. The 10-year-old ferret during physical examination that presented with anorexia and lethargy.

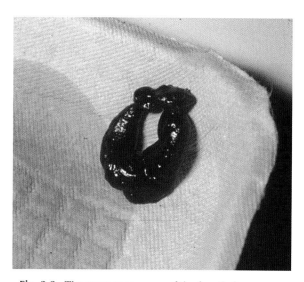

Fig. 2.2. The gross appearance of the ferret's feces.

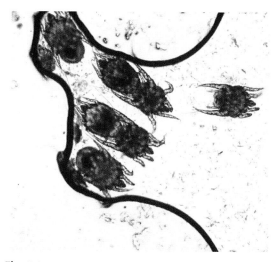

Fig. 2.3. A microscopic image of the material collected from the ferret's ear.

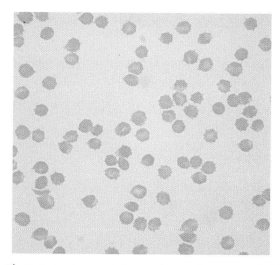

Fig. 2.4. A microscopic image of the erythrocytes on the blood film from the ferret (Wright–Giemsa stain, 100×).

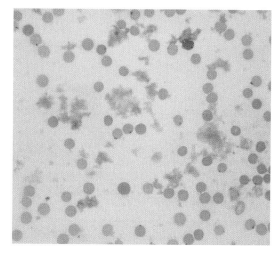

Fig. 2.5. A microscopic image of the erythrocytes on the blood film from the ferret (methylene blue stain, 100×).

Table 2.1. Hematology results.

	Day 1	Day 6	Reference[a]	Reference[b]	Reference[c]
WBC (10^3/μL)	5.2	5.2	4.0–9.0	4.4–19.1	7.7–15.4 (11.3)
Neutrophils (10^3/μL)	4.5	4.6	1.5–3.5	—	—
Neutrophils (%)	86	88	—	11–82	24–78 (40)
Lymphocytes (10^3/μL)	0.6	0.5	0.5–5.0	—	—
Lymphocytes (%)	11	9	—	12–54	28–69 (50)
Monocytes (10^3/μL)	0.2	0.3	0–0.5	—	—
Monocytes (%)	3	3	—	0–9	3.4–8.2 (6.6)
Eosinophils (10^3/μL)	0	0	0–0.5	—	—
Eosinophils (%)	0	0	—	0–7	0–7 (2)
Basophils (10^3/μL)	0	0	0	—	—
Basophils (%)	0	0	—	0–2	0–2.7 (0.7)
Plasma protein (g/dL)	3.5	7.7	5.0–6.5	—	—
RBC (10^6/μL)	3.7	9.4	7.0–11.0	7.3–12.2	—
Hb (g/dL)	7.1	18.1	12–18	16.3–18.2	12.0–16.3 (14.3)
PCV (%)	20	54	35–53	44–61	36–50 (43)
MCV (fL)	54.0	58.0	47–52	—	—
MCHC (g/dL)	36	33.0	33–55	—	—
Reticulocytes per microliter	7,360	46,110	—	—	—
Reticulocytes (%)	0.2	4.9	—	1–12	—
RDW	12.5	12.3	—	—	—
Platelets (10^3/μL)	73.0	475	—	297–730	—
MPV (fL)	9.3	8.5	—	—	—
Clumped platelets	Yes	No	—	—	—
Howell–Jolly bodies	Few	Few	—	—	—
Echinocytes	Moderate	Few	—	—	—

[a]Colorado State University reference ranges.
[b]Fox (1988).
[c]Carpenter (2005).

Table 2.2. Plasma biochemical results.

		Reference[a]	Reference[b]	Reference[c]
Glucose (mg/dL)	132	95–140	94–207	63–134 (101)
BUN (mg/dL)	23	10–26	10–45	12–43 (28)
Creatinine (mg/dL)	0.3	0–0.5	0.4–0.9	0.2–0.6 (0.4)
Phosphorus (mg/dL)	3.8	3.0–5.5	4.0–9.1	5.6–8.7 (6.5)
Calcium (mg/dL)	8.8	8.0–9.7	8.0–11.8	8.6–10.5 (9.3)
Total protein (g/dL)	7.4	5.0–6.4	5.1–7.4	5.3–7.2 (5.9)
Albumin (g/dL)	3.0	2.9–4.1	2.6–3.8	3.3–4.1 (3.7)
Globulin (g/dL)	4.4	1.8–3.0	—	2.0–2.9 (2.2)
A/G ratio	0.7	1.0–2.2	—	1.3–2.1 (1.8)
Cholesterol (mg/dL)	259	70–200	64–296	—
Total bilirubin (mg/dL)	0.3	0–0.3	<1	—
CK (IU/L)	136	80–400	—	—
ALP (IU/L)	25	10–60	9–84	30–120 (53)
ALT (IU/L)	207	80–270	—	82–289 (170)
AST (IU/L)	68	30–75	28–120	—
GGT (IU/L)	5	1–15	—	5
Sodium (mg/dL)	142	147–153	137–162	146–160 (152)
Potassium (mg/dL)	3.5	3.3–4.5	4.5–7.7	4.3–5.3 (4.9)
Chloride (mg/dL)	109	114–120	106–125	102–121 (115)
Bicarbonate (mg/dL)	16.3	15–23	—	—
Anion gap	20	14–21	—	—
Calculated osmolality	28.5	—	—	—
Lipemia (mg/dL)	0	—	—	—
Hemolysis (mg/dL)	13	—	—	—
Icterus (mg/dL)	0	—	—	—

[a]Colorado State University reference ranges.
[b]Fox (1988).
[c]Carpenter (2005).

Heinz bodies in this case has disappeared. Heinz bodies are caused by oxidative damage to hemoglobin. A common cause for this condition in domestic cats is ingestion of onions or onion products. Other plants, such as garlic, *Brassica*, and red maple (*Acer rubrum*) leaves, may also cause Heinz body formation. Drugs such as acetaminophen, phenazopyridine, phenothiazine, and propylene glycol, to name a few, will also cause Heinz body formation. No history of exposure to any of these materials was revealed in this case. Heinz body formation can occur without exposure to oxidant chemicals or drugs with medical conditions, such as lymphoma, diabetes mellitus, and hyperthyroidism.

Summary

The ferret's overall condition improved after 5 days of treatment for *Helicobacter*-induced gastrointestinal ulcers and hemorrhage, which continued for a total of 21 days. This treatment consisted of amoxicillin (20 mg/kg PO BID), doxycycline (5 mg/kg PO BID), omeprazole (0.7 mg/kg PO daily), and sucralfate (25 mg/kg PO every 8 hours). He was also successfully treated for an ear mite infestation using ivermectin (0.3 mg/kg) subcutaneously once every 10 days for three treatments.

A 6-Year-Old Ferret with Anorexia and Lethargy

3

Signalment

A 6-year-old female ferret (*Mustela putorius furo*) was presented for anorexia and lethargy.

History

This adult female ferret had a 2-day history of anorexia. The client had not observed her eating or drinking during this period and reported that the ferret has been sleeping more than usual. The owner did observe that although her stool production was less than normal, it appeared dark. During the past year, the ferret has been given oral melatonin for suspected adrenal disease. The ferret was normally fed a diet of kibbled ferret food.

Physical Examination Findings

The ferret was thin (body score of 3/9) and weighed 500 g. She was lethargic and at least 10% dehydrated. She was weak and reluctant to move. Her body temperature was 98°F and she had tachypnea. Black tarry stools were found adherent to the hair around the anus. A large ulcer was found during examination of the oral cavity. See Figures 3.1 and 3.2 and Tables 3.1 and 3.2 .

Other Diagnostic Findings

A radiographic evaluation of the ferret (Fig. 3.3) indicated a diffuse, unstructured interstitial to alveolar pattern in the caudal dorsal lungs. Because the radiographs were not centered over the thorax, specific thoracic radiographs were recommended for further evaluation. The cardiac silhouette appears to be within normal limits and the pulmonary vasculature appears to be within normal limits. The serosal detail of the abdomen is poor. There is very little falciform fat (back fat), suggesting an overly thin animal. What can be visualized in the abdomen appears to be otherwise normal. On the lateral image, the abdomen appears mildly pendulous. There is a large spleen, although this is typical for a ferret; however, splenomegaly cannot be entirely ruled out. The findings of the thorax and lungs could be indicative of hematogenous pneumonia in the caudal dorsal lungs. Alternatively, diffuse neoplasia cannot be entirely ruled out. Repeat imaging with computed radiography would be recommended to try to further evaluate these caudal dorsal lung lobes. The appearance of the loss of serosal detail in the abdomen could be the result of poor body condition score, although peritoneal effusion or carcinomatosis cannot be entirely ruled out. The remainder of the abdomen is unremarkable. An ultrasound examination was recommended, but declined by the client owing to the cost of the procedure.

Interpretive Discussion

Figure 3.2a shows a marked number of polychromatophilic erythrocytes and echinocytes. Figure 3.2b shows a toxic neutrophil among erythrocytes, exhibiting significant polychromasia. Figure 3.2c shows a monocyte among erythrocytes, exhibiting significant polychromasia and many echinocytes. Figure 3.2d shows a lymphocyte with a moderate amount of dark blue cytoplasm, indicating a reactive lymphocyte as well as a significant polychromasia and many echinocytes.

In general, the hematology of ferrets resembles that of domestic carnivores. In this case, the ferret has a marked regenerative anemia based on the marked polychromasia on the blood film, presence of nucleated erythrocytes, and marked number of reticulocytes. The cause of the anemia is likely to be associated with blood loss as indicated by the low total protein and a low platelet count that indicates excessive consumption of platelets. The blood loss is likely from gastrointestinal

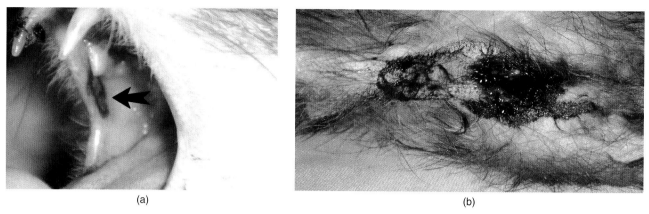

(a)

(b)

Fig. 3.1. The 6-year-old ferret during physical examination that presented with anorexia and lethargy. (a) Oral cavity examination reveals an ulcer (arrow). (b) The Ferret in left lateral recumbency (the tail is on the left side of image and legs are on the right side). Melena seen on perianal region.

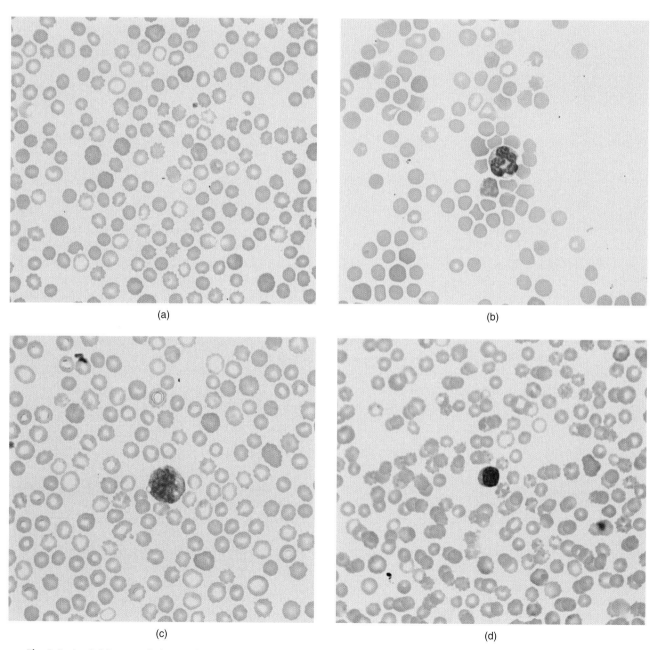

(a)

(b)

(c)

(d)

Fig. 3.2. (a–d) Microscopic images from the blood film (Wright–Giemsa stain, 100×).

Table 3.1. Hematology results.

		Reference[a]	Reference[b]	Reference[c]
WBC ($10^3/\mu L$)	2.4	4.0–9.0	4.4–19.1	2.5–8.6 (5.9)
Neutrophils ($10^3/\mu L$)	1.6	1.5–3.5	—	—
Neutrophils (%)	67	—	11–82	12–41 (31)
Band cells ($10^3/\mu L$)	0	0.5–5.0	0	—
Band cells (%)	1	—	0	0–4.2 (1.7)
Lymphocytes ($10^3/\mu L$)	0.3	0–0.5	—	—
Lymphocytes (%)	14	—	12–54	25–95 (58)
Monocytes ($10^3/\mu L$)	0.1	0–0.5	—	—
Monocytes (%)	4	—	0–9	1.7–6.3 (4.5)
Eosinophils ($10^3/\mu L$)	0	0	—	—
Eosinophils (%)	0	—	0–7	1–9 (4)
Basophils ($10^3/\mu L$)	0	5.0–6.5	—	—
Basophils (%)	0	7.0–11.0	0–2	0–2.9 (0.8)
nRBC ($10^3/\mu L$)	0.3	12–18	0	—
nRBC (%)	14	35–53	0	—
Plasma protein (g/dL)	4.4	47–52	—	—
RBC ($10^6/\mu L$)	6.5	33–55	7.3–12.2	—
Hb (g/dL)	11.1	—	16.3–18.2	15.2–17.4 (15.9)
PCV (%)	34	—	44–61	47–51 (48)
MCV (fL)	53	—	—	—
MCHC (g/dL)	33	—	—	—
Reticulocytes ($10^3/\mu L$)	712	—	—	—
Reticulocytes (%)	11	—	1–12	—
RDW	17.2	—	—	—
Platelets ($10^3/\mu L$)	6.9	—	297–730	—
MPV (fL)	7.9	—	—	—
Polychromasia	Marked			
Howell–Jolly bodies	Few			
Echinocytes	Moderate			

[a]Colorado State University reference ranges.
[b]Fox (1988).
[c]Carpenter (2005).

Table 3.2. Plasma biochemical results.

		Reference[a]	Reference[b]	Reference[c]
Glucose (mg/dL)	88	95–140	94–207	63–134 (101)
BUN (mg/dL)	50	10–26	10–45	12–43 (28)
Creatinine (mg/dL)	0	0–0.5	0.4–0.9	0.2–0.6 (0.4)
Phosphorus (mg/dL)	7.2	3.0–5.5	4.0–9.1	5.6–8.7 (6.5)
Calcium (mg/dL)	8.1	8.0–9.7	8.0–11.8	8.6–10.5 (9.3)
Total protein (g/dL)	4.2	5.0–6.4	5.1–7.4	5.3–7.2 (5.9)
Albumin (g/dL)	2.6	2.9–4.1	2.6–3.8	3.3–4.1 (3.7)
Globulin (g/dL)	1.6	1.8–3.0	—	2.0–2.9 (2.2)
A/G ratio	1.6	1.0–2.2	—	1.3–2.1 (1.8)
Cholesterol (mg/dL)	112	70–200	64–296	—
Total bilirubin (mg/dL)	0.7	0–0.3	<1	—
CK (IU/L)	820	80–400	—	—
ALP (IU/L)	26	10–60	9–84	30–120 (53)
ALT (IU/L)	290	80–270	—	82–289 (170)
AST (IU/L)	346	30–75	28–120	—
GGT (IU/L)	49	1–15	—	5
Sodium (mg/dL)	145	147–153	137–162	146–160 (152)
Potassium (mg/dL)	4.7	3.3–4.5	4.5–7.7	4.3–5.3 (4.9)
Chloride (mg/dL)	115	114–120	106–125	102–121 (115)
Bicarbonate (mg/dL)	12.4	15–23	—	—
Anion gap	22	14–21	—	—
Calculated osmolality	301	—	—	—
Lipemia (mg/dL)	14	—	—	—
Hemolysis (mg/dL)	24	—	—	—
Icterus (mg/dL)	0	—	—	—

[a]Colorado State University reference ranges.
[b]Fox (1988).
[c]Carpenter (2005).

hemorrhage as indicated by the presence of melena on the physical examination.

Neutrophil concentrations are generally higher than lymphocyte concentrations in normal ferrets and they tend to increase in concentration, while lymphocytes decrease in concentration with increasing age. The total leukocyte count of healthy ferrets can be as low as 3,000/μL; therefore, ferrets are unable to develop a marked leukocytosis with inflammatory disease, and concentrations greater than 20,000/μL are unusual and a left shift is rare. In this case, the ferret has a leukopenia with slightly toxic neutrophils and a left shift indicative of a degenerative left shift. She has also a severe lymphopenia.

The increased serum blood urea nitrogen (BUN) concentration can be associated with dehydration, renal failure, or gastrointestinal hemorrhage. The nonexistent creatinine supports the idea of gastrointestinal hemorrhage; however, one must consider that in normal and azotemic ferrets, the plasma creatinine concentration is lower than that in dogs and cats. The mean plasma creatinine concentration of healthy ferrets is 0.4–0.6 mg/dL with a range of 0.2–0.9 mg/dL. As a result, a moderate increase in the plasma creatinine concentration (i.e., 1–2 mg/dL) in a ferret is significant and suggestive of renal disease. This, however, is not an issue in this case.

Evaluation of the liver in ferrets by laboratory testing is the same as that for those in dogs and cats. The plasma alanine aminotransferase (ALT) activity, which appears elevated in this case, is a sensitive and specific test for hepatocellular disease in ferrets. Ferrets with hepatocellular disease commonly have increased aspartate aminotransferase (AST) activity as well. Those with cholestasis likely have increased plasma alkaline phosphatase and γ-glutamyl transferase (GGT) activities. Ferrets rarely become icteric or have plasma bilirubin concentrations greater than 2.0 mg/dL, even when hepatobiliary disease is severe. In this case, the ferret likely has hepatocellular disease.

The causes of hypoproteinemia in ferrets are the same as those in dogs and cats. In this case, it is likely associated with significant blood loss from gastrointestinal hemorrhage.

The prognosis for survival in this ferret based on the physical examination, hemogram, and plasma biochemical profile is poor.

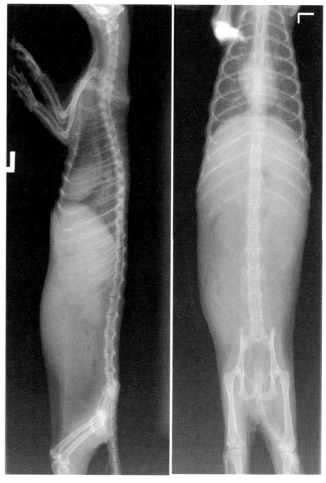

Fig. 3.3. The radiograph of dorsoventral position (right image) and left lateral position (left image).

Summary

The ferret was immediately transferred to the critical care unit for intravenous fluid therapy, correction of hypothermia, and treatment for *Helicobacter*-induced gastrointestinal ulcers. The treatment plan included doxycycline (2.5 mg PO BID), amoxicillin (11 mg PO TID), sucralfate (125 mg PO QID), and two beads from a 20 mg omeprazole capsule (PO daily). The ferret died within 12 hours following presentation. Gross necropsy findings revealed a large perforated ulcer at the gastric pylorus, associated with a marked amount of hemorrhage.

4

A 2-Year-Old Ferret with Weight Loss and Lethargy

Signalment

A 2-year-old castrated male Fitch ferret (*Mustela putorius furo*) was presented for weight loss and lethargy.

History

The ferret was presented with a complaint of weight loss and lethargy despite having a good appetite during the past 11 months. The client recently (within the past 30 days) moved into the area from out of state. There are five other ferrets in the household along with six cats and two dogs. All the pets were healthy except for this ferret. The other ferrets included a 4-year-old castrated male obtained at 8 months of age, a $2^1/_2$-year-old spayed female obtained when she was 8 months of age, a $1^1/_2$-year-old castrated male obtained at 6 months of age, an 8-month-old spayed female obtained at 6 months of age, and a 4-month-old castrated male obtained at $3^1/_2$ months of age. The only vaccination that the ferret had received was a canine distemper vaccine given at the pet store when the ferret was first obtained.

The ferret was seen by a veterinarian 2 months prior to presentation and at the onset of the clinical signs of weight loss and lethargy. A blood profile was part of the medical records that the client accompanied (Tables 4.1 and 4.2). According to the medical records, the only abnormality found on the physical examination was slightly thickened intestines on abdominal palpation. The whole body radiographic images were within normal limits. At that time the ferret weighted 1.1 kg and was treated with amoxicillin (7.5 mg PO BID) and metronidazole (0.5 mg PO BID) for 10 days. According to the medical records, the ferret's overall condition had improved following the antibiotic treatments; however, according to the client, the ferret showed no improvement.

Physical Examination Findings

The 670 g ferret appeared extremely thin (body score of 2/9); otherwise, he was alert, active, and appeared normal with a respiratory rate of 33 breaths/minute and heart rate of 240 beats/minute. Feces passed in the examination room appeared normal, and a cytological examination later revealed normal cytodiagnosis. The ferret was not painful on abdominal palpation and no abnormalities were found.

An abdominal ultrasound examination revealed multiple enlarged cranial mesenteric lymph nodes. The liver was heterogeneous with ill-defined hyperechoic areas in the right quadrant. The appearance of the liver was likely related to benign hyperplasia or possibly an infiltrative process or lymphoma. Although the size and the shape of the kidneys were within normal limits, there was poor corticomedullary distinction on the ultrasound examination. The appearance of the kidneys could be a result of a normal variant, glomerulonephritis, or an infiltrative process. Both adrenal glands were visualized and appeared normal. Likewise, the stomach, spleen, small intestine, and urinary bladder were within normal limits. The multiple enlarged cranial mesenteric lymph nodes correlated with a reactive or neoplastic process; therefore, lymphoma was considered. There was no evidence of abnormalities in the intestinal tract. An ultrasound-guided fine-needle aspiration biopsy of an enlarged mesenteric lymph node was performed to obtain a sample for cytodiagnosis in an effort to evaluate the cause of the lymphadenopathy (Figs. 4.2 and 4.3).

A blood sample was obtained via jugular venipuncture and submitted for a blood profile (Tables 4.1 and 4.2 and Fig. 4.1).

Interpretive Discussion

The blood profile 2 months prior to presentation revealed a marked eosinophilia on the hemogram and a

Table 4.1. Hematology results.

		Two months earlier	Reference[a]	Reference[b]	Reference[c]
WBC (10^3/μL)	9.0	8.9	4.0–9.0	4.4–19.1	7.7–15.4 (11.3)
Neutrophils (10^3/μL)	4.8	2.9	1.5–3.5		—
Neutrophils (%)	53	33		11–82	24–78 (40)
Lymphocytes (10^3/μL)	2.5	2.9	0.5–5.0		—
Lymphocytes (%)	28	33		12–54	28–69 (50)
Monocytes (10^3/μL)	0.7	0.4	0–0.5		—
Monocytes (%)	8	5		0–9	3.4–8.2 (6.6)
Eosinophils (10^3/μL)	1.0	2.3	0–0.5		—
Eosinophils (%)	10	26		0–7	0–7 (2)
Basophils (10^3/μL)	0	0.3	0		—
Basophils (%)	0	3		0–2	0–2.7 (0.7)
Plasma protein (g/dL)	5.1	—	5.0–6.5	—	—
RBC (10^6/μL)	8.99	10.6	7.0–11.0	7.3–12.2	—
Hb (g/dL)	15.6	17.2	12–18	16.3–18.2	12.0–16.3 (14.3)
PCV (%)	45	53	35–53	44–61	36–50 (43)
MCV (fL)	50	50	47–52	—	—
MCHC (g/dL)	35	32	33–55	—	—
Reticulocytes per microliter	17,980	—	—	—	—
Reticulocytes (%)	0.2	—	—	1–12	—
RDW	11.5	—	—	—	—
Platelets (10^3/μL)	482	762	—	297–730	—
MPV (fL)	7.2	—	—	—	—
Clumped platelets	Present	—			

[a]Colorado State University reference ranges.
[b]Fox (1988).
[c]Carpenter (2005).

Table 4.2. Plasma biochemical results.

		Two months earlier	Reference[a]	Reference[b]	Reference[c]
Glucose (mg/dL)	109	114	95–140	94–207	63–134 (101)
BUN (mg/dL)	31	32	10–26	10–45	12–43 (28)
Creatinine (mg/dL)	0.2	0.5	0–0.5	0.4–0.9	0.2–0.6 (0.4)
Phosphorus (mg/dL)	3.3	2.4	3.0–5.5	4.0–9.1	5.6–8.7 (6.5)
Calcium (mg/dL)	8.4	9.2	8.0–9.7	8.0–11.8	8.6–10.5 (9.3)
Total protein (g/dL)	4.2	5.5	5.0–6.4	5.1–7.4	5.3–7.2 (5.9)
Albumin (g/dL)	2.1	3.0	2.9–4.1	2.6–3.8	3.3–4.1 (3.7)
Globulin (g/dL)	2.1	2.5	1.8–3.0	—	2.0–2.9 (2.2)
A/G ratio	1.0	1.2	1.0–2.2	—	1.3–2.1 (1.8)
Cholesterol (mg/dL)	226	279	70–200	64–296	—
Total bilirubin (mg/dL)	0.1	0.1	0–0.3	<1	—
CK (IU/L)	197	150	80–400	—	—
ALP (IU/L)	163	128	10–60	9–84	30–120 (53)
ALT (IU/L)	118	150	80–270	—	82–289 (170)
AST (IU/L)	56	53	30–75	28–120	—
GGT (IU/L)	9	—	1–15	—	5
Sodium (mg/dL)	151	163	147–153	137–162	146–160 (152)
Potassium (mg/dL)	4.4	4.6	3.3–4.5	4.5–7.7	4.3–5.3 (4.9)
Chloride (mg/dL)	121	120	114–120	106–125	102–121 (115)
Bicarbonate (mg/dL)	24.2	—	15–23	—	—
Anion gap	10	—	14–21	—	—
Calculated osmolality	307	—	—	—	—
Lipemia (mg/dL)	0	—	—	—	—
Hemolysis (mg/dL)	0	—	—	—	—
Icterus (mg/dL)	0	—	—	—	—

[a]Colorado State University reference ranges.
[b]Fox (1988).
[c]Carpenter (2005).

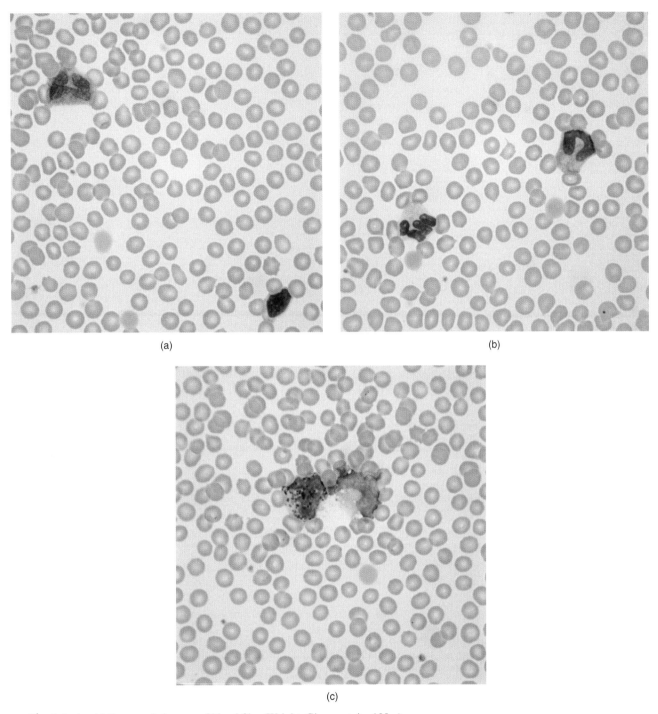

Fig. 4.1. (a–c) Microscopic images of blood film (Wright–Giemsa stain, 100×).

hypophosphatemia and increased plasma alkaline phosphatase on the biochemistry profile. The eosinophilia can be associated with parasitism, hypersensitivity, or inflammation of epithelial surfaces with high mast cell content. The hypophosphatemia is likely related to a dietary deficiency or intestinal malabsorption of phosphorus. Other causes such as an increased cellular up-take of phosphorus when high-energy phosphorylated intermediates are formed or renal tubular phosphate reabsorption are also possible. Alkaline phosphatase is synthesized by the liver, osteoblasts, intestinal epithelium, and renal epithelium; however, the normal alkaline phosphatase activity in the blood of domestic carnivores originates from hepatocytes. Increases in this activity in

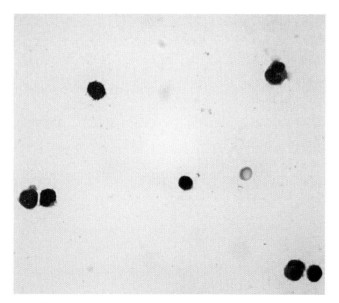

Fig. 4.2. A microscopic image of lymph node aspirate (Wright–Giemsa stain, 100×).

these animals can occur with cholestasis, osteoblastic activity, and a variety of neoplasms.

The current blood biochemistry profile reveals a hypoproteinemia, hypoalbuminemia, and a persistent increase in alkaline phosphatase activity. The hypoalbuminemia with a normal globulin concentration has resulted from either a decrease in albumin production (such as hepatic failure, starvation, intestinal malabsorption, or exocrine pancreatic insufficiency) or a loss of albumin (such as glomerular disease). The hemogram reveals a neutrophilia and a persistent eosinophilia.

Figure 4.1a shows an eosinophil and small mature lymphocyte among normal-appearing erythrocytes. Figure 4.1b shows a neutrophil (leukocyte on the left) and an eosinophil (leukocyte on the right) among normal erythrocytes. Figure 4.1c reveals a basophil and a monocyte.

Figures 4.2 and 4.3 reveal a heterogeneous population of lymphocytes predominated by small, mature lymphocytes. There appears to be a mild increase in the number of eosinophils observed. No microorganisms or evidence of neoplasia is present. Neutrophils and plasma cells are present in low numbers; however, this is not demonstrated in the figures. These findings are

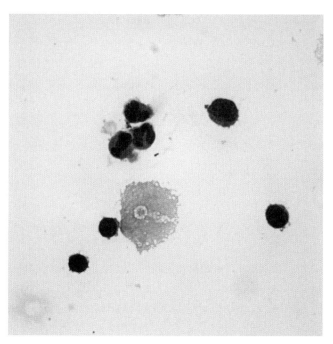

Fig. 4.3. A microscopic image of the moderately cellular lymph node aspirate (Wright–Giemsa stain, 100×).

consistent with a reactive lymph node associated with an increase in the number of eosinophils.

Summary

A presumptive diagnosis for inflammatory bowel disease, specifically an eosinophilic gastroenteritis, was made based on the diagnostic findings. An offer of obtaining a definitive diagnosis by obtaining an intestinal biopsy was declined by the client. Instead, the client elected to try medical treatment for that disease with an assessment of the ferret's response.

The ferret was given oral prednisone (0.9 mg BID) for 30 days. In addition, the client was instructed to change the ferret's diet to a different brand of food. A hypoallergenic diet for ferrets or cats was recommended.

At the 1-month recheck examination, the ferret appeared less thin and weighed 782 g. According to the client, the ferret had regained its normal energy level and was no longer lethargic. The client declined a follow-up blood profile because of the cost of the tests.

A 3-Year-Old Rabbit with Anorexia

Signalment

A 3-year-old intact female domestic rabbit (*Oryctolagus cuniculus*) was presented for anorexia.

History

The rabbit was presented with 3-day duration of anorexia. The normal diet consisted of pellets, vegetables, and fruit (kale, carrots, apple, banana), and a small amount of alfalfa hay given twice weekly. She also received two to three treats daily. She lived with another intact female rabbit in the house, and the owners reported that she was exhibiting increased nesting behavior. According to the client, there were no changes in the home that may have caused a stressful situation that may account for the anorexia. It was also noted that the rabbit produced small, dry, scant feces and was drinking less water than usual.

Physical Examination Findings

On physical examination, the rabbit was bright, alert, and responsive and weighed 2.25 kg. The abdomen was distended and firm. The feces were small, dry, and scant. The heart rate was greater than 200 beats/minute and the respiratory rate was greater than 88 breaths/minute, although this was difficult to assess due to sniffing.

Blood was collected from the left saphenous vein for a complete blood count and diagnostic profile (Tables 5.1 and 5.2 and Figs. 5.1a–5.1d).

Other Diagnostic Information

Radiographs were taken (Figs. 5.2 and 5.3).

The radiographs revealed multiple 3–5 mm in length, smoothly marginated, mineral opaque calculi located in the urinary bladder. There was also an 11 mm in length, oblong, smoothly marginated, mineralized structure located in the fat within the left inguinal region. There was a large amount of fat identified within the midventral abdomen, likely within the broad ligament of the uterus. There was also an ill-defined oblong soft tissue opacity identified on the caudal aspect of this intra-abdominal fat dorsal to the bladder, most likely representing the uterus. The remaining abdominal structures were displaced cranially secondary to the large amount of intra-abdominal fat. The right kidney contained several 3–4 mm in length linear mineral opacities within the renal pelvis and cortex.

The interpretation of the radiographs included multiple cystic calculi and multifocal right renal mineralization consistent with nephroliths or diverticular mineralization. The left inguinal mineralized structure likely represented a benign structure such as mineralized fat. The uterus appeared mildly enlarged, which may be due to hydrometra, mucometra, pyometra, or uterine neoplasia.

Interpretive Discussion

Figure 5.1a shows two heterophils and a basophil. The echinocytes are likely an artifact associated with crenation; however, they have been associated with renal disease and lymphoma in dogs (Thrall, 2004). Figure 5.1b shows an eosinophil and a moderate number of polychromatic erythrocytes. Figure 5.1c shows a lymphocyte and two monocytes. Figure 5.1d shows a heterophil and a giant platelet. The platelets in the background of the images indicate that there is an adequate number.

The hemogram indicates a mild leukocytosis that could be associated with a physiological leukocytosis associated with handling or possible mild inflammation. The heterophil morphology appears normal. Although the rabbit is not anemic, the erythrocytes exhibit a

Table 5.1. Hematology results.

	Results	Reference[a]
WBC ($10^3/\mu$L)	13.6	6.3–11.0
Neutrophils ($10^3/\mu$L)	6.9	1.5–3.2
Lymphocytes ($10^3/\mu$L)	4.9	3.4–7.0
Monocytes ($10^3/\mu$L)	0.8	0.1–0.5
Eosinophils ($10^3/\mu$L)	0.5	0–0.2
Basophils ($10^3/\mu$L)	0.3	0.1–0.4
Plasma protein (g/dL)	7.8	—
RBC ($10^6/\mu$L)	5.87	4–8
Hb (g/dL)	13.1	8–15
PCV (%)	42	30–50
MCV (fL)	72	58–76.2
MCHC (g/dL)	31	29–34
RDW	12.3	—
Platelets ($10^3/\mu$L)	507	290–650
MPV (fL)	7.2	—
Reticulocytes	0.1	—

[a]Campbell and Ellis (2007).

Table 5.2. Plasma biochemical results.

	Results	Reference[a]
Glucose (mg/dL)	219	75–150
BUN (mg/dL)	18	15–30
Creatinine (mg/dL)	2.1	0.8–2.5
Phosphorus (mg/dL)	4.5	2.3–6.9
Calcium (mg/dL)	15.2	8–14
Total protein (g/dL)	7.4	5.4–7.5
Albumin (g/dL)	3.6	2.5–4.5
Globulin (g/dL)	3.8	1.9–3.5
A/G ratio	0.9	—
Cholesterol (mg/dL)	68	35–60
Total bilirubin (mg/dL)	0.1	0–0.75
CK (IU/L)	618	—
ALP (IU/L)	27	4–16
ALT (IU/L)	44	14–80
AST (IU/L)	32	14–113
GGT (IU/L)	4	—
Sodium (mEq/dL)	154	138–155
Potassium (mEq/dL)	4.4	3.7–6.8
Chloride (mEq/dL)	100	92–112
Bicarbonate (mEq/dL)	7.4	16.2–31.8
Anion gap	51	—
Calculated osmolality	313	—
Lipemia (mg/dL)	27	—
Hemolysis (mg/dL)	23	—
Icterus (mg/dL)	0	—

[a]Carpenter (2005).

regenerative response (macrocytosis and moderate poly-chromasia).

The plasma biochemical profile shows hyperglycemia that is likely associated with a stress response and increased corticosteroid release. The high calcium concentration is a common finding in rabbits, especially those with high calcium content in their diet (i.e., alfalfa pellets) as rabbits are highly efficient in extracting calcium from their diet. The low bicarbonate concentration could be compensation for a respiratory alkalosis associated with the rabbit's rapid breathing. The low bicarbonate concentration is also associated with an apparent increase in the anion gap, suggestive of an anion gap acidosis. The number of unmeasured anions in the blood of healthy dogs and cats generally exceeds the number of unmeasured cations by 8–27 mEq/L (Fettman, 2004). This number, however, is likely to be different in the healthy rabbit. A blood gas evaluation is required to better evaluate the acid–base status of this rabbit.

Summary

The rabbit underwent general anesthesia for a cystotomy and ovariohysterectomy. The rabbit was given terbutaline (0.02 mg), glycopyrrolate (0.017 mg), hydromorphone (0.23 mg), and midazolam (0.63 mg) subcutaneously for preanesthetic medications 30 minutes before induction. For induction, she was given ketamine (11.3 mg) and midazolam (0.63 mg) intravenously. Intubation of rabbits is often difficult because of the angle of the pharynx and lack of visualization of the larynx. Intubation of this rabbit proved to be more difficult than expected, but was successful after several attempts.

The rabbit was placed in dorsal recumbency and a 7 cm ventral midline abdominal incision was made caudal to the umbilicus, using a #15 blade. The body wall was opened with a stab incision and the incision was extended cranially and caudally with the blade and then further extended with Metzenbaum scissors.

The urinary bladder was exteriorized and a stay suture was placed near the apex using 4-0 glycomer 631 suture. The urinary bladder was isolated with lap sponges and a 3 cm incision was made. Urine was removed via suction, and an 8 French feeding tube was advanced normograde 8 cm into the bladder and urethra. The bladder and urethra were flushed to dislodge any calculi. Two small pieces, 1 mm in diameter, were recovered. The bladder was closed using a simple continuous full thickness pattern with 5-0 glycomer 631 suture.

The uterus was identified and exteriorized. A mass was identified on the distal right horn (Fig. 5.4). Two encircling ligatures were placed around the left ovarian vessels using 4-0 glycomer 631 suture, and the ovarian pedicle was transected. This was repeated on the right side. Two encircling ligatures were placed around the left and right uterine arteries with 3-0 glycomer 631 suture. Each artery was transected between the ligatures. Two transfixing sutures using 3-0 polytrimethylene carbonate suture were placed in the midbody of the vaginal vault, and forceps were placed distally. The vagina was

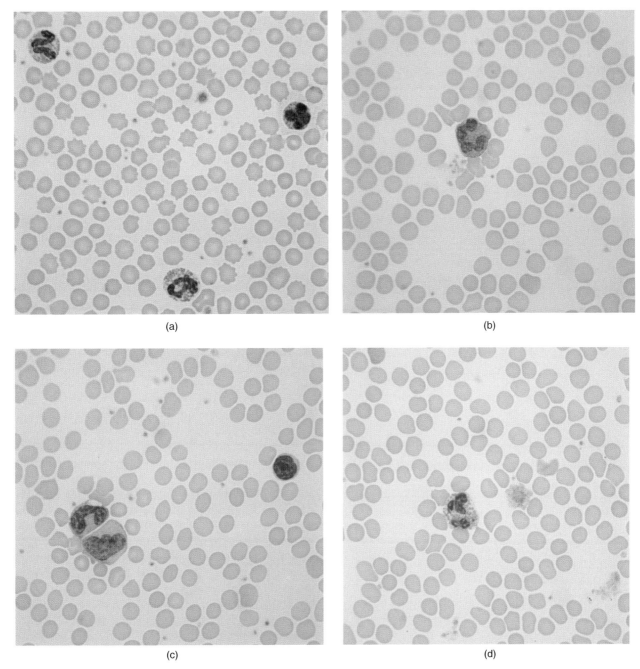

(a)

(b)

(c)

(d)

Fig. 5.1. (a–d) Blood films (Wright–Giemsa stain, 100×).

transected just proximal to the forceps. The reproductive tract was removed and submitted for histopathologic examination.

The body wall was closed with a simple continuous pattern using 3-0 glycomer 631 suture, and the skin was closed with a Ford interlocking pattern using 4-0 nylon suture. Recovery was uneventful.

The rabbit remained hospitalized overnight for observation. The following day the cranial half of the suture line was opened and the rabbit was given midazolam (0.5 mg) and hydromorphone (0.1 mg) in order to re-

pair the dehiscence. The area was prepared for surgery and closed with staples. Other findings on physical examination included increased respiratory sounds over the trachea, clear lung auscultation, and no fecal output. The increased respiratory sounds over the trachea were attributed to the increased difficulty during intubation and presumably laryngeal inflammation. The lack of fecal output was attributed to ileus, likely a result of mild discomfort postoperatively along with the use of opioid medication during anesthesia. Treatment for the postoperative ileus included force feedings with a

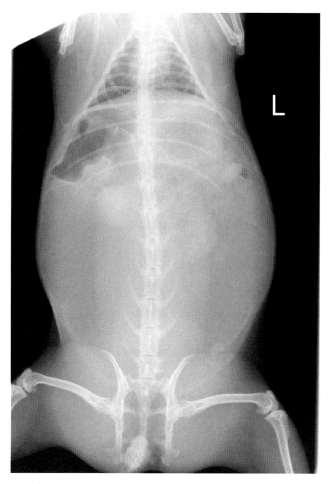

Fig. 5.2. The radiograph (ventrodorsal position).

critical care feed (45 mL PO), subcutaneous fluids (250 mL lactated Ringer's solution), and pain management with meloxicam (0.5 mg/kg PO BID for 5 days). It was also suspected that the meloxicam would resolve the inflammation associated with the larynx.

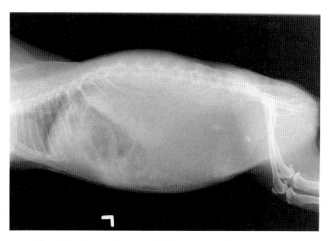

Fig. 5.3. The radiograph (left lateral position).

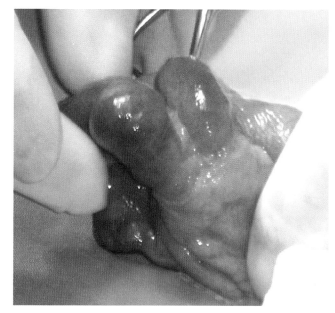

Fig. 5.4. A gross image of the uterus during surgery.

Histology results of the reproductive tract revealed both ovaries expanded by a noncapsulated mass. The mass was composed of sheets of well-differentiated luteal cells. The cells were round to oval with distinct cell borders and a moderate amount of lightly eosinophilic cytoplasm. Nuclei were round with finely stippled chromatin and a single prominent nucleolus. There was some normal-appearing stroma, which contained normal follicular tissue. The right and left uterine horns showed that the endometrium was diffusely expanded by large cystic structures. There was mild smooth muscle hyperplasia and minimal inflammation was present. The diagnosis of the uterus was moderate cystic endometrial hyperplasia, and the right and left ovaries were bilateral luteomas.

The rabbit returned 2 days later due to dyspnea. The owners reported the rabbit had breathing difficulties since they brought her home after surgery, but her condition worsened during the past 24 hours. The rabbit was having difficulty swallowing the medications, and she was still not eating on her own. According to the client, the rabbit appeared more anxious and was producing a small amount of feces and urinating normally. There was no problem with the incision. On physical examination, the rabbit was orthopneic and open-mouth breathing. She was exhibiting an increased inspiratory effort. The respiratory sounds over the trachea were increased with normal lung sounds. The skin over dewlap was fluctuant. The skin incision appeared to be healing. It was suspected that the irritated larynx was edematous and causing her to have difficulty breathing and swallowing. She was given one injection of dexamethasone (0.2 mg/kg IM), one injection of famotidine

(1 mg/kg SC), 250 mL of lactated Ringer's solution subcutaneously, and was sent home with trimethoprim-sulfa (30 mg/kg PO BID for 10 days) and ranitidine (2 mg/kg PO BID for 5 days).

The rabbit worsened over the next 24 hours and returned the following day for euthanasia. When she was presented, she was agonal and the skin around her ventral neck moved synchronously with her difficult breathing pattern. A tracheal rent was suspected. The rabbit was euthanized and submitted for a necropsy.

The necropsy showed that the mucosa of the oral esophagus contained a 0.25 cm × 0.5 cm focal lesion that communicated aborally with at least a 3 cm abscess in the tissue adjacent to the trachea and the esophagus. There was a large amount of thick caseous material in the abscess. The right lung lobe was heavy, dark red, and consolidated. Bilaterally, the kidneys contained multifocal areas of depression that were mottled red and white, ranging in size from 1 to 5 mm. The left kidney had a loss of corticomedullary junction. The lower molars had lingual points ranging in size from 1 to 2 mm. Histopathologically, there was a moderate amount of pulmonary edema and the abscess incorporating the esophagus, and trachea was composed of neutrophils (heterophils), lymphocytes, plasma cells, and a few macrophages. The abscess appeared to be associated with the esophagus and extended into the trachea. The abscess was surrounded by dense fibrous connective tissue. The lesion diagnoses were pneumonia and an esophageal perforation with associated fascial abscesses and communication into the trachea. The esophageal abscess appeared to be a chronic process that most likely was not related to the intubation of the patient according to the pathology report.

A 6-Year-Old Hedgehog with Anorexia and Ataxia

Signalment

A 6-year-old intact African female pygmy hedgehog (*Atelerix albiventris*) was presented for anorexia and ataxia.

History

The client owned the hedgehog for approximately 2 years and thought she was always small and not able to "ball up" all the way. The hedgehog had not been eating well for the past $1^1/_2$ weeks, and according to the clients, she had not eaten anything at all for the past 5 days. It was also noted that she was not drinking as much as usual and was having trouble walking since she had stopped eating. They described the ataxia as wobbling on her hind legs and falling to one side. The hedgehog was also defecating less often and the consistency of her feces had changed from a usually diarrhea-like consistency to a solid.

Her normal diet consisted of hedgehog mix and treats that included pastrami, roast beef, and hardboiled egg yolk. The hedgehog was normally housed in a clear plastic basket, with solid sides containing recycled paper as substrate. She also had a water bowl in the basket and a plastic ball to get around the house, both of which she had not been using much lately.

Physical Examination Findings

The 235 g hedgehog appeared lethargic but alert and responsive. She was thin with a body condition score of 2/5 with a prominent pelvis and spine. She exhibited a plantigrade stance and was reluctant to move. She was ataxic in the hind end when she did walk.

Blood was collected for a complete blood count and diagnostic profile (Figs. 6.1 and 6.2 and Tables 6.1 and 6.2).

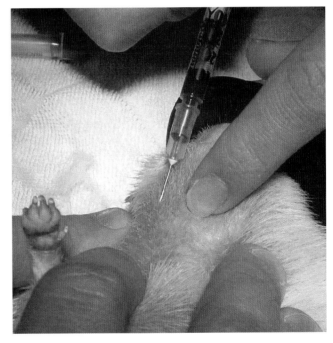

Fig. 6.1. Venipuncture (right jugular vein).

Interpretive Discussion

The images show an eosinophil (Fig. 6.2a), a lymphocyte (Fig. 6.2b), a monocyte (Fig. 6.2c), a basophil (Fig. 6.2d), and neutrophils (Figs. 6.2b–6.2d). The erythrocytes in the images show increased polychromasia, 3+ anisocytosis, spherocytes, and schistocytes. Giant platelets can also be seen.

The hemogram indicates a relative neutrophilia and lymphopenia, indicative of a stress leukogram and normal red blood cell indices. The blood film indicates increased polychromasia and anisocytosis. The appearance of schistocytes suggests intravascular shearing of erythrocytes as would be seen in dogs with vascular neoplasia (hemangiosarcomas), disseminated intravascular coagulopathy, or possibly iron deficiency. Spherocytes

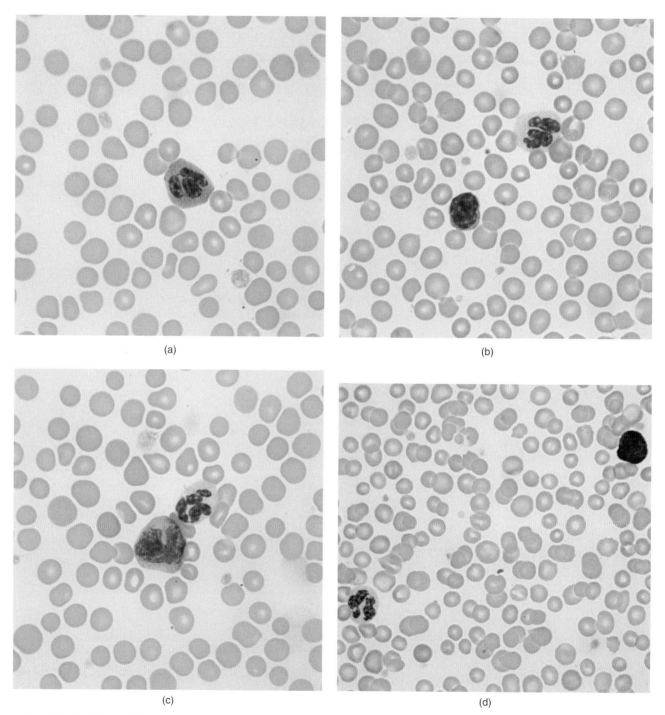

(a)

(b)

(c)

(d)

Fig. 6.2. (a–d) Blood films (Wright–Giemsa stain, 100×).

suggest immune-mediated destruction of erythrocytes (immune-mediated hemolytic anemia). The hedgehog is not currently anemic; therefore, the regenerative appearance of the erythron suggests either recovery from anemia or anemia has yet to occur. A second hemogram in 48 hours would be helpful in evaluation of the erythron.

The plasma biochemistry profile indicates that the hedgehog is in renal failure based on the marked increase in blood urea nitrogen (BUN) and creatinine along with increased phosphorus. The increased plasma aspartate aminotransferase (AST) activity is likely associated with skeletal muscle injury as indicated by the increased plasma creatine kinase (CK) activity.

Table 6.1. Hematology results.

		Reference[a]
WBC ($10^3/\mu$L)	13.1	11 (3–43)
Neutrophils ($10^3/\mu$L)	10.9	5.1 (0.6–37.4)
Neutrophils (%)	83	—
Lymphocytes ($10^3/\mu$L)	0.9	4.0 (0.9–13.1)
Lymphocytes (%)	7	—
Monocytes ($10^3/\mu$L)	0.8	0.3 (0–1.6)
Monocytes (%)	6	—
Eosinophils ($10^3/\mu$L)	0.3	1.2 (0–5.1)
Eosinophils (%)	2	—
Basophils ($10^3/\mu$L)	0.1	0.4 (0–1.5)
Basophils (%)	1	—
Plasma protein (g/dL)	6.8	—
RBC ($10^6/\mu$L)	5.59	6 (3–16)
Hb (g/dL)	11.3	12.0 (7.0–21.1)
PCV (%)	36	36 (22–64)
MCV (fL)	65	67 (41–94
MCHC (g/dL)	31	34 (17–48)
Reticulocytes per microliter	0.1	—
Reticulocytes (%)	1	—
RDW	21.5	—
Platelets ($10^3/\mu$L)	215	226 (60–347)
MPV (fL)	16.2	—

[a]Carpenter (2005).

Table 6.2. Plasma biochemical results.

		Reference[a]
Glucose (mg/dL)	116	89 (59–119)
BUN (mg/dL)	142	27 (13–54)
Creatinine (mg/dL)	4.2	0.4 (0–0.8)
Phosphorus (mg/dL)	9.9	5.3 (2.4–12.0)
Calcium (mg/dL)	9.4	8.8 (5.2–11.3)
Total protein (g/dL)	6.5	5.8 (4.0–7.7)
Albumin (g/dL)	3.1	2.9 (1.8–4.2)
Globulin (g/dL)	3.4	2.7 (1.6–3.9)
A/G ratio	0.9	—
Cholesterol (mg/dL)	124	131 (86–189)
Total bilirubin (mg/dL)	0.1	0.3 (0–1.3)
CK (IU/L)	8,064	863 (333–1964)
ALP (IU/L)	68	51 (8–92)
ALT (IU/L)	61	53 (16–134)
AST (IU/L)	82	34 (8–137)
GGT (IU/L)	7	4 (0–12)
Sodium (mg/dL)	141	141 (120–165)
Potassium (mg/dL)	3.3	4.9 (3.2–7.2)
Chloride (mg/dL)	116	109 (92–128)
Bicarbonate (mg/dL)	6.5	—
Anion gap	22	—
Calculated osmolality	326	—
Lipemia (mg/dL)	6	—
Hemolysis (mg/dL)	16	—
Icterus (mg/dL)	0	—

[a]Carpenter (2005).

Summary

The client elected not to pursue further diagnostic testing or treatment of the hedgehog in the hospital, but wanted to try treatment at home in spite of a poor prognosis for a hedgehog in renal failure. Other rule-outs included a gastric ulcer and possible wobbly hedgehog syndrome, although it was unlikely that this geriatric hedgehog was suffering from wobbly hedgehog syndrome, a neurodegenerative disease of the spinal cord and brain that typically affects hedgehogs less than 3 years of age (Graesser et al., 2006). The hedgehog was treated at home with 7 mL of lactated Ringer's solutions, given subcutaneously twice daily, ranitidine (3 mg/kg PO BID), trimethoprim-sulfa (15 mg/kg PO BID), and aluminum hydroxide (25 mg/kg PO with feeding up to TID). The owners were also instructed to decrease the protein in the diet.

The hedgehog's condition continued to decline and the client returned 6 days later to euthanize her pet. A necropsy was not performed.

A 7-Year-Old Guinea Pig with Anorexia and Decreased Water Intake

Signalment

A 7-year-old castrated male guinea pig (*Cavia porcellius*) was presented with a 3-day history of partial anorexia and decreased water intake (Fig. 7.1).

History

The guinea pig was housed alone in a commercial guinea pig cage kept in a bedroom. He was fed primarily a grass hay diet supplemented with a variety of leafy vegetables and a limited amount of commercial guinea pig pellets. During the past 3 days, the guinea pig was noted to be eating and drinking less and producing fewer than normal feces during that time. The guinea pig had no previous health problems.

Physical Examination Findings

On physical examination, the 698 g guinea pig appeared thin and lethargic. He had a pulse rate greater than 250 beats/minute and a respiratory rate of 32 breaths/minute. His temperature was 100°F. A blood sample was collected via jugular venipuncture and submitted for a complete blood cell count and plasma biochemistry profile (Tables 7.1 and 7.2 and Figs. 7.2a–7.2f).

Interpretive Discussion

Figure 7.2a shows erythrocytes exhibiting a mild anisocytosis. One polychromatic erythrocyte is shown. There are three heterophils exhibiting hypersegmen-

tation of the nucleus. A number of platelets are also present. Figure 7.2b shows a monocyte and four heterophils with nuclear hypersegmentation. A few platelets are present. The erythrocytes show no polychromasia. Figure 7.2c shows a heterophil and an eosinophil. The erythrocytes exhibit no polychromasia and a few platelets can be seen. Figure 7.2d shows a heterophil and a basophil. One polychromatic erythrocyte is seen as well as a few platelets. Figure 7.2e shows a heterophil and two lymphocytes. Two polychromatic

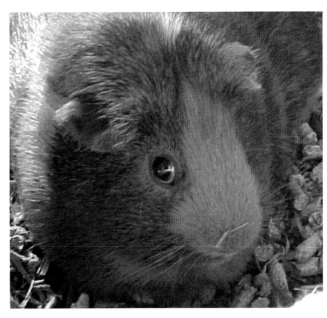

Fig. 7.1. The 7-year-old guinea pig that was presented for partial anorexia.

Table 7.1. Hematology results.

		Reference[a]
WBC ($10^3/\mu$L)	14.0	5.5–17.5
Neutrophils ($10^3/\mu$L)	11.8	—
Neutrophils (%)	84	22–48
Lymphocytes ($10^3/\mu$L)	2.0	—
Lymphocytes (%)	14	39–72
Monocytes ($10^3/\mu$L)	0.1	—
Monocytes (%)	1	1–10
Eosinophils ($10^3/\mu$L)	0.1	—
Eosinophils (%)	0	0–7
Basophils ($10^3/\mu$L)	0	—
Basophils (%)	0	0–2.7
RBC ($10^6/\mu$L)	4.16	3.2–8.0
Hb (g/dL)	10.0	10–17.2
PCV (%)	30	32–50
MCV (fL)	73	71–96
MCHC (g/dL)	33	26–39
Reticulocytes per microliter	—	—
Reticulocytes (%)	—	—
RDW	12.1	—
Platelets ($10^3/\mu$L)	364	260–740
MPV (fL)	7.5	—

[a]Quesenberry et al. (2006).

erythrocytes are seen as well as a few platelets. Figure 7.2f shows a heterophil and a large lymphocyte with a Kurloff body. No polychromatic erythrocytes are seen. A few platelets are present.

The leukogram, which reveals a normal total leukocyte count with a relative heterophilia and lymphopenia, likely reflects a stress response. This is also supported by the appearance of heterophils with nuclear hypersegmentation. A nonregenerative, normocytic, normochromic anemia is indicated by the relative lack of polychromasia in the blood film and the normal mean cell volume (MCV) and mean cell hemoglobin concentration (MCHC). The number of platelets is normal. The erythron, therefore, indicates an anemia associated with either a defective marrow dysfunction or a lack of erythropoietin, which can be associated with renal failure, inflammatory disease (anemia of chronic disorders), or an endocrine disorder, such as hypothyroidism.

Table 7.2. Plasma biochemical results.

		Reference[a]
Glucose (mg/dL)	122	60–125
BUN (mg/dL)	150	9.0–31.5
Creatinine (mg/dL)	2.7	0.6–2.2
Phosphorus (mg/dL)	1.5	3.0–7.6
Calcium (mg/dL)	15.6	8.2–12.0
Total protein (g/dL)	3.5	4.2–6.8
Albumin (g/dL)	1.6	2.1–3.9
Globulin (g/dL)	1.9	1.7–2.6
A/G ratio	0.8	—
Cholesterol (mg/dL)	14	16–43
Total bilirubin (mg/dL)	0.1	0–0.9
CK (IU/L)	672	—
ALP (IU/L)	56	55–108
ALT (IU/L)	29	25–59
AST (IU/L)	58	26–68
GGT (IU/L)	6	—
Sodium (mg/dL)	126	120–152
Potassium (mg/dL)	10.2	3.8–7.9
Chloride (mg/dL)	91	90–115
Bicarbonate (mg/dL)	29.7	—
Anion gap	15	—
Calculated osmolality	314	—
Amylase (IU/L)	6,547	—
Iron (ug/dL)	110	—
Lipemia (mg/dL)	0	—
Hemolysis (mg/dL)	17	—
Icterus (mg/dL)	0	—

[a]Quesenberry et al. (2006).

The plasma biochemical profile reveals a significant azotemia, indicating renal failure. The hypercalcemia and hypophosphatemia are common findings in the blood profile of horses suffering from renal failure (Fettman, 2004). Guinea pigs have hindgut fermentation like the horse; therefore, they likely have a similar physiology. Likewise, a markedly elevated plasma amylase activity (a common finding in dogs with renal failure) is also seen in horses with renal failure and is a logical explanation for the increase in this guinea pig (Lassen, 2004). The hypoalbuminemia with a normal globulin concentration occurs with decreased production or

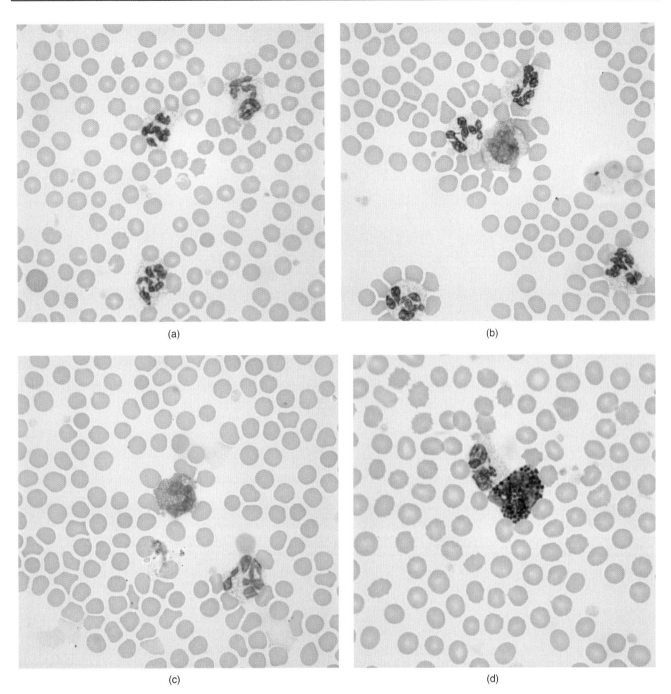

Fig. 7.2. (a–f) Blood films (Wright–Giemsa stain, 100×).

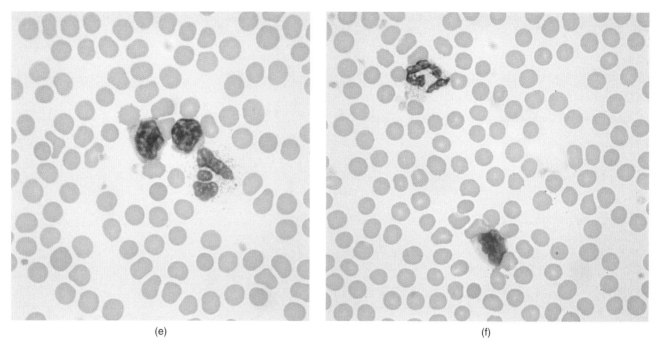

(e)   (f)

Fig. 7.2. (*Continued*)

increased loss of albumin. On the basis of the clinical signs and other plasma biochemical findings, it is likely that the hypoalbuminemia is associated with albumin loss associated with glomerular disease. The hyperkalemia is likely associated with decreased urinary excretion of potassium.

Summary

Because of the poor prognosis of renal failure, the client elected not to pursue further diagnostic testing and treatment. The guinea pig was euthanized; however, no necropsy was performed.

A 3¹/₂-Year-Old Ferret with Lethargy and Weight Loss

Signalment

A 3¹/₂-year-old castrated male ferret (*Mustela putorius furo*) was presented with a history of mild lethargy and weight loss over the past several weeks.

History

The ferret was one of four ferrets in the household. Two of the ferrets were young and newly adopted (as of 1 month prior to the initial presentation of this ferret). The two new ferrets developed a green, mucoid diarrhea soon after arrival. One of the adult ferrets, possibly this ferret, also developed the green diarrhea at the same time. All the ferrets were treated with amoxicillin and metronidazole as part of the supportive care for suspect epizootic catarrhal enteritis. All the ferrets returned to normal after 2 weeks of treatment; however, this patient began to lose weight and became lethargic; therefore, he was presented for evaluation.

Findings from Previous Visits

During physical examination, the ferret was behaving normally and appeared healthy. A small, firm mass in the abdominal cavity was palpated during the examination.

An abdominal ultrasound performed at that time revealed a hypoechoic, well-delineated, 7.9 mm × 5.6 mm, ovoid nodule in the caudal abdomen, presumably within the mesentery. The hypoechoic nodule noted in the caudal mesentery was likely a lymph node, in which case it was mildly enlarged and could be metastatic or reactive in nature. Clinical correlation was recommended. There was mild loss of corticomedullary distinction of the kidneys, bilaterally; however, the kidneys were normal in size and shape. This may be a normal variant; however, mild renal degenerative changes could not be entirely ruled out. The small bowel was noted to be within normal limits. These findings were most consistent with inflammatory bowel disease when correlated with the clinical findings according to the radiologist performing the ultrasonography. A fine-needle aspiration biopsy of the lymph nodes was not obtained at that time because the ferret was not under sedation. Also, it was not indicated at that time because of other diagnostic findings.

The ferret's feces had a "bird seed"-like appearance, which was suggestive of a malabsorption/maldigestion disorder. Furthermore, the cytology of the feces revealed numerous eosinophils, indicating an eosinophilic inflammation. The ferret was treated for eosinophilic gastroenteritis, considered to be an inflammatory bowel disease associated with food allergies. The client was recommended to switch the ferret to another brand of ferret food. The ferret was treated with prednisolone (0.5 mg/kg PO BID) for 14 days.

The ferret returned 2 weeks following initial visit for reevaluation of his gastroenteritis. During that visit, the ferret had lost weight (~10% of the body weight) in spite of having a normal appetite. The client had not switched the ferret to a new food, but had been giving him the prednisolone treatments. Besides appearing thin, the ferret exhibited normal behavior. His feces at that time still had the "bird seed"-like appearance as the previous visit. The client was instructed to return the ferret in 1 month for reevaluation, unless his condition changed.

Physical Examination Findings

The current visit was 1 month following the second visit. The ferret's behavior appeared normal in the examination room; however, the client complained that the ferret was not as active as the other ferrets at home. The ferret had gained a small amount of weight (819 g from a previous 805 g), but still weighed less than he did during his initial visit (860 g). He still produced the

Table 8.1. Hematology results.

		Reference[a]	Reference[b]	Reference[c]
WBC (10^3/μL)	2.7	4.0–9.0	4.4–19.1	7.7–15.4 (11.3)
Neutrophils (10^3/μL)	1.1	1.5–3.5	—	—
Neutrophils (%)	40	—	11–82	24–78 (40)
Lymphocytes (10^3/μL)	1.5	0.5–5.0	—	—
Lymphocytes (%)	54	—	12–54	28–69 (50)
Monocytes (10^3/μL)	0.2	0–0.5	—	—
Monocytes (%)	6	—	0–9	3.4–8.2 (6.6)
Eosinophils (10^3/μL)	0	0–0.5	—	—
Eosinophils (%)	0	—	0–7	0–7 (2)
Basophils (10^3/μL)	0	0	—	—
Basophils (%)	0	—	0–2	0–2.7 (0.7)
Plasma protein (g/dL)	8.3	5.0–6.5	—	—
RBC (10^6/μL)	5.4	7.0–11.0	7.3–12.2	—
Hb (g/dL)	10.1	12–18	16.3–18.2	12.0–16.3 (14.3)
PCV (%)	30	35–53	44–61	36–50 (43)
MCV (fL)	56	47–52	—	—
MCHC (g/dL)	34	33–55	—	—
Reticulocytes per microliter	0	—	—	—
Reticulocytes (%)	0	—	1–12	—
RDW	14.2	—	—	—
Platelets (10^3/μL)	264	—	297–730	—
MPV (fL)	10	—	—	—

[a]Colorado State University reference ranges.
[b]Fox (1988).
[c]Carpenter (2005).

abnormal-appearing feces as during his previous visits. The fecal cytology revealed an increased number of clostridium-like bacteria, but no eosinophils. Enlarged mesenteric lymph nodes were still palpable on physical examination. A blood sample was obtained via jugular venipuncture for a blood profile (Tables 8.1 and 8.2).

A bone marrow aspiration biopsy was performed along with the second hemogram obtained 72 hours following the initial blood profile. The bone marrow sample was obtained while the ferret was under general anesthesia using isoflurane delivered by face mask. The marrow sample was obtained by inserting a 20-gauge spinal needle into the proximal femur and gently aspirating the specimen into the needle's lumen using gentle suction on an attached 3-cc syringe. The bone marrow sample had moderate cellularity. The myeloid cell line was represented by all stages of maturation and appeared to be developing normally. The myeloid/erythroid ratio was 2:1, and 5% of the nucleated cells were small lymphocytes and 2% were plasma cells (Figs. 8.1–8.5).

Interpretive Discussion

Figure 8.1 shows images from the ferret's blood film. Figure 8.1a shows a neutrophil. Figure 8.1b shows an eosinophil. Figure 8.1c shows a cell with a pyknotic nucleus. This cell is likely a monocyte owing to the color

of the cytoplasm. Corticosteroids cause leukocytes to stay in circulation longer resulting in hypersegmentation in neutrophils and cells with pyknotic nuclei. Figure 8.1d shows a lymphocyte. Figure 8.1e shows a monocyte. Figure 8.1f shows a giant platelet.

Figure 8.2 show an image of the blood film stained with a stain designed to reveal reticulocytes. The image shows no reticulocytes are present as indicated in the hemogram report.

The initial hemogram reveals an anemia and leukopenia. The anemia is associated with a macrocytosis based on the increased MCV; however, this is likely not associated with a regenerative response owing to the lack of polychromasia and reticulocytes. The cause of the nonregenerative anemia requires further investigation. The leukopenia and neutropenia are unusual owing to the ferret's corticosteroid treatments. In the dog, a corticosteroid leukogram is generally characterized by a moderate mature neutrophilia, lymphopenia, and eosinopenia (Schultze, 2000). This, however, may not be unusual since healthy ferrets often present with low white blood cells and neutrophil counts. Further investigation into the cause is required to rule out the possibility of neutrophil consumption by inflammatory disease or decreased bone marrow production of neutrophils. A neutropenia with coexisting nonregenerative anemia is suspicious for bone marrow injury.

Table 8.2. Plasma biochemical results.

		Reference[a]	Reference[b]	Reference[c]
Glucose (mg/dL)	118	95–140	94–207	63–134 (101)
BUN (mg/dL)	27	10–26	10–45	12–43 (28)
Creatinine (mg/dL)	0.3	0–0.5	0.4–0.9	0.2–0.6 (0.4)
Phosphorus (mg/dL)	4.6	3.0–5.5	4.0–9.1	5.6–8.7 (6.5)
Calcium (mg/dL)	9.3	8.0–9.7	8.0–11.8	8.6–10.5 (9.3)
Total protein (g/dL)	8.1	5.0–6.4	5.1–7.4	5.3–7.2 (5.9)
Albumin (g/dL)	3.2	2.9–4.1	2.6–3.8	3.3–4.1 (3.7)
Globulin (g/dL)	4.6	1.8–3.0	—	2.0–2.9 (2.2)
A/G ratio	0.7	1.0–2.2	—	1.3–2.1 (1.8)
Cholesterol (mg/dL)	150	70–200	64–296	—
T. Bilirubin (mg/dL)	0.1	0–0.3	<1	—
CK (IU/L)	204	80–400	—	—
ALP (IU/L)	29	10–60	9–84	30–120 (53)
ALT (IU/L)	102	80–270	—	82–289 (170)
AST (IU/L)	60	30–75	28–120	—
GGT (IU/L)	10	1–15	—	5
Sodium (mg/dL)	150	147–153	137–162	146–160 (152)
Potassium (mg/dL)	3.8	3.3–4.5	4.5–7.7	4.3–5.3 (4.9)
Chloride (mg/dL)	117	114–120	106–125	102–121 (115)
Bicarbonate (mg/dL)	20.9	15–23	—	—
Anion gap	15	14–21	—	—
Calculated osmolality	302	—	—	—
Lipemia (mg/dL)	3	—	—	—
Hemolysis (mg/dL)	21	—	—	—
Icterus (mg/dL)	0	—	—	—

[a]Colorado State University reference ranges.
[b]Fox (1988).
[c]Carpenter (2005).

The plasma biochemistry profile reveals hyperproteinemia and hyperglobulinemia, likely indicating an immune response. A protein electrophoresis would aid in determining which specific globulin fractions are elevated.

The repeat hemogram confirmed the nonregenerative anemia, leukopenia, and neutropenia. A hemogram obtained at the same time as the bone marrow aspiration biopsy is necessary for evaluation of the bone marrow cytology.

Figure 8.3 shows images of the bone marrow aspiration biopsy. Figure 8.3a shows a neutrophil and an early eosinophil myelocyte. Figure 8.3b shows a plasma cell, a neutrophil, and a neutrophil metamyelocyte. Figure 8.3c shows three neutrophils, a lymphocyte, an early neutrophil myelocyte, three neutrophil metamyelocytes, an early progranulocyte, and a rubriblast. Figure 8.3d shows three myeloblasts progressing to progranulocytes, two neutrophil metamyelocytes, and a mitotic figure.

Figure 8.4 also shows images of the bone marrow aspiration biopsy. Figure 8.4a shows two neutrophils, three early neutrophil myelocytes, a neutrophil metamyelocyte, a plasma cell, and a prorubricyte. Figure 8.4b shows three neutrophils, two lymphocytes, a neutrophil metamyelocyte, and a neutrophil myelocyte. Figure 8.4c shows a rubriblast, three neutrophils, and a mitotic figure. It is unclear what the vacuolated cell adjacent to the rubriblast might be, but it appears to be in the early myeloid series. Figure 8.4d shows two rubriblasts, a neutrophil, a myeloblast, and two mitotic figures.

Figure 8.5 shows images of the bone marrow sample. Figure 8.5a shows two neutrophils, two band cells, a metamyelocyte, a lymphocyte, a prorubricyte, and a basophilic rubricyte. Figure 8.5b shows four rubriblasts, a neutrophil, a neutrophil early metamyelocyte, and two distorted cells. Figure 8.5c shows a normal progression in the maturation of the neutrophils by showing a myeloblast, a myelocyte, a metamyelocyte, two band cells, and a segmented neutrophil. A lymphocyte and a macrophage exhibiting erythrophagocytosis can also be seen. Figure 8.5d shows a neutrophil, a neutrophil band cell, two lymphocytes, and a macrophage that has phagocytized a cell that appears to be a nucleated erythrocyte.

The bone marrow aspiration biopsy revealed that the myeloid cell line was present at all stages and appeared to be progressing to maturity in an orderly fashion. The erythroid series was well-represented at the early stages (rubriblast and prorubricyte); however,

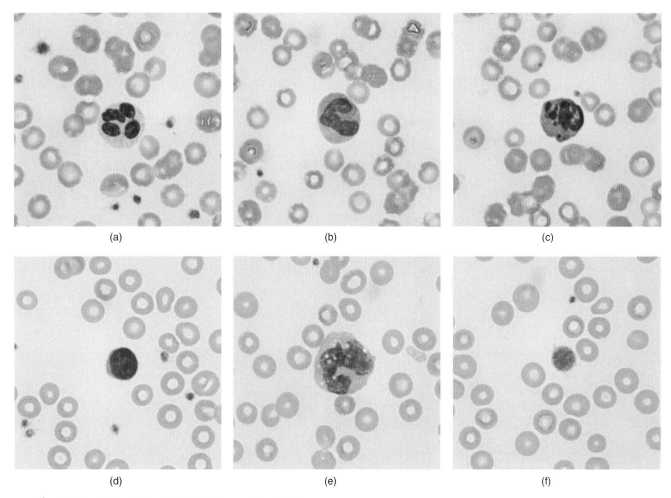

Fig. 8.1. (a–f) Blood films (Wright–Giemsa stain, 100×).

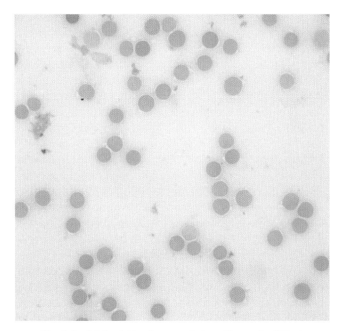

Fig. 8.2. A blood film (new methylene blue stain, 100×).

there were rare cells seen that had progressed further. Small numbers of macrophages containing phagocytized erythrocytes, rubricytes, and leukocytes were noted. The bone marrow indicates an abrupt "maturation arrest" of the erythroid series, which is compatible with immune-mediated clearance of erythroid precursors. The slight decrease in peripheral neutrophil numbers and cytophagia could also be a result of hemophagocytic syndrome secondary to an underlying neoplastic process.

Summary

The ferret was released from the hospital with instructions to continue the prednisolone treatment for the presumed continuation of the eosinophilic gastroenteritis. The client had not changed the ferret's diet as recommended and was asked to do so. The ferret was also treated with metronidazole (25 mg PO BID) for 10 days for the clostridial overgrowth. The results of the blood profile were pending at that time. Once the hemogram

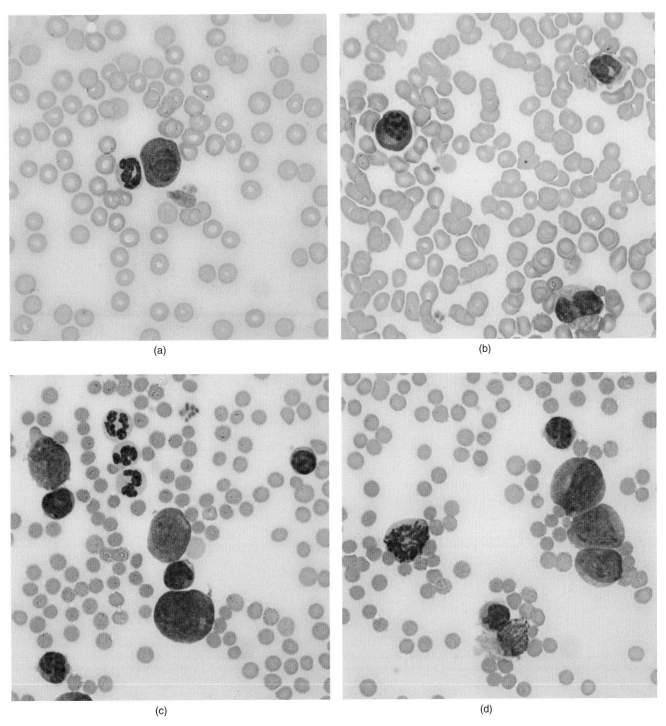

Fig. 8.3. (a–d) The bone marrow aspirate (Wright–Giemsa stain, 100×).

was obtained indicating an anemia with no reticulocytes, the client was asked to return the ferret for a bone marrow evaluation. The bone marrow findings indicated an immune-mediated hemolytic anemia with a maturation arrest of erythrocytes before the metarubricyte stage. This was supported by the presence of macrophages containing phagocytized erythrocytes, rubricytes, and leukocytes. The ferret's oral prednisolone dose was adjusted to from 0.5 to 1.5 mg/kg twice daily to treat this condition.

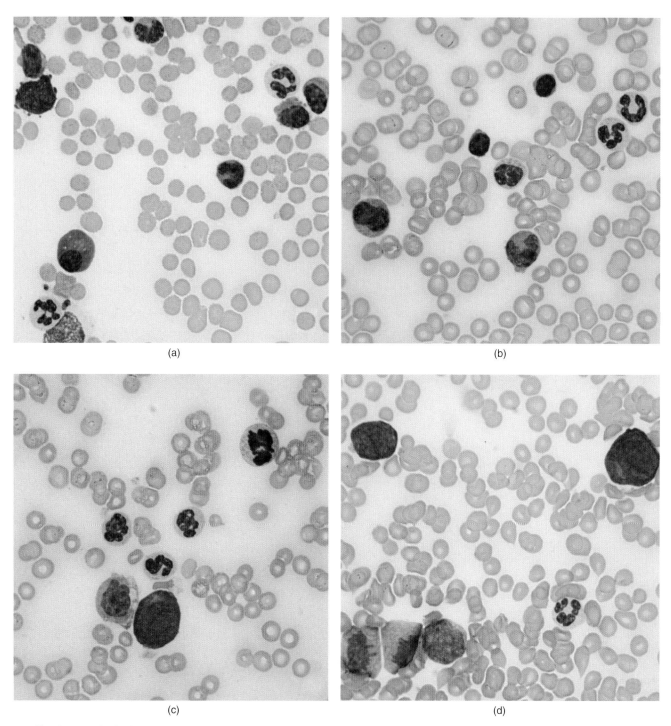

Fig. 8.4. (a–d) The bone marrow aspirate (Wright–Giemsa stain, 100×).

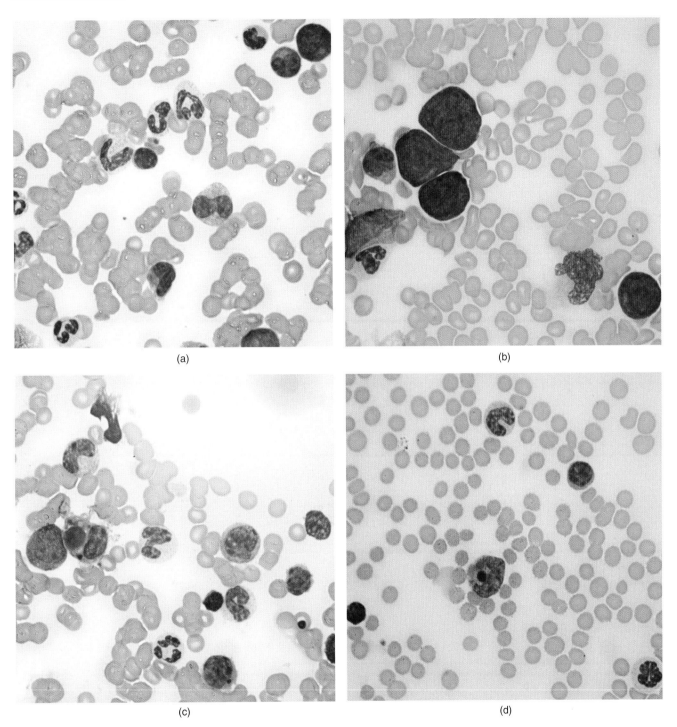

(a)

(b)

(c)

(d)

Fig. 8.5. (a–d) The bone marrow aspirate (Wright–Giemsa stain, 100×).

At the time of this writing, the client was asked to return the ferret for evaluation of the anemia in 5 days. Because there was suspicion that the underlying cause of the inflammatory bowel disease and the immune-mediated disease may be related to a neoplastic condition, evaluation of the mesenteric lymph node by fine-needle aspiration biopsy would be performed at that time.

Section 2
Avian Hematology Case Studies

A 1-Year-Old Parrot with an Acute Onset of Severe Illness

Signalment

A 1-year-old intact male Eclectus parrot (*Eclectus roratus*) was presented with an acute onset of severe illness. The bird appeared normal just 2 hours prior to being found on the floor of the aviary (Fig. 9.1).

History

The bird was housed in a 5 ft × 6 ft cage with five other Eclectus parrots. This cage was inside a larger aviary that at times was open to the public. This bird's wings were clipped so that it could be taken out of its cage for handling. A large number of visitors walked through the aviary the day before presentation, and the bird may have been handled a great deal at that time. The bird had runny droppings, according to the aviculturalist.

Physical Examination Findings

The bird was weak on presentation and unable to hold his head upright in a normal position. He rested his beak on the floor. The bird appeared to be in normal body condition although it weighed 310 g (normal 347–512 g for adult birds). His respiratory rate was rapid at 70 breaths/minute (normal 40–50 breaths/minute), but not labored. The bird demonstrated vertical nystagmus that worsened with positional change of the head. See Figures 9.2–9.4 and Tables 9.1 and 9.2.

Interpretive Discussion

Figures 9.2–9.4a reveal red blood cell agglutination. A marked polychromasia is also shown in the images. Figure 9.4b reveals a binucleated vacuolated lymphocyte and a normal-appearing lymphocyte. Figure 9.4c reveals marked polychromasia and two large lymphocytes. One lymphocyte is vacuolated.

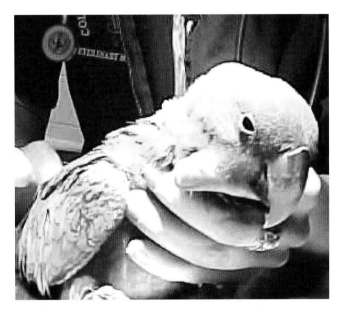

Fig. 9.1. The male Eclectus parrot on presentation.

The erythron reveals a severe regenerative anemia with a positive agglutination that also occurred with exposure to isotonic saline, helping to differentiate agglutination from rouleaux formation. Species-specific antiglobulin reagent (Coomb's serum) is not available for this species; however, a Coomb's test is not indicated owing to the presence of red blood cell agglutination. It is likely that nonpathogenic, naturally occurring cold agglutinin is responsible for the erythrocyte agglutination; otherwise, cold-reactive antibodies would cause red blood cell agglutination of small vessels, causing obstruction and necrosis in the distal extremities that were not observed in this patient.

The leukogram reveals a marked leukopenia with a relative lymphocytosis and monocytosis with heteropenia and immature heterophils. This is indicative of a degenerative left shift. Vacuolated lymphocytes are

45

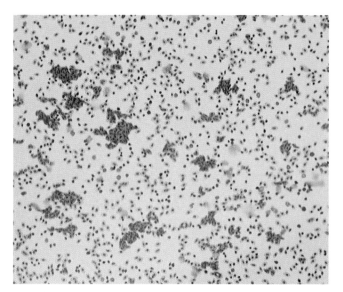

Fig. 9.2. A blood film from the parrot (Wright–Giemsa stain, 10×).

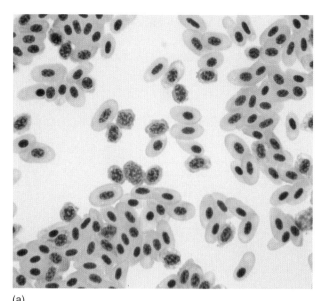

(a)

Fig. 9.4. (a–c) Blood films from the parrot (Wright–Giemsa stain, 100×).

atypical and indicative of either degeneration and/or lymphoid leukemia.

The chemistry profile revealed a marked hypoglycemia that is not compatible with life. This could be a result of a severe septicemia, increased insulin production, hepatic or cardiac failure, or extreme exertion based on the clinical findings. The elevated uric acid value can occur with renal failure, starvation, severe tissue necrosis, or unlikely in this case, postprandial hyperuricemia. The elevated total protein along with marked hypoalbuminemia and hyperglobu-

linemia can occur with either decreased albumin production or increased albumin loss along with increased globulin production. A protein electrophoresis would be beneficial in the evaluation of the gammopathy. Chronic liver disease, lymphoma, and glomerular disease may explain these findings. Except for low bicarbonate suggestive of a metabolic acidosis, the remainder of the chemistry profile appears within normal limits.

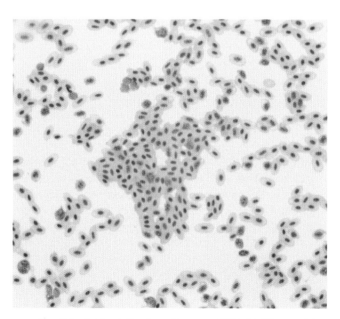

Fig. 9.3. A blood film from the parrot (Wright–Giemsa stain, 50×).

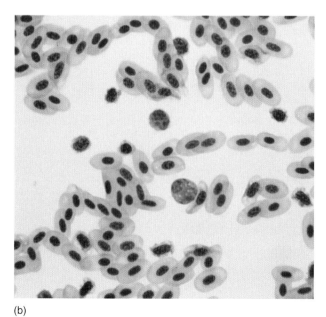

(b)

Fig. 9.4. (*Continued*)

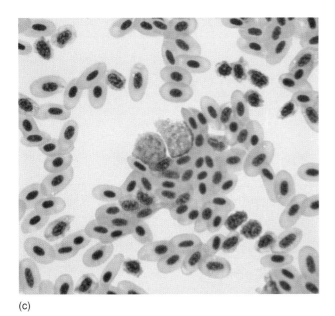

(c)

Fig. 9.4. (*Continued*)

Summary

The bird died within 3 hours of presentation. The gross necropsy revealed an enlarged dark red to black spleen (2 cm diameter) with a gelatinous parenchyma that exuded from the capsule on cut surface. All other organs were found to be within normal limits grossly; however, histopathologic examination revealed multi-centric lymphoma (leukemic stage). Death of this bird was likely caused by bacterial septicemia secondary to lymphoma. A heavy growth of Group B *Salmonella* was isolated from multiple sites. Fluorescent antibody testing of the liver and spleen was negative for *Chlamydophila*.

Table 9.1. Hematology results.

		Reference[a]
PCV (%)	30	45–55
Hb (g/dL)	—	14–16
Erythrocytes (10^6/μL)	—	2.7–3.8
MCV (fL)	—	125–175
MCHC (g/dL)	—	29–32
Leukocytes		
WBC (10^3/μL)	3.5	9.0–20.0
Heterophils (10^3/μL)	0	—
Heterophils (%)	0.75	35–50
Immature (10^3/μL)	0	Rare
Immature (%)	0.25	—
Lymphocytes (10^3/μL)	2.5	—
Lymphocytes (%)	70	45–65
Monocytes (10^3/μL)	1.0	—
Monocytes (%)	28	0–2
Eosinophils (10^3/μL)	0	—
Eosinophils (%)	0	0–1
Basophils (10^3/μL)	0	—
Basophils (%)	1	0–3
Thrombocytes		
Estimated number	Adequate	1–5/1,000× field
Morphology	Normal, clumped	
Plasma protein (refractometry) (g/dL)	5.8	3–5

[a]Campbell and Ellis (2007).

Table 9.2. Plasma biochemical results.

		Reference[a]
Glucose (mg/dL)	12	227–425
BUN (mg/dL)	3	3.0–5.5
Uric acid (mg/dL)	14.3	2.5–11
Total protein (biuret) (g/dL)	5.1	4.0–4.4
Albumin (g/dL)	<1.0	2.3–2.6
Globulin (g/dL)	4.1	1.7–1.8
Aspartate aminotransferase (IU/L)	218	120–370
Creatine kinase (IU/L)	732	100–500
Calcium (mg/dL)	9.2	7.0–13
Phosphorus (mg/dL)	6.1	2.9–6.5
Sodium (mEq/L)	151	130–145
Potassium (mEq/L)	3.2	3.5–4.3
Chloride (mEq/L)	118	100–120
Bicarbonate (mEq/L)	8.6	20–30
Anion gap (calculated)	28	—
Cholesterol (mg/dL)	—	130–350
Calculated osmolality	289	—
Lipemia (mg/dL)	—	—
Hemolysis (mg/dL)	—	—
Icterus (mg/dL)	—	—

[a]Johnston-Delaney and Harrison (1996).

10

A 2-Year-Old Chicken with Lethargy, Inappetence, and Lack of Egg Laying

Signalment

A 2-year-old Ameraucana hen (*Gallus gallus*) was presented with a 2-day history of lethargy, inappetence, and no egg laying (Fig. 10.1).

History

The hen lived in a heated hen house with about 30 other hens. The other hens had been healthy, except for one that died suddenly a week earlier. A necropsy of that hen revealed an ovarian adenocarcinoma. Another hen from the flock started to show the same signs as this hen the morning prior to presentation of this patient.

Physical Examination Findings

On physical examination, the hen appeared to be slightly underweight, lethargic, weak, and fluffed. During the examination, she frequently kept her eyes closed and was reluctant to move. Her droppings revealed a watery yellow urinary component. See Tables 10.1 and 10.2 and Figs. 10.2a and 10.2b.

Interpretive Discussion

Figure 10.2a reveals from top to bottom, a normal heterophil, a basophil, a lymphocyte, and a thrombocyte among the normal-appearing erythrocytes. Figure 10.2b reveals a normal heterophil, a monocyte, and a lymphocyte with normal erythrocytes. Both images suggest an elevated leukocyte count based on the white blood cell density in the oil-immersion images; however, based on published reference values, the total leukocyte count is normal for this species. In other avian species, such as psittacine birds, the total leukocyte count would indicate a moderate leukocytosis. The normal heterophil morphology is important to note, because regardless of the cell count, the presence of heterophils exhibiting toxic changes would indicate a severe inflammatory response. In this case, the slight increase in heterophils with normal morphology is not significant.

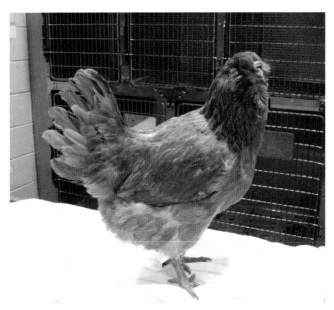

Fig. 10.1. The appearance of the patient on initial physical examination.

49

Table 10.1. Hematology results.

	Day 1	Day 10	Reference[a]
PCV (%)	26	37	22–35
Hb (g/dL)	—	—	7–13
Erythrocytes ($10^6/\mu$L)	—	—	2.5–3.5
MCV (fL)	—	—	90–140
MCH (pg)	—	—	33–47
MCHC (g/dL)	—	—	26–35
Leukocytes			
WBC ($10^3/\mu$L)	21.6	17.4	12.0–30.0
Heterophils ($10^3/\mu$L)	6.5	4.7	3.0–6.0
Heterophils (%)	30	27	—
Bands ($10^3/\mu$L)	—	—	Rare
Bands (%)	—	—	—
Lymphocytes ($10^3/\mu$L)	13.4	11.5	7.0–17.5
Lymphocytes (%)	62	66	—
Monocytes ($10^3/\mu$L)	1.1	0.7	0.1–2.0
Monocytes (%)	5	4	—
Eosinophils ($10^3/\mu$L)	0	0.3	0–1.0
Eosinophils (%)	0	2	—
Basophils ($10^3/\mu$L)	0.6	0.2	Rare
Basophils (%)	3	1	—
Thrombocytes			
Estimated number	Adequate	Adequate	1–5/1,000× field
Morphology	Normal, clumped	Normal	
Plasma protein (refractometry) (g/dL)	8.1	5.5	3–5

[a]Zinkl (1986).

Table 10.2. Plasma biochemical results.

	Day 1	Day 10	Reference[a]
Glucose (mg/dL)	250	—	227–300
BUN (mg/dL)	3.0	—	< 5
Uric acid (mg/dL)	9.6	—	2.5–8.1
Total protein (biuret) (gm/dL)	7.8	5.3	3.3–5.5
Albumin (g/dL)	2.3	1.6	1.3–2.8
Globulin (g/dL)	5.5	3.7	1.5–4.1
Aspartate aminotransferase (IU/L)	363	299	<275
Creatine kinase (IU/L)	510	—	100–500
Calcium (mg/dL)	13.4	—	13.0–23.0
Phosphorus (mg/dL)	3.1	5.5	6.2–7.9
Sodium (mEq/L)	157	—	131–171
Potassium (mEq/L)	3.6	—	3.0–7.3
Chloride (mEq/L)	122	—	100–120
Bicarbonate (mEq/L)	18.1	—	20–30
Anion gap (calculated)	21	—	—
Cholesterol (mg/dL)	176	—	86–211
Calculated osmolality	314	—	—
Lipemia (mg/dL)	0	—	—
Hemolysis (mg/dL)	57	—	—
Icterus (mg/dL)	1	—	—

[a]Johnston-Delaney and Harrison (1996).

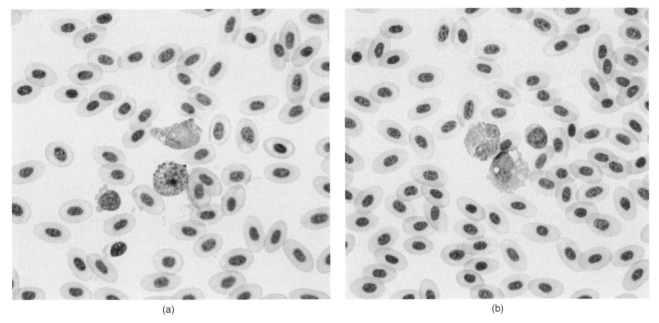

(a)
(b)

Fig. 10.2. (a and b) Blood films from the hen (Wright–Giemsa stain, 100×).

Summary

The yellow urinary component of the droppings found on physical examination could represent bilirubinuria, suggestive of either hepatobiliary disease or hemolysis. Because birds lack biliverdin reductase enzyme in their livers, biliverdin, a green pigment, is their main bile pigment; therefore, hepatobiliary disease or hemolysis would expect to result in green urine. Some birds, however, do produce a yellow urine with these conditions. This is likely caused by posthepatic reduction of biliverdin to bilirubin by other enzymes.

The plasma biochemistry panel revealed a mildly elevated aspartate aminotransferase (AST), which is suggestive of hepatocellular disease; however, this enzyme is not specific for the liver. It is also possible that the elevated AST has resulted from the previous skeletal muscle injury or exertion that has yet to return to normal. The diagnostic testing that may have provided further evidence for hepatobiliary disease that included whole body radiographs, ultrasound, plasma bile acid concentration, and liver biopsy was offered but declined by the client.

The hypophosphatemia is likely the result of poor dietary intake of phosphorus. The hyperproteinemia could be explained by hemoconcentration or inflammation.

The mild heterophilia could represent mild inflammation or a stress response; however, the elevated total protein and globulins likely result from an inflammatory response. A protein electrophoresis that was offered but declined by the client would have added to the understanding of the increased total protein.

Although the packed cell volume (PCV) on day 1 is normal when compared to published values for chickens, this bird would be considered to be moderately anemic when compared to many other species of birds where a PCV less that 35% is generally considered to be low.

A weak presumptive diagnosis of hepatobiliary disease based on the yellow urates and elevated plasma AST was considered. There are many causes of hepatobiliary disease in chickens; however, a viral hepatitis was considered due to a high incidence of chickens in the area with hepatitis caused by an adenovirus according to a local poultry specialist. Also, another chicken in the patient's flock apparently began to show similar symptoms suggestive of a contagious etiology.

Without a definitive or stronger presumptive diagnosis and no specific treatment for the weaker viral hepatitis diagnosis, the chicken was placed on supportive care. The chicken was given subcutaneous fluids and sent home with treatments that included continuation of subcutaneous fluids, an oral antibiotic (trimethoprim-sulfa at 25 mg/kg twice daily), and milk thistle (9 mg given orally once daily). She was to be kept isolated from the other chickens for 10 days when she was to return for reexamination.

An examination of the chicken 9 days later revealed that the bird had greatly improved. Her presenting clinical signs had disappeared 5 days following her initial examination. Plasma chemistries that were abnormal on the initial visit were repeated and demonstrated a return to normal, except for the plasma AST activity, which had dropped, but had not yet returned to normal.

Clinical cases such as this are common in exotic animal practice where clients often decline diagnostic testing, usually because of the cost of the procedures. Evaluation of the blood film alone or in combination with a few other tests often provides valuable information to aid in case management.

11

A 14-Year-Old Macaw with Feather-Picking Behavior and Weight Loss

Signalment

A 14-year-old Blue and Gold macaw (*Ara ararauna*) of unknown gender was presented for a weeklong history of feather picking and weight loss.

History

According to the owner, the bird recovered from liver disease $1^1/_2$ years earlier where she exhibited similar signs to what she was showing now. The client, although she did not weigh the bird, believed the bird had lost weight. The bird was still eating and drinking well except for a decreased appetite for pellets. The macaw also had a history of getting bitten on the left wing by a raccoon a year earlier resulting in limited use of the wing.

Physical Examination Findings

The 825 g macaw appeared bright, alert, and responsive on physical examination. The droppings appeared normal. The bird had picked many of the covert feathers along the breast and under the wings.

The bird was placed under a general anesthetic (isoflurane via face mask) to obtain a blood sample for a blood profile via jugular venipuncture (Tables 11.1 and 11.2 and Figs. 11.1a–11.1c) and whole body radiographs (Figs. 11.2 and 11.3). A second radiographic study using contrast in the gastrointestinal tract was performed 2 hours later when the bird had recovered from the initial anesthetic. This was performed by delivery of 10 mL of a 60% weight by volume suspension of barium via feeding tube into the crop, followed 45 minutes later with acquisition of the radiographic images (Figs. 11.4 and 11.5).

Interpretive Discussion

The hemogram reveals a low packed cell volume (PCV) according to the reference values for macaws;

however, in general, birds have a normal PCV that ranges between 35 and 55%. The leukogram reveals a significant leukocytosis with a heterophilia, relative lymphopenia, and monocytosis. These findings support an inflammatory leukogram and possibly an anemia.

Figure 11.1a shows a heterophil with increased cytoplasmic basophilia indicative of toxicity (1+). The erythrocytes reveal an increase in polychromasia. Figure 11.1b shows two heterophils, one with cytoplasmic basophilia indicating 1+ toxicity and a fragment of cytoplasm from another heterophil. Two lymphocytes (upper left and lower left) are also present. Erythrocytes exhibit increased polychromasia. Figure 11.1c shows a monocyte and erythrocytes showing polychromasia.

Radiographic images (Figs. 11.2 and 11.3) reveal a large soft tissue opaque mass within the coelomic cavity. The mass appears to originate in the caudodorsal portion of the coelomic cavity, causing cranioventral and leftward displacement of the grit-filled ventriculus. Several loops of gas-filled small intestine can be seen protruding to the ventral margin of the coelomic cavity caudal to the keel. The normal reticular pattern of the pulmonary parenchyma can be seen on the lateral view. The examination repeated 45 minutes postadministration of the barium suspension revealed positive contrast within the gastrointestinal tract, being displaced cranially and ventrally by the above-described soft tissue mass. The differentials for this caudal coelomic mass include neoplasia of the kidney, neoplasia of the gonad, or enlargement of the oviduct. This could be better characterized with an ultrasound evaluation.

Summary

Ultrasound evaluation of the liver was performed and the portions visualized were within normal limits. There was a moderate amount of fluid within the coelomic cavity. In the caudal coelomic cavity, there

53

Table 11.1. Hematology results.

		Reference[a]
PCV (%)	41	47–55
Leukocytes		
WBC (10^3/µl)	30.7	7.0–22.0
Heterophils (10^3/µL)	27.0	—
Heterophils (%)	88	40–60
Lymphocytes (10^3/µL)	2.5	—
Lymphocytes (%)	8	35–60
Monocytes (10^3/µL)	1.2	—
Monocytes (%)	4	0–3
Eosinophils (10^3/µL)	0	—
Eosinophils (%)	0	0–1
Basophils (10^3/µL)	0	—
Basophils (%)	0	0–1
Thrombocytes		
Estimated number	Adequate	1–5/1,000× field
Morphology	Normal, clumped	
Plasma protein (refractometry) (g/dL)	3.5	3–5

[a]Campbell and Ellis (2007).

was an echo complex, slightly hyperechoic mass-like lesion. The mass had blood flow primarily around the periphery, although some blood flow was noted within the central portion of the mass. Adjacent to the vascular mass, there was a fluid-filled, tubular-shaped structure with echogenic material in the lumen. The examination was abbreviated due to patient stress. The vascular mass in the caudal abdomen was likely arising from the reproductive tract. The tubular structure with echogenic debris is thought to represent a dilated oviduct with remnants of eggs or neoplastic cells within. Surgical exploration was recommended.

The macaw was anesthetized using atropine (0.03 mg), butorphanol (0.83 mg), and midazolam (0.17 mg) given intramuscularly as preanesthetic agents 10 minutes prior to anesthesia induction with isoflurane. A 4.0 Cole tube was used to intubate the bird for anesthetic maintenance with isoflurane (1–2%).

The bird was placed in dorsal recumbency, and radiocautery was used to create a skin incision extending from the cranial extent of the left pubis to just dorsal to the uncinate process of the left eighth rib. The radiosurgical body wall incision was initiated just caudal to the last rib and extended caudally to the cranial extent of the

Table 11.2. Plasma biochemical results.

		Reference[a]
Glucose (mg/dL)	261	290–750
BUN (mg/dL)	3	—
Uric acid (mg/dL)	7.4	1–6
Total protein (biuret) (gm/dL)	2.9	3.4–4.2
Albumin (g/dL)	0.9	1.3–1.7
Globulin (g/dL)	2.0	1.3–1.9
Aspartate aminotransferase (IU/L)	84	90–180
Creatine kinase (IU/L)	237	180–500
Calcium (mg/dL)	12.7	9.5–10.5
Phosphorus (mg/dL)	4.8	4.6–6.4
Sodium (mEq/L)	140	148–156
Potassium (mEq/L)	2.4	2.2–3.9
Chloride (mEq/L)	97	105–113
Bicarbonate (mEq/L)	32.7	—
Anion gap (calculated)	13	—
Cholesterol (mg/dL)	107	100–300
Calculated osmolality	281	—

[a]Pollack et al. (2005).

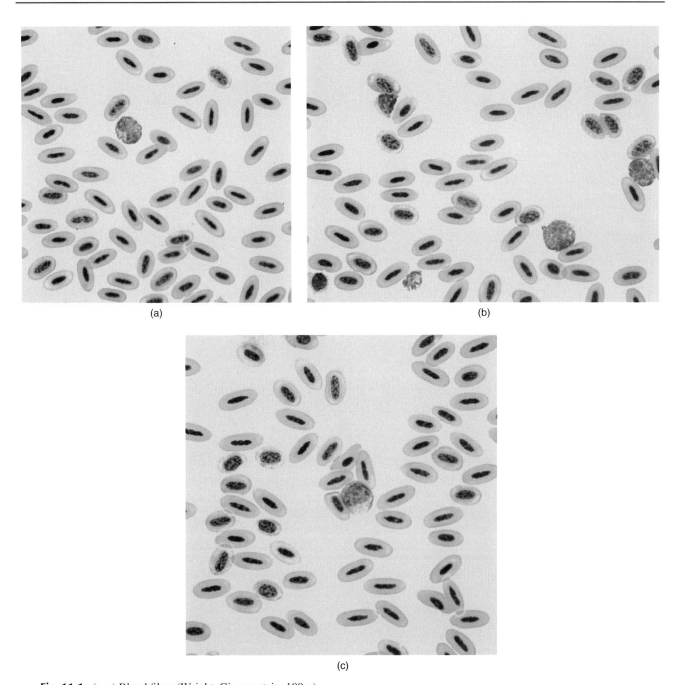

(a)

(b)

(c)

Fig. 11.1. (a–c) Blood films (Wright–Giemsa stain, 100×).

pubis. Radiocautery was also used to incise the skin and body wall from the cranial extent of the previous incision, along the caudal border of the sternum to approximately midline, creating a flap, which was retracted medially and caudally to increase exposure. Exposure was also increased by transection of the last rib using Mayo scissors. Radiosurgery and hemoclips were utilized in transecting the chronically inflamed and highly vascular peritoneum, and in freeing the oviduct from numerous gastrointestinal adhesions. A large (4 cm × 3 cm) mass of suspected yolk material was discovered

free in the ventral coelom and was removed. The oviduct was distended with fluid, fragments of inspissated yolk material, and a second large mass of inspissated yolk material. The ovary appeared small and inactive. The oviduct was elevated from the caudal vena cava, and the dorsal and ventral ligaments as well as the dorsal suspensory ligament were dissected utilizing radiocautery and hemoclips. The left abdominal air sac was entered during the procedure, and suction was utilized to prevent fluid entry into the respiratory tract. An absorbable gelatin compressed sponge and polyanhydroglucuronic

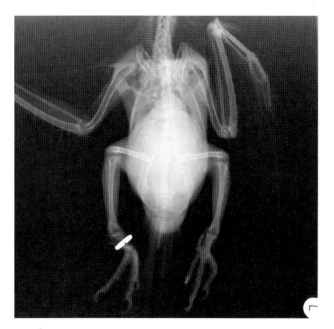

Fig. 11.2. The whole body ventral–dorsal radiograph.

acid were used to control intracoelomic hemorrhage. Two encircling ligatures were placed on the uterus near its entry into the cloaca using a 2-0 polytrimethylene carbonate suture, and the uterus was transected proximally. A 3-0 polytrimethylene carbonate suture was used to close the body wall in a simple continuous pattern, while a 4-0 glycomer 631 suture was used to close the skin in a Ford interlocking pattern. Both the ectopic inspissated yolk material and oviduct and associated material were submitted for histopathologic evaluation.

Histology revealed that the lumen of the oviduct was filled with abundant macrophages, heterophils, and necrotic debris. The mucosal epithelium was intact and

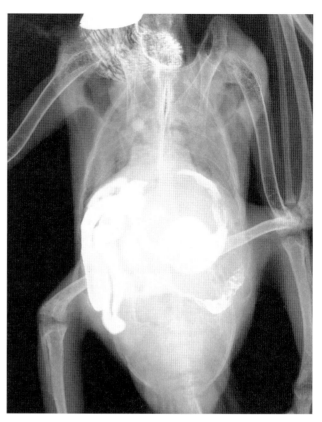

Fig. 11.4. The whole body ventral–dorsal radiograph 45 minutes after delivery of barium sulfate.

the lamina propria contained a moderately increased population of lymphocytes and plasma cells. At the serosal surface, there was accumulation of fibrin, mixed inflammatory cells, and necrotic debris. Histology of the egg revealed necrosis and chronic inflammation with intralesional bacterial colonies. These histologic findings were consistent with a severe chronic-active salpingitis and serositis associated with an ectopic egg.

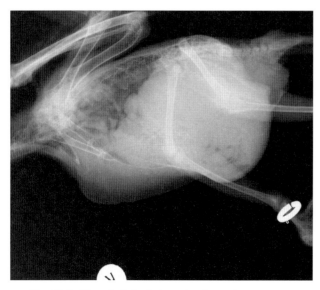

Fig. 11.3. The whole body lateral radiograph.

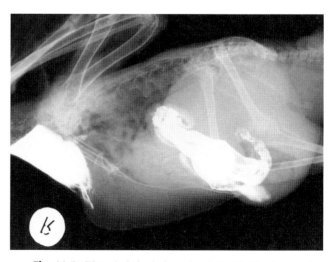

Fig. 11.5. The whole body lateral radiograph 45 minutes after delivery of barium sulfate.

A 14-Year-Old Parrot with Weakness, Anorexia, and Labored Breathing

Signalment

A 14-year-old female Quaker parrot (*Myiopsitta monachus*) was presented for weakness, anorexia, and labored breathing (Fig. 12.1).

History

She was the only bird in the household and was housed in a commercial birdcage. She was fed a seed mixture diet supplemented with fruits and vegetables. The client had been away from home for 3 days and just returned to find the bird weak with labored breathing.

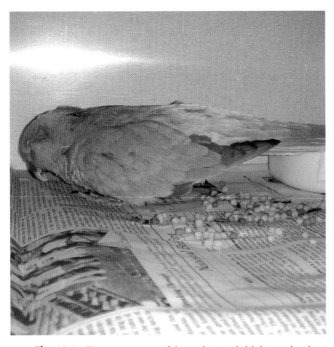

Fig. 12.1. The appearance of the patient on initial examination.

Physical Examination

On initial physical examination, the bird appeared thin and exhibited an increased respiratory effort with prolonged respiratory recovery time. She was placed immediately inside an oxygen cage for respiratory support. As soon as she appeared stable, a quick physical examination was performed and blood was collected via jugular venipuncture for testing (Tables 12.1 and 12.2 and Figs. 12.2a–12.2c).

Table 12.1. Hematology results.

		Reference[a]	Decision level[b]
PCV (%)	74	30–58	35–55
Leukocytes			
WBC (10^3/μL)	14.3	8–17	5.0–20.0
Heterophils (10^3/μL)	9.0	—	2.1–10.0
Heterophils (%)	63	0–24	—
Lymphocytes (10^3/μL)	5.0	—	1.7–10.0
Lymphocytes (%)	35	74–90	—
Monocytes (10^3/μL)	0.3	—	0–0.7
Monocytes (%)	2	1–4	—
Eosinophils (10^3/μL)	0	—	0–0.4
Eosinophils (%)	0	0–2	—
Basophils (10^3/μL)	0	—	0–0.4
Basophils (%)	0	0–6	—
Thrombocytes			
Estimated number	Adequate		1–5/1,000
Morphology	Normal, clumped		× field
Plasma protein (refractometry) (g/dL)	—		3–5

[a]Carpenter (2005).
[b]Decision levels used by authors when reference values are unavailable.

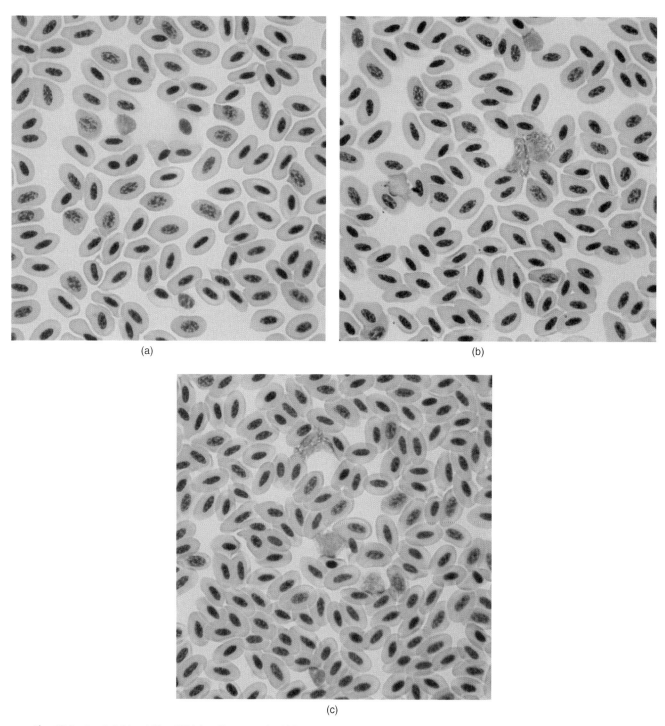

Fig. 12.2. (a–c) A blood film (Wright–Giemsa stain, 100×).

Interpretive Discussion

The hemogram reveals either a relative or an absolute polycythemia (erythrocytosis). The plasma chemistries reveal a mild hypoglycemia and hypophosphatemia that are likely associated with prolonged starvation or anorexia. The increase in the plasma CK

and AST activities are likely associated with skeletal muscle exertion or injury.

Figure 12.2a reveals normal-appearing erythrocytes with a slightly increased degree of polychromasia (8% from the blood film). Figure 12.2b reveals two normal-appearing heterophils and erythrocytes. Figure 12.2c

Table 12.2. Plasma biochemical results.

		Reference[a]	Decision level[b]
Glucose (mg/dL)	194	200–350	200–500
Uric acid (mg/dL)	2.1	3.5–11.5	<15
Total protein (biuret) (g/dL)	—	3.8–5.0	2.5–4.0
Aspartate aminotransferase (IU/L)	300	150–380	<275
Creatine kinase (IU/L)	3269	—	<500
Calcium (mg/dL)	8.7	7–12	8–11
Phosphorus (mg/dL)	3.3	—	5–7
Sodium (mEq/L)	151	—	130–160
Potassium (mEq/L)	3.7	—	2.0–4.0
Bile acid (μmol/L)	35	—	<75

[a]Carpenter (2005).
[b]Decision levels used by authors when reference values are unavailable.

shows a normal heterophil and two small, mature lymphocytes among normal erythrocytes.

Summary

The initial complete blood count revealed a marked increase in the packed cell volume (PCV) and total solid that were too high to be measured. The bird was treated orally with 0.05 mL of 50% dextrose solution for her hypoglycemia. At the same time, 6 mL of lactated Ringer's solution was given subcutaneously. She received more subcutaneous fluids and was fed by gavage a nestling bird diet 4 hours later when she became more stable. A radiographic examination was postponed until she became stronger. An intraosseous catheter was placed in the left ulna for fluid delivery at this time because her overall condition had improved. She spent the night in the critical care unit for monitoring and fluid support. The next morning, she appeared quiet, but was alert and responsive. She also appeared stronger with reduced dyspnea. At this time, her PCV was 44%, supporting the diagnosis of a relative erythrocytosis on presentation. Since her overall condition had improved, radiographs were obtained. The radiographs revealed a slightly larger than pea-sized opacity within the caudal lungs, suggesting the possible presence of a granuloma (fungal or bacterial) or neoplasia. Additional diagnostic testing that included a tracheal wash for cytology and culture, laparoscopy with possible biopsy for histology and culture, or an MRI was offered. Later that day, the bird was taken off the oxygen support for 20 minutes to evaluate her ability to breathe and recover without oxygen supplementation. Although she maintained a slightly increased respiratory rate, the lack of oxygen did not exacerbate the respiratory effort. The client elected to take the bird home for monitoring and nursing care to return the next day for further diagnosis. The client did not return for the scheduled appointment because the bird was behaving normally at home. It was discovered that the bird had been deprived of food and water for 3 days while her owner was out of town.

A 4-Year-Old Parrot with Anorexia, Weakness, and Lethargy

13

Signalment

A 4-year-old male Eclectus parrot (*Eclectus roratus*) was presented with anorexia, weakness, and lethargy.

History

This bird was a chronic feather picker and had been picking his feathers for the past 4 years. During the past 2 years, the bird was examined every 6 months. The examinations included blood profiles, whole body radiographs, and skin biopsy histology. All tests had been within normal limits. A laparoscopic examination performed 2 years prior revealed no gross abnormalities. Based on these findings, the feather-picking disorder was considered to result from a behavior disorder that started when the client and the bird moved into a new house just prior to the onset of the feather-picking behavior. The bird was fed a commercial pelleted diet for psittacines supplemented with fruits, vegetables, beans, corn, rice, pasta, nuts, and occasional sunflower seeds. He was the only bird in the household. He did not respond to various treatments for the feather-picking behavior that included amitriptyline and acupuncture therapy.

Physical Examination Findings

The bird was extremely weak on presentation and was poorly responsive. He was given a poor prognosis for survival. The bird weighed 350 g (during the past 2 years, his body weight would fluctuate between 340 and 370 g). Very few feathers were present on the bird's body and wings and mostly head feathers remained. There were a few wing feathers present in various stages of growth. A blood sample was obtained via jugular venipuncture for blood profiling (Tables 13.1 and 13.2 Fig. 13.1).

Table 13.1. Hematology results.

		Reference[a]	Reference[b]
PCV (%)	51	45–55	45–50
Leukocytes			
WBC ($10^3/\mu$L)	17.5	9.0–20.0	8.1–11.4
Heterophils ($10^3/\mu$L)	14.0	—	5.1–7.4
Heterophils (%)	80	35–50	63–65
Lymphocytes ($10^3/\mu$L)	2.5	—	3.0–3.5
Lymphocytes (%)	14	45–65	31–37
Monocytes ($10^3/\mu$L)	0.5	—	0–0.3
Monocytes (%)	3	0–2	0–3
Eosinophils ($10^3/\mu$L)	0.4	—	0
Eosinophils (%)	2	0–1	0
Basophils ($10^3/\mu$L)	0.2	—	0–0.1
Basophils (%)	1	0–3	0–1
Thrombocytes			
Estimated number	Adequate	1–5/1,000 × field	1–5/1,000 × field
Morphology	Normal, clumped		
Plasma protein (refractometry) (g/dL)	3.6	3–5	4.7–5.3

[a]Campbell and Ellis (2007).
[b]Ranges from three previous blood profiles from wellness examinations.

Interpretive Discussion

The hemogram reveals a mild leukocytosis with a heterophilia, lymphopenia, and mild monocytosis and eosinophilia. This likely reflects a stress leukogram.

Figure 13.1a reveals three normal heterophils and two thrombocytes. Two erythrocytes exhibiting polychromasia can be seen.

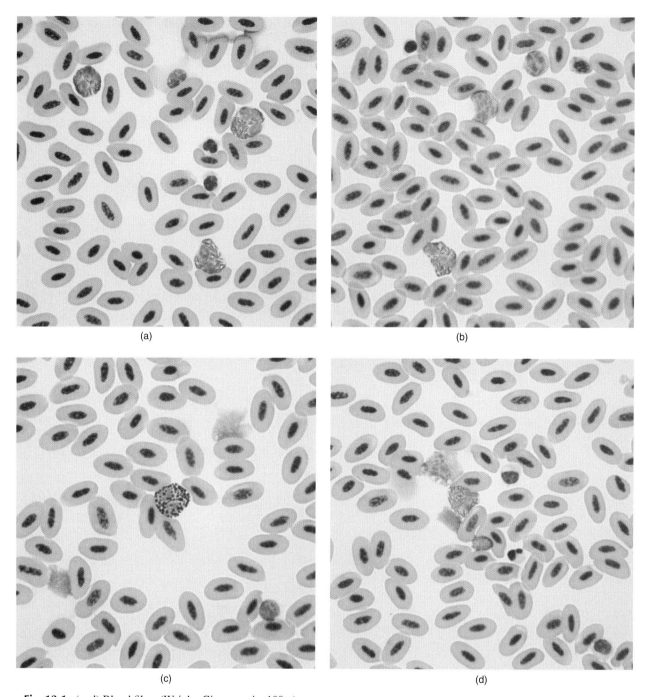

(a)   (b)

(c)   (d)

Fig. 13.1. (a–d) Blood films (Wright–Giemsa stain, 100×).

Figure 13.1b shows a normal heterophils and two lymphocytes. This image shows little polychromasia.

Figure 13.1c reveals a basophil and two polychromatic erythrocytes.

Figure 13.1d shows a heterophil, a monocyte with a vacuolated cytoplasm, and three thrombocytes. There is little polychromasia present.

The plasma biochemical profile reveals a severe hypoglycemia, one that is not compatible with life. The bird also has hypoproteinemia and hypoalbuminemia, although a protein electrophoresis may provide better clarification of the status of albumin. The plasma creatine kinase is elevated, indicating skeletal muscle involvement. The low bicarbonate value reflects the metabolic component of the acid–base status of the bird and likely indicates a metabolic acidosis rather than compensation for a respiratory alkalosis as the bird was breathing normally.

Table 13.2. Plasma biochemical results.

		Reference[a]	Reference[b]
Glucose (mg/dL)	105	220–284	227–425
BUN (mg/dL)	3.0	1.0–4.0	3.0–5.5
Uric acid (mg/dL)	5.3	2.1–5.5	2.5–11
Total protein (biuret) (gm/dL)	2.3	3.9–4.2	4.0–4.4
Albumin (g/dL)	0.9	1.4	2.3–2.6
Globulin (g/dL)	1.4	2.5–2.8	1.7–1.8
Aspartate aminotransferase (IU/L)	125	120–170	120–370
Creatine kinase (IU/L)	813	219–525	100–500
Calcium (mg/dL)	8.2	8.1–8.7	7.0–13
Phosphorus (mg/dL)	4.9	1.6–5.5	2.9–6.5
Sodium (mEq/L)	154	152–155	130–145
Potassium (mEq/L)	4.0	2.4–4.0	3.5–4.3
Chloride (mEq/L)	118	116–120	100–120
Bicarbonate (mEq/L)	14.4	15.2–20.0	20–30
Anion gap (calculated)	26	23–26	—
Cholesterol (mg/dL)	—	375	130–350
Calculated osmolality	301	299–303	—
Lipemia (mg/dL)	0	—	—
Hemolysis (mg/dL)	42	—	—
Icterus (mg/dL)	4	—	—

[a]Ranges from three previous blood profiles from wellness examinations.
[b]Johnston-Delaney and Harrison (1996).

Summary

The bird was hospitalized for fluid support via an intraosseous catheter, treatment for hypoglycemia, and antibiotics for possible infection. The bird died within 12 hours of presentation and was submitted for necropsy. The gross necropsy findings revealed a slightly thickened crop wall. The mucosa of the proventriculus was pale, rough in texture, and proliferative with prominent irregular folds.

Histopathologic examination revealed patchy congestion of the spleen, marked autolysis of the duodenum, cloacal, and lower gastrointestinal tract. The liver exhibited diffuse congestion. Multiple 0.5 to 1.0 mm tubular nematode parasites were present in the submucosa of the proventriculus. These parasites had a distinct body cavity with prominent reproductive organs and a thick connective tissue outer capsule. They were surrounded by a keratinizing proventricular epithelial layer. The proventriculus exhibited a mild hyperkeratosis. The pathological diagnosis was proventricular mucosal hyperplasia, associated with nematodiasis and severe feather picking. The proventricular nematodes were likely to be either a *Spiroptera* sp. or a *Dispharynx* sp.

An Adult Vulture with Generalized Weakness

14

Signalment

An adult Turkey vulture (*Cathartes aura*) was presented for generalized weakness (Fig. 14.1).

History

An adult Turkey vulture was presented to a local raptor rehabilitation facility. It was one of several birds that had recently returned to their summer roost in early spring. This bird was found lying on the ground apparently unable or unwilling to move. The bird was easily approached and captured.

Physical Examination Findings

The bird was presented with generalized weakness. It sat with its feet clenched. The bird was in excellent body condition and there was no indication of trau-

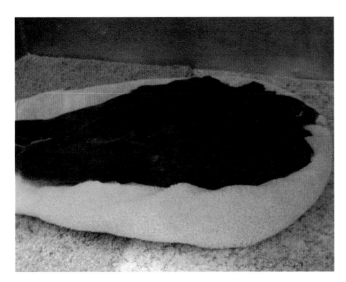

Fig. 14.1. The Turkey vulture with generalized weakness.

matic injury. A blood sample was obtained by venipuncture of the basilic vein for hematology (Table 14.1 and Fig. 14.2).

Interpretive Discussion

The hemogram indicates a mild to moderate leukocytosis with a marked heterophilia and slight to moderate monocytosis. The packed cell volume (PCV) and plasma total protein are normal. These findings indicate an inflammatory leukogram predominated by a heterophilia without an associated anemia, suggesting this is an acute response.

Figure 14.2 reveals two heterophils and a thrombocyte. The remainder of the cells are represented by erythrocytes, mature erythrocytes, and rubricytes. There are nine rubricytes in the image. Basophilic rubricytes have dark blue cytoplasm (the round erythroid cell in the center). Early polychromatic rubricytes have a gray cytoplasm owing to an increased hemoglobin concentration (the four round erythroid cell at the top of the image). Rubricytes represent approximately 10% of the erythrocyte population. The number of cells is inappropriate in regard to the normal PCV and lack of polychromatic erythrocytes.

The presence of rubricytes in a nonanemic bird and absence of significant polychromasia are suggestive of lead poisoning; however, myelodysplasia or myeloproliferation can also be considered.

Summary

This bird had a blood lead concentration of 23.9 ppm on presentation. Two other birds from the same roost presented with identical clinical signs as this bird during the same week. The two additional birds also had elevated blood lead levels and demonstrated an inappropriate release of rubricytes on their blood film.

Table 14.1. Hematology results.

		Reference[a]	Reference[b]	Decision level[c]
PCV (%)	50	40–60	51–58	35–55
Leukocytes				
WBC ($10^3/\mu L$)	37.1	7–34	11–32	5–20
Heterophils ($10^3/\mu L$)	33.0	2.9–15.4	6.7–19.8	2.1–10.0
Heterophils (%)	89	—	—	—
Lymphocytes ($10^3/\mu L$)	1.9	1.1–14.7	0.8–5.6	1.7–10.0
Lymphocytes (%)	5	—	—	—
Monocytes ($10^3/\mu L$)	1.5	0.2–1.2	0–0.4	0–0.7
Monocytes (%)	4	—	—	—
Eosinophils ($10^3/\mu L$)	0	0.3–1.0	1.5–7.5	0–0.4
Eosinophils (%)	0	—	—	—
Basophils ($10^3/\mu L$)	0.7	0.1–1.0	0–2.3	0–0.4
Basophils (%)	2	—	—	–
Thrombocytes				
Estimated number	Adequate			1–5/1,000× field
Morphology	Normal, clumped			
Plasma protein (refractometry) (g/dL)	4.9	3.5–4.2		3–5

[a]Ranges from International Species Information System, Apple Valley, MN, 1999.
[b]Hawkey and Samour (1988).
[c]Decision levels used by authors when reference values are unavailable.

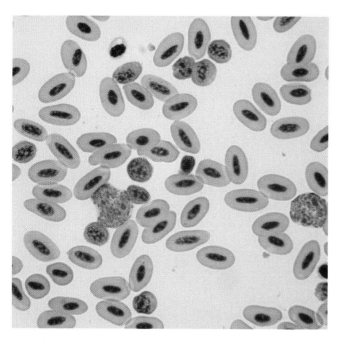

Fig. 14.2. A blood film (Wright–Giemsa stain, 100×).

All three birds were given supportive care and treated with the chelating agent calcium EDTA (edentate calcium disodium) at a dose of 30 mg/kg intramuscularly twice daily for 5 days. Following 3 days off the chelating treatment, the vultures were again treated for 5 days. The birds were also treated with fluorinated chloramphenicol (30 mg/kg intramuscularly daily for 10 days) to protect them from secondary bacterial infections and metoclopramide (2 mg/kg intramuscularly twice daily for 10 days) because gastrointestinal stasis is a common disorder in vultures with lead poisoning. This vulture patient's condition improved slightly after two treatments with the chelating agent and the plasma lead concentration dropped to 1.5 ppm. The other two vultures died within 2 weeks of treatment.

Ingestion of lead results in variable types of anemia (normochormic or hypochromic, macrocytic, or normocytic) in mammals. Nucleated erythrocytes (immature erythrocytes such as metarubricytes), basophilic stippling, and Howell–Jolly bodies are frequently seen in dogs (Walker, 1999). A significant number of nucleated red blood cells out of proportion to the apparent need as indicated by the PCV are often seen in dogs with lead poisoning (Thrall, 2004). In the dog, lead interferes with hemoglobin synthesis leading to an accumulation of metarubricytes in the bone marrow, which are released and account for the high nucleated erythrocyte count in the peripheral blood with no other signs of erythrogenesis, such as increased polychromasia and anisocytosis (Coles, 1986).

A 2-Year-Old Tragopan with Wounds

Signalment

A 2-year-old male Satyr tragopan (*Tragopan satyra*), a type of pheasant, was presented with wounds on his back.

History

The tragopan was housed in a free-flight aviary with a female tragopan and domestic geese. The birds were fed a commercial diet for game birds supplemented with a variety of fruits. The bird received wounds from an unknown attacker 5 days prior to presentation. He had been treated for 5 days with a systemic antibiotic (enrofloxacin) and a topical antibiotic (nitrofurazone). The tragopan was presented because his overall condition had deteriorated to the point that he no longer was able to walk during the past 24 hours.

Physical Examination Findings

The 2.65 kg bird was presented with three large open necrotic wounds on his back. The bird was markedly depressed and unable or unwilling to stand. Blood was collected by venipuncture of the medial metatarsal vein for a blood profile (Tables 15.1 and 15.2 and Figs. 15.1a and 15.1b).

Interpretive Discussion

The hemogram revealed a marked leukocytosis with a marked heterophilia, lymphopenia, and monocytosis.

Table 15.1. Hematology results.

		Reference[a]	Reference[b,c]
PCV (%)	40	22–35	23–55
Leukocytes			
WBC (10^3/μL)	56.1	12.0–30.0	9.0–32.0
Heterophils (10^3/μL)	48.8	3.0–6.0	
Heterophils (%)	87		15–50
Lymphocytes (10^3/μL)	0.6	7.0–17.5	
Lymphocytes (%)	1		29–84
Monocytes (10^3/μL)	6.7	0.1–2.0	
Monocytes (%)	12		0.1–7
Eosinophils (10^3/μL)	0	0–1.0	
Eosinophils (%)	0		0–16
Basophils (10^3/μL)	0	Rare	
Basophils (%)	0		0–8
Thrombocytes			
Estimated number	Adequate	1–5/1,000× field	
Morphology	Normal, clumped		
Plasma protein (refractometry) (g/dL)	5.4	3–6	

[a]Reference for galliformes (Zinkl, 1986).
[b]Pollack et al. (2005).
[c]Cray (2000).

Table 15.2. Plasma biochemical results.

		Reference[a]
Glucose (mg/dL)	267	227–300
BUN (mg/dL)	3	<5
Uric acid (mg/dL)	6.9	2.5–8.1
Total protein (biuret) (g/dL)	5.1	3.3–5.5
Albumin (g/dL)	1.2	1.3–2.8
Globulin (g/dL)	3.9	1.5–4.1
Aspartate aminotransferase (IU/L)	412	<275
Creatine kinase (IU/L)	1,936	100–500
Calcium (mg/dL)	16.2	13.0–23.0
Phosphorus (mg/dL)	6.0	6.2–7.9
Sodium (mEq/L)	157	131–171
Potassium (mEq/L)	3.3	3.0–7.3
Chloride (mEq/L)	115	100–120
Bicarbonate (mEq/L)	29	20–30

[a]Johnston-Delaney and Harrison (1996).

Figures 15.1a and 15.1b reveal the morphology of the heterophils in the blood film. The heterophils exhibit deep cytoplasmic basophilia, reduction of the number of rod-shaped eosinophilic granules, and cytoplasmic vacuolization; these are features of toxic heterophils. The bird has a severe inflammatory leukogram.

The plasma biochemical profile suggests a hypoalbuminemia; however, a protein electrophoresis would provide a better assessment of the protein profile. The plasma creatine kinase (CK) activity is markedly increased, indicating skeletal muscle injury or exertion. The degree of increased plasma aspartate aminotransferase (AST) activity is also a likely indication of skele-tal muscle involvement rather than hepatocellular disease. A much higher degree of AST activity would be expected with hepatocellular disease; however, one cannot completely rule out coexisting hepatocellular disease based on the plasma CK and AST activities alone.

Summary

Because of the bird's physical condition, blood profile results, and poor prognosis for survival, the client elected to euthanize the bird. A necropsy revealed multifocal puncture wounds with gangrenous cellulitis and myositis.

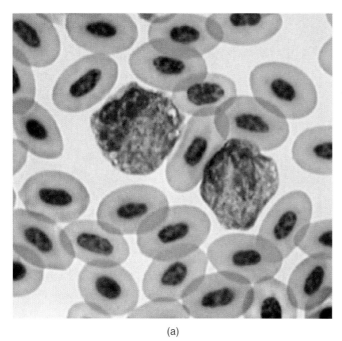

(a)

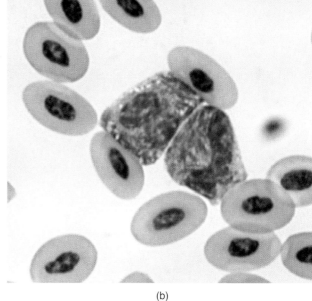

(b)

Fig. 15.1. (a and b) Blood films (Wright–Giemsa stain 100×).

A 5-Month-Old Chicken with Lethargy

16

Signalment

A 5-month-old female chicken (*Gallus gallus*) was presented with a complaint of lethargy (Fig. 16.1).

History

The hen was purchased as a chick along with eight other chicks. All had been healthy, except the rooster disappeared several days earlier. The chickens lived in a coop with a fenced area for foraging and exercise. They were fed a diet of layer pellets and cracked corn. None of the birds had been vaccinated or treated for internal parasites. This patient began acting lethargic and depressed 3 days prior to presentation. She had not

been eating during that period. The client thought the chickens had been attacked by a dog 3 days prior to presentation; however, no one witnessed such an event.

Physical Examination Findings

The 1.43 kg hen was fluffed and obtunded on physical examination. She tended to lean to the right when standing or walking. She appeared thin with a body score of 2/5. No other significant findings were observed on the physical examination. A blood sample was obtained via venipuncture of the medial metatarsal vein for a complete blood count and plasma biochemical profile (Tables 16.1 and 16.2 and Figs. 16.2a–16.2e). Whole body radiographs were also obtained.

Interpretive Discussion

The hemogram reported from the laboratory reveals a heterophilia, a lymphopenia, and a marked monocytosis likely indicating a stress response with an inflammatory response consisting primarily of monocytes. The plasma biochemistry profile indicates a hyperproteinemia with a hyperglobulinemia that also supports an inflammatory response. A protein electrophoresis would provide a better assessment of the protein profile. The plasma creatine kinase (CK) activity shows a marked increase, indicating skeletal muscle injury or exertion. The degree of increase in the plasma aspartate aminotransferase (AST) activity is likely a reflection of skeletal muscle involvement rather than hepatocellular disease. A much higher degree of AST activity would be expected with hepatocellular disease; however, one cannot completely rule out coexisting hepatocellular disease based on the plasma CK and AST activities alone. The hypophosphatemia is likely associated with decrease dietary intake owing to the recent anorexia.

Monocytosis in birds has been reported in association with infection with *Mycobacterium* spp.,

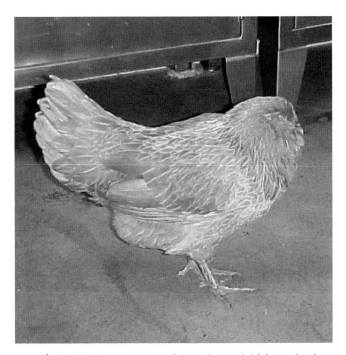

Fig. 16.1. The appearance of the patient on initial examination.

69

Table 16.1. Hematology results.

	Reference[a]	Reference[b,c]
PCV (%)	35	22–35	23–55
Leukocytes			
WBC ($10^3/\mu L$)	27.6	12.0–30.0	9.0–32.0
Heterophils ($10^3/\mu L$)	11.3	3.0–6.0	
Heterophils (%)	41		15–50
Lymphocytes ($10^3/\mu L$)	6.1	7.0–17.5	
Lymphocytes (%)	22		29—84
Monocytes ($10^3/\mu L$)	10.0	0.1–2.0	
Monocytes (%)	36		0.1–7.0
Eosinophils ($10^3/\mu L$)	0	0–1.0	
Eosinophils (%)	0		0–16
Basophils ($10^3/\mu L$)	0.3	Rare	
Basophils (%)	1		0–8
Thrombocytes			
Estimated number	Adequate		1–5/1,000× field
Morphology	Normal, clumped		
Plasma protein (refractometry) (g/dL)	7.0		3–6

[a]Reference for galliformes (Zinkl, 1986).
[b]Pollack et al. (2005).
[c]Cray (2000).

Table 16.2. Plasma biochemical results.

		Reference[a]
Glucose (mg/dL)	249	227–300
BUN (mg/dL)	2	<5
Uric acid (mg/dL)	5.9	2.5–8.1
Total protein (biuret) (g/dL)	7.1	3.3–5.5
Albumin (g/dL)	1.6	1.3–2.8
Globulin (g/dL)	5.5	1.5–4.1
Aspartate aminotransferase (IU/L)	324	<275
Creatine kinase (IU/L)	1,813	100–500
Calcium (mg/dL)	13.1	13.0–23.0
Phosphorus (mg/dL)	3.3	6.2–7.9
Sodium (mEq/L)	158	131–171
Potassium (mEq/L)	3.1	3.0–7.3
Chloride (mEq/L)	124	100–120
Bicarbonate (mEq/L)	28.8	20–30
Anion gap (calculated)	15	—
Cholesterol (mg/dL)	—	86–211
Calculated osmolality	316	—
Lipemia (mg/dL)	13	—
Hemolysis (mg/dL)	0	—
Icterus (mg/dL)	1	—

[a]Johnston-Delaney and Harrison (1996).

Chlamydophila psittaci, and *Aspergillus* spp. A monocytosis can also be associated with egg-related coelomitis or coccidiosis.

Figure 16.2a shows a heterophil, a basophil, a lymphocyte (the distorted cell with blue cytoplasm), and two thrombocytes. The erythrocytes appear normal. Figure 16.2b reveals an eosinophil and two thrombocytes (small nonerythroid cells at the top). Figure 16.2c shows a heterophil, two large lymphocytes, and a thrombocyte (cell to the right of the heterophil). Figure 16.2d shows a monocyte and a thrombocyte. Figure 16.2e shows a heterophil, three lymphocytes (cells with the light blue cytoplasm), and two thrombocytes.

It is likely that the laboratory reported the large lymphocytes in the blood film as monocytes, therefore artificially creating the monocytosis. With this in mind, a review of the blood film revealed a different differential: 42% heterophils, 47% lymphocytes, 9% monocytes, 1% eosinophils, and 1% basophils. The new leukocyte differential supports a different leukogram of a heterophilia and slight monocytosis that supports a different set of rule-outs, making traumatic injury with secondary bacterial infection higher on the list.

Summary

On the basis of the original hemogram findings, whole body radiographs were obtained and revealed normal radiographic findings for a chicken. The negative radiographic findings led to the performance of an exploratory laparoscopic examination in search of the cause of a severe monocytosis. The laparoscopic examination was performed following mask induction and maintenance (after intubation) with isoflurane anesthesia. Laparoscopy (entering on the left flank area) revealed a normal coelomic cavity with normal ovary, left kidney, left adrenal gland, left lung, air sacs, spleen, proventriculus, intestines, and left lobe of liver. There was no evidence for egg-related peritonitis, granulomatous airsacculitis/pneumonia, or intestinal disorders. The coelomic cavity contained a moderate amount of fat.

A presumptive diagnosis of traumatic injury possibly associated with a dog attack was made. The bird was provided intravenous bolus fluid therapy (20 mL lactated Ringer's solution) and subcutaneous fluid therapy (70 mL lactated Ringer's solution). The bird was treated at home with 43 mg fluorinated chloramphenicol intramuscularly daily for ten treatments for possible bacterial infection. Meloxicam (0.5 mg PO daily) was also given. The bird was to be syringe-fed a gruel made from her pelleted diet for nutritional support.

According to the client, the hen made a remarkable recovery within 48 hours following the initiation of the antibiotic and anti-inflammatory treatment. She began eating on her own and her behavior returned to normal.

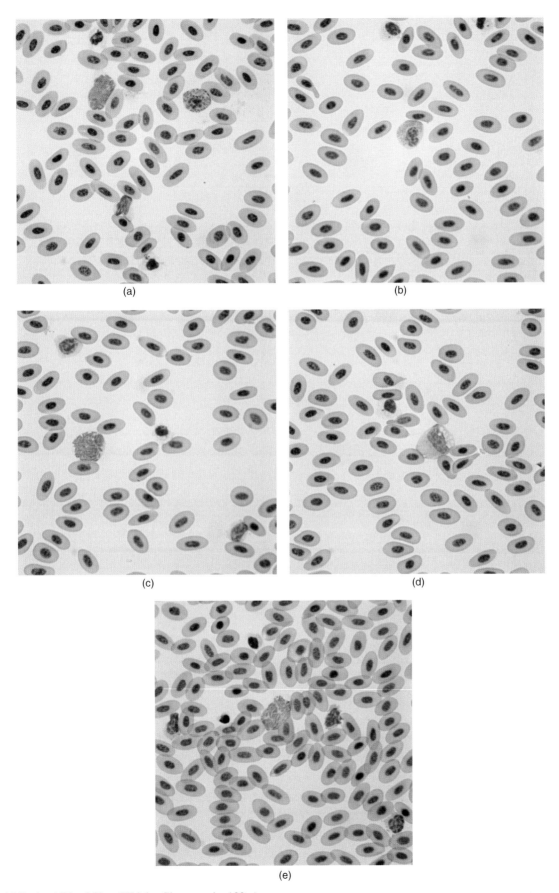

Fig. 16.2. (a–e) Blood films (Wright–Giemsa stain, 100×).

17

A 4-Year-Old Budgerigar with Generalized Weakness and Breathing Heavily

Signalment

A female budgerigar (*Melopsittacus undulatus*) was presented for weakness and breathing heavily.

History

The 4-year-old female budgerigar lived in the same commercial birdcage with another female budgerigar. The birds were fed primarily a commercial seed mixture designed for their species. The client had owned the birds for $1^{1}/_{2}$ years and neither bird has been ill during that time. The birds were housed in a room on the second floor of the house; however, the cage door had been left open and this bird was found on the first floor 24 hours earlier exhibiting heavy breathing. Other pets in the house included two cats and three frogs. The family also keeps ten chickens outside the house.

Physical Examination Findings

The 33 g female budgerigar was in good body condition; however, she was weak and tended to keep her eyes closed. She sat quietly with her feathers fluffed on the examination table. The bird exhibited noticeable breathing movements. Bruising associated with a small scab that was associated with a small puncture wound was found in the right axillary area. A drop of blood was obtained via jugular venipuncture for evaluation of a blood film (Fig. 17.1).

Interpretive Discussion

Figure 17.1 reveals erythrocytes exhibiting polychromasia. One mid polychromatic rubricyte can be seen. More importantly, however, is the presence of rod-shaped bacteria on the blood film indicating a bacteremia.

Summary

The puncture wound was likely associated with a cat bite resulting in the bacteremia. *Pasteurella multocida*, a common organism associated with cat bites, was most likely the cause of the bacteremia. The bird was given a poor prognosis for survival based on her clinical presentation and the presence of bacteria in the blood film. The bird was immediately given enrofloxacin (10 mg/kg subcutaneously) and ceftiofur (100 mg/kg intramuscularly) and placed in an oxygen-enriched cage. The patient died 3 hours after delivery of the antibiotics. This case demonstrates the importance of treatment with an antibiotic that targets *P. multocida* immediately following a cat bite in a bird as this organism commonly causes a fatal bacteremia.

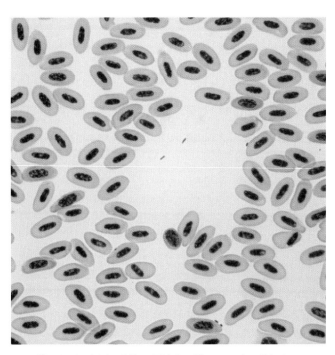

Fig. 17.1. A blood film (Wright–Giemsa stain, 100×).

73

A 4 $^1/_2$-Year-Old Duck with Acute Dyspnea

Signalment

A Pekin duck (*Anas platyrhynchos domestica*) was presented during the winter with acute dyspnea.

History

A 4$^1/_2$-year-old Pekin duck was presented with an acute onset of dyspnea. The bird had a history of degenerative joint disease in the right hip and stifle following survival of a fox attack. The owner noticed the dyspnea the night before presentation and believed the duck had lost a significant amount of weight during the past 2 weeks.

The duck was housed in a barn with the other ducks during the winter and spent much of her time outside during the warmer months. She was the only duck show-ing signs of illness. The ducks were fed a commercial duck feed.

Physical Examination Findings

The 1.9 kg duck appeared moderately thin (body score of 2/5) and dehydrated. She was bright, alert, and responsive, but was in severe respiratory distress on presentation and could not vocalize. The duck was immediately placed into an oxygen-enriched cage that provided noticeable respiratory relief.

Once the bird appeared stable, a tracheal wash for cytodiagnosis was performed. A small blood sample via venipuncture of the medial metatarsal vein was collected for a complete blood cell count (Table 18.1 and Figs. 18.1–18.2).

Table 18.1. Hematology results.

		Reference[a]	Reference[b]
PCV (%)	36	46–51	34–44
Leukocytes			
WBC ($10^3/\mu L$)	47.3	23–25	23–25
Heterophils ($10^3/\mu L$)	40.2	—	—
Heterophils (%)	85	35–40	27–31
Lymphocytes ($10^3/\mu L$)	2.4	—	—
Lymphocytes (%)	5	52–56	64–68
Monocytes ($10^3/\mu L$)	4.3	—	—
Monocytes (%)	9	0–6	0–3
Eosinophils ($10^3/\mu L$)	0.5	—	—
Eosinophils (%)	1	0–1	0–1
Basophils ($10^3/\mu L$)	0	—	—
Basophils (%)	0	0–4	0–3
Thrombocytes			
Estimated number	Adequate	1–5/1,000× field	1–5/1,000× field
Morphology	Normal, clumped		
Plasma protein (refractometry) (g/dL)	6.0	—	—

[a]Reference range for Mallard ducks (*A. platyrhynchos*) in January (Campbell and Ellis, 2007).
[b]Reference range for Mallard ducks (*A. platyrhynchos*) in June (Campbell and Ellis, 2007).

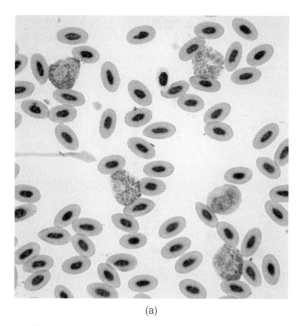
(a)

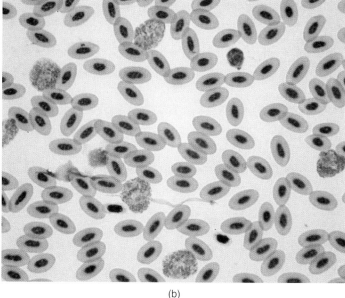
(b)

Fig. 18.1. (a–b) Blood films (Wright–Giemsa stain, 100×).

Interpretive Discussion

The hemogram reveals a marked leukocytosis with a heterophilia and monocytosis. The bird is considered to be anemic based on reference values for Mallard ducks during the winter and that most birds have a normal packed cell volume (PCV) between 35 and 55%. The refractometric total protein appears increased based on most birds having a refractometric total protein ranging between 3.5 and 5.5 g/dL. This value is either increased because of dehydration, as noted on the physical examination findings, or the bird has hyperproteinemia associated with a hyperglobulinemia as part of the inflammatory response.

The blood film image shown in Fig. 18.1a reveals four normal-appearing heterophils, a monocyte, and a thrombocyte. It also reveals little polychromasia in a bird with a low PCV, indicating no regenerative response to the anemia. Figure 18.1b reveals six normal-appearing heterophils, a thrombocyte, and a small mature lymphocyte. The number of heterophils present in this 100× oil-immersion image provides evidence of a significant leukocytosis and heterophilia. This figure also reveals little polychromasia, indicating the nonregenerative appearance of the anemia.

The tracheal wash image shown in Fig. 18.2a reveals numerous ciliated respiratory epithelial cells (columnar ciliated cells with a nucleus situated at the opposite pole of the cell from the ciliated end). The presence of these cells in the sample confirms that the tube used to collect the sample was indeed within the upper respiratory tract. Figure 18.2b reveals seven nondegenerate heterophils (the one at the top right-hand corner is com-

pletely degranulated) and two macrophages (one is exhibiting leukophagocytosis). Figure 18.2c reveals five nondegenerate heterophils, two macrophages, a squamous epithelial cell, and a goblet cell (the columnar epithelial cell with a nucleus at one end and cytoplasmic granules between the squamous epithelial cell and the two heterophils in the upper left-hand corner). The tracheal wash cytology indicates a mixed cell inflammation associated with the trachea, syrinx, and/or primary bronchi, but no etiologic agent could be found.

Although no etiologic agent was found, the marked inflammatory leukogram with a heterophilia and monocytosis and the mixed cell inflammation found in the tracheal wash sample provides a strong presumptive diagnosis for aspergillosis. The definitive diagnosis would have been provided by the presence of septate, branching hyphae or a positive culture of *Aspergillus* sp. (usually *A. fumigatus*).

Summary

The prognosis for survival of a bird with a severe inflammatory leukogram and a nonregenerative anemia associated with lower respiratory tract disease and weight loss is poor regardless of the etiology. The client was informed that a granuloma often forms in the syrinx that partially occludes the upper airway requiring removal via surgery or endoscopy. Hospitalization of the bird was offered to provide oxygen therapy as well as other supportive care along with the necessary systemic antimicrobial medication and topical treatment of the respiratory tract in the form of nebulization therapy;

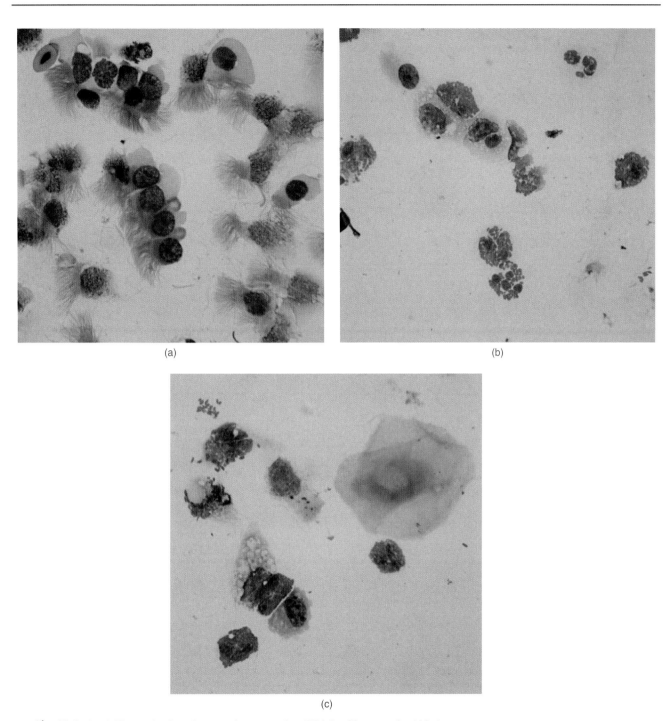

(a)

(b)

(c)

Fig. 18.2. (a–c) The tracheal wash, cytospin preparation (Wright–Giemsa stain, 100×).

however, the client elected to treat the bird at home. The bird was treated at home for the presumed diagnosis of aspergillosis with itraconazole (10 mg PO daily). Enrofloxacin (20 mg PO daily) and meloxicam (0.6 mg PO BID for 3 days) were also prescribed. The bird died 36 hours later.

The necropsy revealed a granular to fibrinous, slightly firm (0.4 cm × 0.2 cm × 0.2 cm), brown/gray mass at the tracheal–syrinx interface occupying approximately 30% of the lumen. Histopathologic examination revealed an ulcerated, pedunculated, round mass composed of a thick layer of degenerate polymorphonuclear and mononuclear cells, ghost cells, and karyorrhectic debris within a bright, eosinophilic granular to fibrillar substance flanked to each side by stratified squamous epithelium. The mass extended from the wall of the trachea to occupy approximately 30% of the tracheal lumen. Within this region (most prominently in the periphery), there were large numbers of dimorphic parallel-walled hyphae that have frequent septae and regular branching consistent with those of *Aspergillus* spp. Underlying the serocellular crusts of the mass, there was a short stalk composed of marked pyogranulomatous inflammation within a highly vascular fibrous stroma that extended transmurally between highly mineralized tracheal rings. Smaller areas of tracheal ulceration were also identified. These areas also had mild to moderate subepithelial expansion by pyogranulomatous inflammation. All other organs, except for diffuse congestion of the lungs, were within normal limits grossly.

A 14-Year-Old Falcon with Anorexia

Signalment

A 14-year-old female Prairie falcon (*Falco mexicanus*) was presented with anorexia.

History

This 14-year-old female Prairie falcon was presented with a 4-day history of not eating well. The falconer worried that the bird had vision problems resulting in a decrease in appetite.

The client obtained the bird from the wild when she was young and had been using her for falconry. The falcon had been healthy during the entire time she had been in his care until lately and with the exception of the bird surviving a West Nile virus infection 6 years earlier.

The bird was fed Coturnix quail (*Coturnix coturnix*); however, during the past week, the bird required hand feeding bits of quail. The client was concerned that the falcon had a sour crop as regurgitated quail parts were found in the mews overnight. According to the client, the bird had lost weight. She normally weighed 850 g; however, when he weighed her prior to presentation, she weighed 710 g.

Physical Examination Findings

The 720 g falcon exhibited generalized weakness and required leaning on her handler for stability. It was noted that the bird drooped her wings and had a prominent keel on palpation, indicating significant weight loss. A cataract was found in the right eye; however, the eye appeared to have restricted vision.

A blood sample was obtained via venipuncture of the basilic vein for a blood profile (Tables 19.1 and 19.2 and Fig. 19.1).

Interpretive Discussion

The hemogram reveals an inflammatory leukogram based on the significant leukocytosis and heterophilia. The falcon does not appear anemic based on a normal packed cell volume (PCV) and plasma total protein concentration.

The increased blood urea nitrogen (BUN) and uric acid concentrations in the plasma biochemistry profile support the likelihood of renal failure in this bird. Because birds are uricotelic, they generally have little urea nitrogen in their normal blood biochemistry profile. An elevated urea nitrogen concentration, therefore, would be an indication of renal failure, prerenal azotemia, or postrenal azotemia. Increased uric acid concentrations can be associated with renal failure in birds; however, because it is not a specific test for renal disease, it does not confirm the diagnosis. The reference range for uric acid concentration provided for the Peregrine falcon (*Falco peregrinus*) has a high upper limit that would be considered to be abnormal for most birds. The reason for this may be that nonfasted birds were used to obtain the reference range because postprandial hyperuricemia is a common finding in raptors. Another explanation for this high reference value may be that birds with renal disease may have been included.

The marked increases in plasma aspartate aminotransferase (AST) and alanine aminotransferase (ALT) activities indicated hepatocellular disease. The plasma creatine kinase value is also markedly increased suggesting that the elevated AST and ALT values may also be related to skeletal muscle involvement; therefore, it is not known if these values represent skeletal muscle injury with coexisting hepatocellular disease. However, the degree of ALT and AST activities likely reflects hepatocellular disease as these enzymes are markedly elevated to a degree not typically associated with skeletal muscle injury alone. It should be noted that the bile acid concentration, another potential indicator of

79

Table 19.1. Hematology results.

		Reference[a]	Reference[b]
PCV (%)	46	34–56	35–55
Leukocytes			
WBC ($10^3/\mu$L)	36.7	4.0–23.5	5–20
Heterophils ($10^3/\mu$L)	33.4	2.1–13.5	2.1–10.0
Heterophils (%)	91	—	—
Lymphocytes ($10^3/\mu$L)	2.6	0.6–10.6	1.7–10.0
Lymphocytes (%)	7	—	—
Monocytes ($10^3/\mu$L)	0.7	0.1–2.9	0–0.7
Monocytes (%)	2	—	—
Eosinophils ($10^3/\mu$L)	0	0.1–0.5	0–0.4
Eosinophils (%)	0	—	—
Basophils ($10^3/\mu$L)	0	0.1–1.4	0–0.4
Basophils (%)	0	—	—
Thrombocytes			
Estimated number	Adequate	1–5/1,000× field	1–5/1,000× field
Morphology	Normal, clumped		
Plasma protein (refractometry) (g/dL)	4.6	2.1–4.3	3–5

[a]Ranges for the Peregrine falcon (*F. peregrinus*) from International Species Information System, Apple Valley, MN, 1999.
[b]Decision levels used by authors when reference values are unavailable.

hepatic disease, appears to be normal, indicating a normal enterohepatic circulation of bile acids and not supportive of hepatic disease.

Table 19.2. Plasma biochemical results.

		Reference[a]	Reference[b]
Glucose (mg/dL)	385	237–423	200–500
BUN (mg/dL)	25	1–13	<10
Uric acid (mg/dL)	22.9	2.9–30.8	<15
Total protein (biuret) (g/dL)	3.3	2.1–4.3	2.5–4.0
Albumin (g/dL)	1.1	0.9–1.9	—
Globulin (g/dL)	2.2	1.1–2.1	—
Aspartate aminotransferase (IU/L)	1,471	15–192	<275
Alanine aminotransferase (IU/L)	1,302	4–86	—
Creatine kinase (IU/L)	3,614	283–1,431	<500
Calcium (mg/dL)	13.6	8–12	8–11
Phosphorus (mg/dL)	5.4	0–6	5–7
Sodium (mEq/L)	161	150–171	130–160
Potassium (mEq/L)	4.0	1.0–6.3	2–4
Chloride (mEq/L)	103	113–126	111–120
Bicarbonate (mEq/L)	20.9	13–26	—
Anion gap (calculated)	41	—	—
Bile acids (μmol/L)	14.0	20–118[c]	—
Calculated osmolality	336	309–314	—
Lipemia (mg/dL)	5	—	—
Hemolysis (mg/dL)	39	—	—
Icterus (mg/dL)	3	—	—

[a]Ranges for the Peregrine falcon (*F. peregrinus*) from International Species Information System, Apple Valley, MN, 1999.
[b]Decision levels used by authors when reference values are unavailable.
[c]Carpenter (2005).

The plasma calcium concentration is slightly elevated, but not clinically significant. The hypochloremia without hyponatremia or metabolic alkalosis is likely associated with an acute loss of chloride from loss of gastric secretions during vomiting.

Figure 19.1a reveals three heterophils and a small mature lymphocyte. The heterophil in the middle has increased cytoplasmic basophilia indicating toxicity (1+). The degree of polychromasia is normal. Figure 19.1b shows four heterophils, a thrombocyte, and a monocyte. The heterophils exhibit evidence of toxicity (1+) based on increased cytoplasmic basophilia. Figure 19.1c reveals four toxic heterophils. The heterophil in the center reveals fewer cytoplasmic granules and retention of primary granules along with cytoplasmic basophilia indicating a greater degree of toxicity (2+ toxicity).

The blood profile in this falcon indicates a severe inflammatory process that likely involves multiple organs, such as a systemic infection or associated with multiple organ failure. The bird was given a poor prognosis for survival.

Summary

Because of the severity of systemic illness in the bird that likely involved multiple organs and the associated poor prognosis, the client elected to euthanize the falcon. The body was submitted for a necropsy examination.

On entering the coelomic cavity during necropsy, fibrous adhesions between the caudal ventral aspect of the liver and the body wall, as well as between the ventriculus, spleen, and liver, were noted. Additionally, there

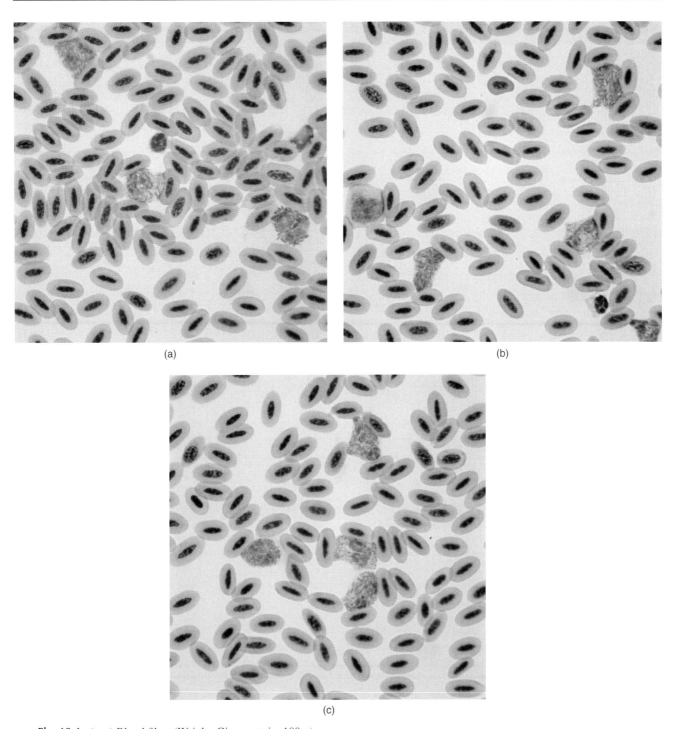

(a)

(b)

(c)

Fig. 19.1. (a–c) Blood films (Wright–Giemsa stain, 100×).

was an abundant amount of a yellow-orange, granular fibrous tissue in the coelomic cavity surrounding the spleen, ventriculus, and caudal pole of the right kidney. The liver was enlarged, firm, and mottled with a diffuse color varying from yellow–green, brown, and black. The mottled appearance extended through the cut surface. The pale tan-colored parenchyma was more

firm compared to the surrounding parenchyma. The 1 cm diameter spleen was grossly enlarged to about three times its normal size and was colored dark red extending through the cut surface. The crop was empty. The ventriculus contained a small amount of dark green–brown fluid that contained fibrinous material. The cranial pole of both kidneys appeared mildly enlarged symmetrically. The caudal pole of the right kidney was entirely encased within the previous-mentioned yellow–orange fibrous tissue. No other significant gross abnormalities were apparent.

Histopathologic examination of the liver revealed diffusely expanding portal regions and sinusoids, coalescing to form focally extensive regions of complete parenchyma effacement by large populations of round cells admixed with fewer atypical red cells and heterophils. These cells were round to polygonal blast cells with distinct cell borders, a high N/C ratio, and scant eosinophilic cytoplasm. Nuclei were round to irregular with closely clumped, frequently marginated chromatin. There was marked anisocytosis and anisokaryosis. The mitotic index was high, averaging eight to ten mitotic figures per $400\times$ field. The cells effaced vessel walls and were found within vessel lumens. Larger vessels occasionally contained fibrin thrombi. There was multifocal hemorrhage and necrosis in the liver.

The spleen was expanded with variable effacement of the parenchyma by a population of cells markedly similar to those described within the liver on histopathologic examination. The cells occasionally extended into the capsule and were found in adjacent adipose tissues. The splenic capsule was expanded by a moderate amount of fibroplasia and a mixture of mononuclear inflammatory cells, predominated by macrophages.

The lungs were diffusely poorly fixed and contained an abundant amount of eosinophilic proteinaceous fluid and loss of cellular detail. A section of air sac tissue adjacent to the lungs was expanded by mixed mononuclear inflammatory cells, predominated by macrophages.

Histopathologic examination of the kidneys revealed a population of abundant round cells markedly similar to those previously described in the liver and spleen, expanding the medulla and effacing the peripelvic area. There were multifocal hemorrhage, necrosis, and occasional dystrophic mineralization within the kidneys. Within the cortex (in the proximal segment of the kidney), there were moderate numbers of macrophages and fewer lymphocytes, plasma cells, and heterophils throughout the interstitium. These were occasionally associated with mild to moderate fibrosis. There was marked ectasia of tubular structures throughout the segment of the kidney.

The pericardium was expanded by an abundant number of mixed mononuclear inflammatory cells, predominated by macrophages with few lymphocytes and plasma cells.

The serosal surface of the stomach was moderately expanded by an abundant amount of mixed mononuclear inflammatory cells, predominated by macrophages.

The final diagnosis based on the necropsy was myeloproliferative disease of the liver, spleen, and kidneys, with histiocytic air sacculitis and coelomitis and lymphoplasmacytic interstitial nephritis.

A bone marrow evaluation would have been helpful in this patient; however, the distribution of histologic lesions affecting multiple organs was suggestive of leukemia. The inflammatory changes were likely secondary.

An 8-Month-Old Hawk with Anorexia, Weakness, and Vomiting

Signalment

An 8-month-old female Ferruginous hawk (*Buteo regalis*) was presented with anorexia, weakness, and vomiting (Fig. 20.1).

History

This juvenile female Ferruginous hawk was obtained as a nestling from the wild to be used in hawking (falconry). The bird had been healthy until the past 3 days. The bird was fed the leg of a jackrabbit (*Lepus* sp.) 4 days prior to presentation. The bird stopped eating and became lethargic. The client became concerned that the bird may have ingested the lead shot that was used to kill the hare. Two days after feeding the jackrabbit, the client fed the hawk half of the breast muscle from a pigeon (*Columba livia*). The next day, the bird was fed two halves of a pigeon breast muscle, which the bird regurgitated.

Physical Examination Findings

The 1.4 kg hawk exhibited generalized weakness on presentation. She had a slight reduction of the pectoral muscle mass. The bird's breath had a foul odor as if she had ingested decaying meat. Ingested food could be palpated in the crop. Bile staining of the vent feathers was noted. The fresh mute (dropping) produced in the transport box revealed formed feces (Fig. 20.2).

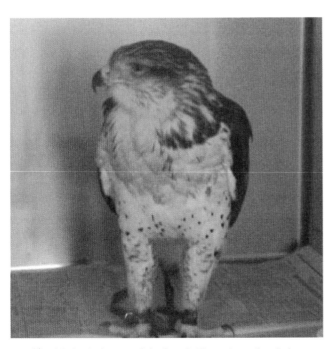

Fig. 20.1. An image of the female Ferruginous hawk that was presented with anorexia, weakness, and vomiting.

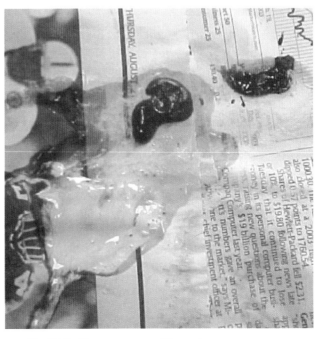

Fig. 20.2. The appearance of the mute.

83

Table 20.1. Hematology results.

		Reference[a]
PCV (%)	19	31–43
Leukocytes		
WBC (10^3/μL)	38.2	19.1–33.4
Heterophils (10^3/μL)	31.3	—
Heterophils (%)	82	—
Lymphocytes (10^3/μL)	3.1	—
Lymphocytes (%)	8	—
Monocytes (10^3/μL)	3.4	—
Monocytes (%)	9	—
Eosinophils (10^3/μL)	0.4	—
Eosinophils (%)	1	—
Basophils (10^3/μL)	0	—
Basophils (%)	0	—
Thrombocytes		
Estimated number	Adequate	1–5/1,000× field
Morphology	Normal, clumped	
Plasma protein (refractometry) (g/dL)	3.0	3–5

[a]Ranges for the Red-tailed hawk (*B. jamaicensis*) (Pollack et al., 2005).

A blood sample was obtained via venipuncture of the basilic vein for a blood profile. Blood was also submitted for blood lead concentration. A fecal smear was obtained for cytology. Before obtaining whole body radiographs to search for any metallic objects (i.e., gun shot) in the gastrointestinal tract, an attempt was made to remove the material from the crop. The hawk managed to regurgitate a necrotic pigeon breast muscle during an attempt to pass a feeding tube (Tables 20.1 and 20.2 and Figs. 20.3–20.7).

Interpretive Discussion

The bird is anemic with a packed cell volume (PCV) of 19% as the PCV of most normal birds generally ranges between 35 and 55%. Although there are no meaningful references, the hemogram also reveals an inflammatory leukogram based on the moderate to marked leukocytosis, marked heterophilia, and monocytosis.

Because birds are uricotelic, they generally have little urea nitrogen in their normal blood biochemistry profile (typically less than 10 mg/dL). Carnivorous birds,

Table 20.2. Plasma biochemical results.

		Reference[a]
Glucose (mg/dL)	342	292–390
BUN (mg/dL)	22	—
Uric acid (mg/dL)	8.2	8.1–16.8
Total protein (biuret) (g/dL)	2.5	3.9–6.7
Albumin (g/dL)	0.6	—
Globulin (g/dL)	1.9	—
Aspartate aminotransferase (IU/L)	474	76–492
Alanine aminotransferase (IU/L)	37	3–50
Creatine kinase (IU/L)	1,107	—
Calcium (mg/dL)	9.2	10.0–12.8
Phosphorus (mg/dL)	5.7	1.9–4.0
Sodium (mEq/L)	150	143–162
Potassium (mEq/L)	3.6	2.6–4.3
Chloride (mEq/L)	117	118–129
Bicarbonate (mEq/L)	18.0	—
Anion gap (calculated)	18	—
Bile acids (μmol/L)	20	—
Calculated osmolality	312	—

[a]Ranges for the Red-tailed hawk (*B. jamaicensis*) (Pollack et al., 2005).

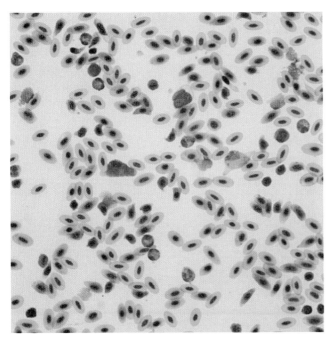

Fig. 20.3. A blood film (Wright–Giemsa stain, 50×).

such as this hawk, generally have higher plasma blood urea nitrogen (BUN) concentrations compared to non-carnivores because of their diet (typically less than 15 mg/dL). An elevated urea nitrogen concentration, therefore, would be an indication of renal failure, prerenal azotemia, or postrenal azotemia. An increase in plasma uric acid concentrations can be associated with renal failure in birds; however, it is neither a sensitive test nor a specific test for renal disease. The plasma uric acid concentration in this bird is normal, suggesting that the increased plasma BUN concentration is possibly associated with prerenal azotemia as uric acid is eliminated by tubular secretion and not glomerular filtration as is urea. Another explanation for the increased plasma BUN concentration is the presence of food in the upper part of the gastrointestinal tract resulting in absorption of urea from the diet.

The increased plasma aspartate aminotransferase (AST) activity is associated with a marked increase in the plasma creatine kinase activity, suggesting that both these enzymes are elevated owing to skeletal muscle injury. One, however, cannot rule out skeletal muscle injury with coexisting hepatocellular disease based on these two enzymes alone. The degree of plasma AST activity appears less than one would expect if hepatocellular disease was present and the plasma ALT activity, another nonspecific indicator of hepatocellular disease, is normal. The bile acid concentration, another potential indicator of hepatic disease, appears to be normal, indicating a normal enterohepatic circulation of bile acids and does not support hepatic disease at this time.

The yellow urate component of the mute is indicative of bile pigment in the urine (Fig. 20.2). Biliverdin, a green pigment, is generally considered to be the primary bile pigment in birds as these animals lack the hepatic biliverdin reductase enzyme needed to convert biliverdin to bilirubin. Some birds, however, manage to produce bilirubin, a yellow pigment, but likely do so by posthepatic means. The yellow urates could be explained by the presence of bilirubin in the urine as a result of either hepatic disease or hemolytic activity. Without other evidence for hepatic disease, hemolysis is the better explanation and is likely the cause of the anemia.

Figure 20.3 is a low magnification of the blood film showing a high leukocyte count, which is reflected by the actual count on the leukogram. The image shows nine heterophils, one large lymphocyte, one small lymphocyte, one monocyte, and increased polychromasia. The image also shows three *Leukocytozoon* gametocytes, two macrogametocytes that stain blue and one microgametocyte that stains colorless or gray. Figure 20.4a is a higher magnification of the blood film and shows one heterophil, one monocyte, and increased polychromasia. There is a *Leukocytozoon* macrogametocyte adjacent to the monocyte that appears round and may be outside its host cell. Figure 20.4b shows a toxic heterophil as indicated by increased cytoplasmic basophilia, two *Leukocytozoon* macrogametocytes that stain blue and one microgametocyte that stains colorless or gray. The image also shows increased polychromasia with the presence of immature erythrocytes. Figure 20.4c shows a heterophil, an eosinophil (to the left of center), a monocyte, two *Leukocytozoon* macrogametocytes, and increased polychromasia with immature erythrocytes. Figure 20.4d shows three toxic heterophils as indicated by increased cytoplasmic basophilia, a monocyte, a *Leukocytozoon* macrogametocyte, and increased polychromasia with immature erythrocytes. No thrombocytes are shown in any of the images, suggesting a thrombocytopenia. Thrombocytes, however, were reported as adequate on the hematologic examination report.

Figure 20.5 is an image of a fecal smear showing increased numbers of *Clostridium*-like bacteria as indicated by their "safety pin" or "tennis racket" shape.

The blood profile in this hawk indicates a severe inflammatory process that is likely associated with the presence of necrotic meat and associated bacterial toxins in the upper gastrointestinal tract. This is in part supported by the presence of a large number of clostridium-like bacteria in the fecal cytology.

The whole body radiographs (Figs. 20.6 and 20.7) reveal an enlarged proventriculus and ventriculus that is likely the result of ingested meat. No metallic object can be seen in the radiograph.

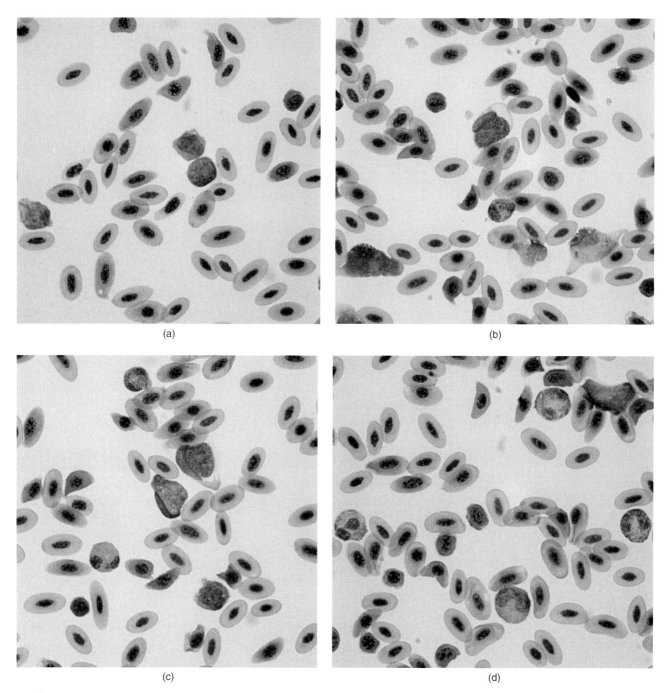

Fig. 20.4. (a–d) Blood films (Wright–Giemsa stain, 100×).

The bird shows a marked regenerative response to her anemia.

Summary

The hawk was tube-fed 100 mg of an activated charcoal solution in an effort to reduce toxin absorption from the gastrointestinal tract. The charcoal appeared in the

feces 20 minutes after dosing, indicating rapid gastrointestinal motility. She was also given an intravenous bolus of 20 mL of a lactated Ringer's solution. Although no metallic object was found on radiographs, 50 mg of calcium ethylenediaminetetraacetic acid (EDTA) was given intramuscular as treatment for lead toxicity since a negative finding on radiographs does not rule out that possibility. The following day, the results of the blood

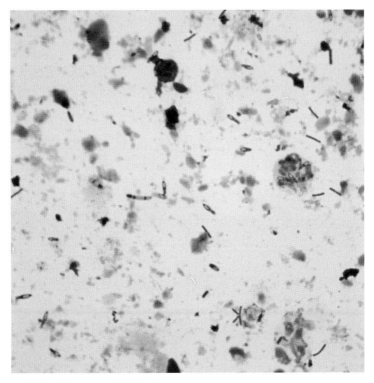

Fig. 20.5. The fecal smear (Wright–Giemsa stain, 100×).

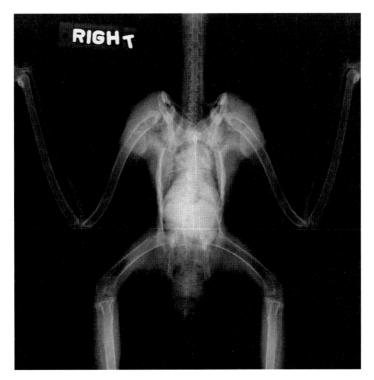

Fig. 20.6. The whole body dorsoventral radiograph.

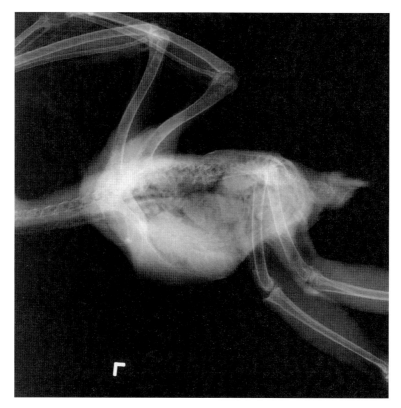

Fig. 20.7. The whole body lateral radiograph.

lead concentration were 0.09 ppm and considered to be negative.

The bird was treated with 48 mg trimethoprim-sulfa orally twice daily for 10 days. According to the client, the bird made a remarkable recovery and had nearly re-turned to her normal behavior the following day. The client did not return the bird for the recommended eval-uation after 5 days of treatment; however, a conversation with the client revealed that the bird was eating well and behaving normally.

A Juvenile Kestrel with a Drooping Right Wing and Blood in the Left Nares

21

Signalment

A juvenile male kestrel (*Falco sparverius*) was presented with a drooping right wing and a small amount of dried blood in the left nares.

History

This young kestrel was presented with a drooping right wing. The bird was found in a yard beside a house and was presented by the person who found him. No other information was available.

Physical Examination Findings

The 91.5 g falcon was presented in good body condition. The bird exhibited a drooping right wing and a small amount of dried blood in his left nares. Palpation of the wing indicated a luxation of the right elbow joint. These findings indicated that the bird was suffering from traumatic injury.

A blood sample was obtained via venipuncture of the basilic vein for a blood profile when the bird was under general anesthesia using isoflurane via face mask for obtaining whole body radiographs. The whole body radiographs confirmed the physical examination findings by revealing a luxation of the right elbow with the radius and ulna displaced dorsally. No other abnormalities were seen on the radiographs (Tables 21.1 and 21.2 and Figs. 21.1a–21.1e).

Interpretive Discussion

The hemogram reveals a marked anemia based on the packed cell volume (PCV). The significant plasma biochemical profile results include an increased blood

Table 21.1. Hematology results.

		Reference[a]	Reference[b]
PCV (%)	19	34–56	35–55
Leukocytes			
WBC ($10^3/\mu$L)	10.1	4.0–23.5	5–20
Heterophils ($10^3/\mu$L)	6.7	2.1–13.5	2.1–10.
Heterophils (%)	66	—	—
Lymphocytes ($10^3/\mu$L)	2.4	0.6–10.6	1.7–10.0
Lymphocytes (%)	24	—	—
Monocytes ($10^3/\mu$L)	0.9	0.1–2.9	0–0.7
Monocytes (%)	9	—	—
Eosinophils ($10^3/\mu$L)	0	0.1–0.5	0–0.4
Eosinophils (%)	0	—	—
Basophils ($10^3/\mu$L)	0.1	0.1–1.4	0–0.4
Basophils (%)	1	—	—
Thrombocytes			
Estimated number	Adequate	1–5/1,000× field	
Morphology	Normal, clumped		
Plasma protein (refractometry) (g/dL)	4.5	2.1–4.3	3–5

[a]Ranges for the Peregrine falcon (*Falco peregrinus*) from International Species Information System, Apple Valley, MN, 1999.
[b]Decision levels used by authors when reference values are unavailable.

urea nitrogen (BUN) concentration that is suggestive of a prerenal azotemia as the bird has no other indications for renal or postrenal azotemia. The marked increase in plasma creatine kinase is likely associated with skeletal muscle injury from the traumatic event that resulted in the injury to the elbow.

Figure 21.1a shows a marked degree of polychromasia, indicating that the bird has a regenerative anemia. The image shows *Hemoproteus* sp. and *Plasmodium* sp. gametocytes within the erythrocytes, indicating a mixed infection of blood parasites and the cause of the apparent hemolytic anemia. Figure 21.1b shows schizogony

89

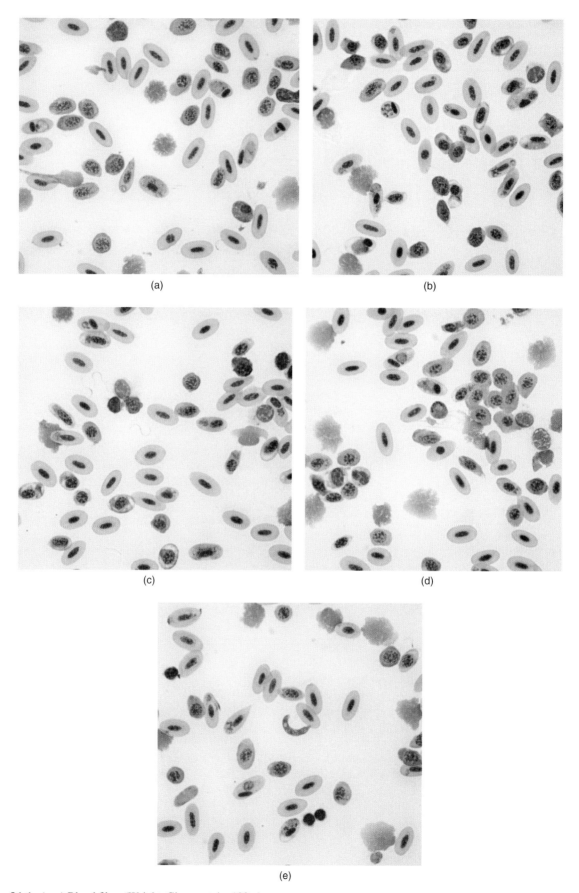

Fig. 21.1. (a–e) Blood films (Wright–Giemsa stain, 100×).

Table 21.2. Plasma biochemical results.

		Reference[a]	Reference[b]
Glucose (mg/dL)	392	237–423	200–500
BUN (mg/dL)	26	1–13	<10
Uric acid (mg/dL)	4.1	2.9–30.8	<15
Total protein (biuret) (g/dL)	3.7	2.1–4.3	2.5–4.0
Albumin (g/dL)	1.5	0.9–1.9	—
Globulin (g/dL)	2.2	1.1–2.1	—
Aspartate aminotransferase (IU/L)	120	15–192	<275
Creatine kinase (IU/L)	1,518	283–1,431	<500
Calcium (mg/dL)	10.4	8–12	8–11
Phosphorus (mg/dL)	4.5	0–6	5–7
Sodium (mEq/L)	155	150–171	130–160
Potassium (mEq/L)	2.3	1.0–6.3	2–4
Chloride (mEq/L)	120	113–126	111–120
Bicarbonate (mEq/L)	25.7	13–26	—
Anion gap (calculated)	12	—	—
Calculated osmolality	317	309–314	—
Lipemia (mg/dL)	33	—	—
Hemolysis (mg/dL)	155	—	—
Icterus (mg/dL)	1	—	—

[a]Ranges for the Peregrine falcon (*F. peregrinus*) from International Species Information System, Apple Valley, MN, 1999.
[b]Decision levels used by authors when reference values are unavailable.

(merozoites within the round erythrocyte) in the peripheral blood indicative of a *Plasmodium* infection. The images also show erythrocytes containing developing trophozoites and gametocytes of both *Plasmodium* and *Hemoproteus*. Figure 21.1c shows increased polychromasia. It also shows three tiny snake-like exflagellated microgametocytes in between the cells (surrounding the lymphocytes near the center of the image). Figure 21.1d shows an extracellular macrogametocyte between the center and the top of the image. Figure 21.1e shows a banana-shaped object near the center of the image. This is an ookinete, the zygote formed by the union of a macrogametocyte and a microgametocyte. Macrogametocytes, microgametocytes, and ookinetes are rarely found in the peripheral blood films of animals, and when this occurs, it is likely associated with a substantial delay between blood collection and preparation of the blood film. It is difficult to determine if the ookinete is from the *Hemoproteus* or *Plasmodium*. A delay between blood collection and blood film preparation also explains the increased number of smudge cells on the blood film.

Summary

The bird was euthanized because of the severity of the elbow luxation and its poor prognosis for eventual release. A necropsy revealed increased laxity of the right elbow when compared to the left elbow. There was appreciable swelling associated with the right elbow, and the joint capsule was thickened. There was no appreciable fluid in the joint space. There was mild roughening of the articular surface of the humerus at the right elbow joint. These findings indicate that it was unlikely the injury to the right elbow was a recent event because of the thickening of the joint capsule and changes on the articular surface. No other significant gross lesions were noted.

Section 3
Herptile Hematology Case Studies

A 20-year-old turtle with lethargy and anorexia

22

Signalment

A 20-year-old intact female Western ornate box turtle (*Terrapene ornata ornata*) was presented with the complaint of lethargy with partial anorexia for the past 2 weeks. According to the client, the turtle spent most of her time sitting in a water bowl lately.

History

The turtle was surrendered to the humane society after spending nearly 20 years in an indoor cage. Little was known about her previous history. Lately, she had been living outside in a pen with other box turtles where she was fed a variety of insects, earthworms, berries, flowers, and eggs. During the past several days, she had been spending much of her time just sitting in a water bowl, even in the middle of the day in direct sunshine.

Physical Examination Findings

The physical examination revealed a 740 g female box turtle (Fig. 22.1). The turtle was active, but not as active as one would expect. No abnormalities were found on the physical examination See Figures 22.2 and 22.3. Because of the difficulty in obtaining a blood sample for a blood profile, only a drop of blood was collected via the subcarapacial sinus for preparation of a blood film (Figs. 22.4 and 22.5).

Interpretive Discussion

Five mineralized ovoid structures are seen within the coelomic cavity on the dorsoventral radiograph (Fig. 22.2). The remaining coelomic structures are difficult to discern secondary to overlying ossified structures. Extra coelomic structures appear within normal limits. The turtle is gravid and the eggs are filling the majority of the body cavity.

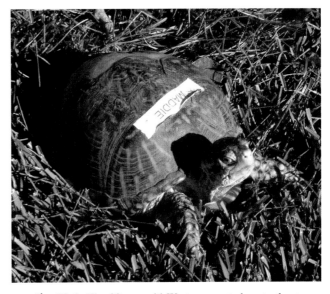

Fig. 22.1. The 20-year-old Western ornate box turtle at presentation.

Figure 22.4 reveals a 10× image of the blood film indicating the presence of numerous leukocytes and a significant leukocytosis. It reveals numerous heterophils and monocytes. Four basophils can be seen. Thrombocytes are easily found and appear adequate in number and are clumped. There is no polychromasia.

Figure 22.5a reveals three heterophils, one monocyte, and a thrombocyte. Figure 22.5b shows four heterophils, one eosinophil, two monocytes, and a lymphocyte. Figure 22.5c reveals thrombocytes among the normal erythrocytes. Figure 22.5d shows a heterophil in the upper part of the image that exhibits a blue cytoplasm with granules that vary in shape, size, and color. These are features of a toxic heterophil compared to the normal-appearing heterophil on the bottom. Four thrombocytes can also be seen between the erythrocytes. Figure 22.5e reveals a toxic heterophil similar to the one in Fig. 22.5d. It has a basophilic cytoplasm with granules

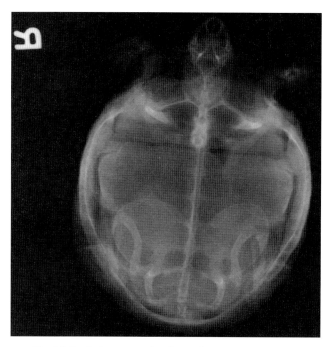

Fig. 22.2. A dorsoventral radiograph.

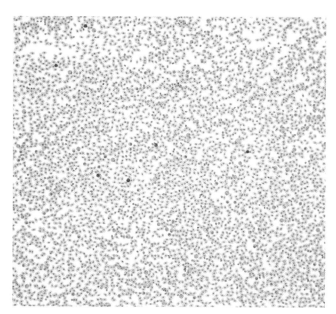

Fig. 22.4. A low magnification (10×) view of the blood film (Wright–Giemsa stain).

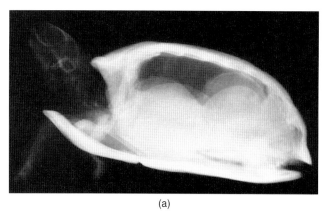

(a)

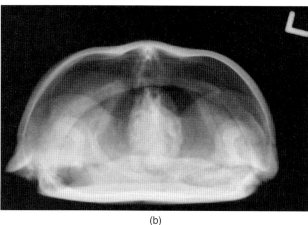

(b)

Fig. 22.3. (a) A lateral radiograph. (b) A craniocaudal (anterior–posterior) radiograph.

that vary in size and color. There are fewer granules than a normal heterophil would have. Figure 22.5f shows a mitotic figure (cell in the middle). It is difficult to tell what type of cell it is. Figure 22.5g indicates a normal basophil (cell to the left of the middle) and a thrombocyte (cell to the right).

This box turtle is likely suffering from chronic egg retention (dystocia). A blood sample was attempted; however, only a small sample volume was obtained owing to the apparent dehydration. This is a common problem with many small exotic animal patients; however, much information about the patient can be obtained by examination of the blood film. The blood film in this case revealed an apparent leukocytosis with toxic heterophils. On the basis of the blood film finding of a severe inflammatory response, it is likely that the turtle is suffering from either a coelomitis or a salpingitis associated with the eggs in the coelomic cavity. The presence of toxic heterophils makes the prognosis guarded at best. An exploratory celiotomy would be recommended in an attempt to evaluate the coelomic contents, remove the eggs, and perform an ovariosalpingohysterectomy.

Summary

The box turtle was given fluids via the subcarapacial sinus prior to anesthetic induction with ketamine and medetomidine. She was maintained on sevoflurane gas anesthesia following intubation. The jugular vein was catheterized for fluid delivery. Prior to surgical closure, she was given butorphanol. A ventral approach through the plastron was performed using a sagittal saw.

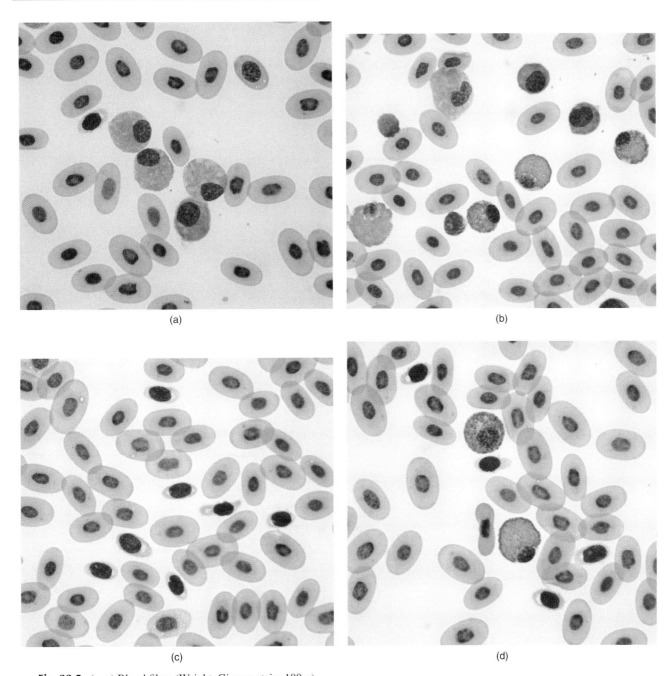

(a)

(b)

(c)

(d)

Fig. 22.5. (a–g) Blood films (Wright–Giemsa stain, 100×).

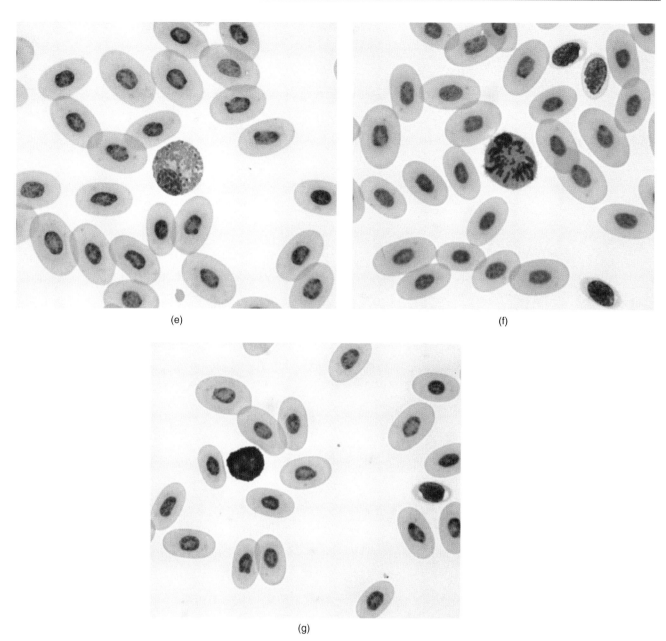

(e)

(f)

(g)

Fig. 22.5. *(Continued)*

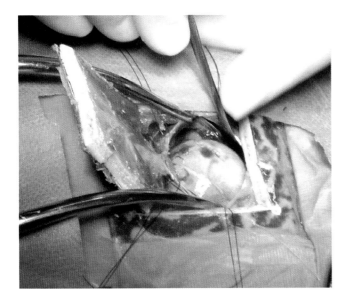

Fig. 22.6. An exploratory coeliotomy revealing a retained egg.

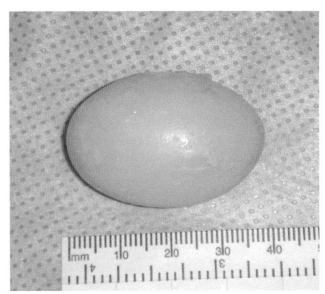

Fig. 22.7. An abnormal egg that was adhered to the oviduct after surgically removed from the coelomic cavity.

The plastron was cut on three sides and scored on the caudal margin. The coelomic membrane was then incised and four stay sutures were placed to hold the membrane open for exposure to the eggs. The eggs were larger than the opening of the plastron, so three of the eggs were deflated using an 18-gauge needle and suction. A total of five eggs were extracted from the oviducts, three from the left side and two from the right. The eggs appeared discolored and some were adhered to the wall of the oviduct. Each ovary was isolated by using electrocautery, and the oviducts were ligated with two encircling ligatures of 3-0 glycomer 631 suture and then amputated. The ends of the oviducts were oversewn with 4-0 glycomer 631 suture to prevent backflow through the oviduct stumps into the coelomic cavity from the cloaca. The stay sutures were removed, and the coelomic membrane was closed with 4-0 glycomer 631 suture. The plastron was then replaced and secured with fiberglass and epoxy. Following surgery, it was noted that the turtle's weight was 435 g, and without the eggs, she was emaciated by using the body weight as a measure.

The turtle died the following day. It is likely that she died from hepatic lipidosis and other complications that occur with prolonged reduction of food intake owing to the space occupying eggs in the coelomic cavity that impact on the amount of food the turtle could actually take in. Also, although no necropsy was performed, it is likely that the retained eggs caused a salpingitis that may have gone systemically based on the presence of the severe inflammatory response. An earlier diagnosis and surgical removal of the eggs may have saved her life (Figs. 22.6 and 22.7).

A 3-Year-Old Lizard with Lethargy and Keeping the Eyes Closed

23

Signalment

A 3-year-old Bearded dragon (*Pogona vitticeps*) was presented with a complaint of lethargy and keeping the eyes closed.

History

The client presented his 3-year-old male Bearded dragon to the emergency hospital with the primary complaint of lethargy and partial anorexia. The lizard had been normal the day before; however, the client was concerned that the lizard had quit eating and was keeping its eyes closed. The lizard normally ate a variety of insects and some fruit and vegetables. It lived alone in a glass terrarium kept at 84°F with access to a basking lamp. The habitat had walnut shell substrate with rocks and branches.

Physical Examination Findings

On physical examination, it was determined that the 400 g Bearded dragon was a female based on the lack of prominent femoral pores and hemipene bulges. She had a respiratory rate of 20 breaths/minute and a heart rate of 52 beats/minute. The lizard was active and her eyes were open. Her coelomic cavity was enlarged, but not painful on palpation (Fig. 23.1).

Whole body radiographs (Fig. 23.3) were obtained for evaluation of the coelomic cavity. Blood was obtained from the caudal vein for a blood profile (Tables 23.1 and 23.2 and Fig. 23.2).

Interpretive Discussion

The hemogram reveals a normal erythron; however, the leukogram reveals a leukopenia with a heteropenia based on published reference values. Figure 23.2a reveals a basophil and normal heterophil; however,

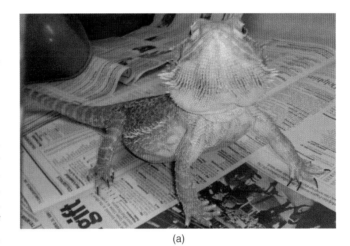

(a)

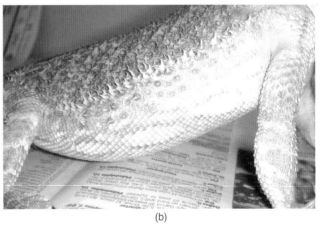

(b)

Fig. 23.1. Bearded dragon on presentation

Fig. 23.2b reveals a toxic heterophil as indicated by increased cytoplasmic basophilia. Fifty percent of the heterophils in the blood film had this toxic appearance. Figure 23.2c reveals a lymphocyte.

The chemistry profile is normal based on published reference values; however, the plasma calcium concentration appears elevated. The upper limit of the published

Table 23.1. Hematology findings.

		Reference[a]
PCV (%)	34	24–36
Leukocytes		
WBC (10^3/μL)	3.0	6–15
Heterophils (10^3/μL)	0.4	—
Heterophils (%)	14	24–46
Lymphocytes (10^3/μL)	2.1	—
Lymphocytes (%)	68	54–76
Monocytes (10^3/μL)	0.4	—
Monocytes (%)	14	0–8
Eosinophils (10^3/μL)	0	—
Eosinophils (%)	0	0–1
Basophils (10^3/μL)	0.1	—
Basophils (%)	4	0–3
Thrombocytes		
Estimated number	Adequate	1–5/1,000× field
Morphology	Normal, clumped	
Plasma protein (refractometry) (g/dL)	6.8	—

[a]Campbell and Ellis (2007).

normal reference values for calcium appears high and may include normal females undergoing active folliculogenesis, which is likely occurring in this patient.

The radiographs (Fig. 23.3) reveal many round soft tissue densities within the coelomic cavity. These likely represent ovarian follicles and are indicative of active folliculogenesis. The bone cortices of the skeleton appear thinner than normal, suggestive of osteopenia.

On the basis of the blood profile that indicated a leukopenia with toxic heterophils, hypercalcemia, and the radiographic findings of ovarian follicles and os-

teopenia, a diagnosis of active folliculogenesis with possible complications with calcium metabolism and yolk-related coelomitis was made.

Summary

On the basis of the diagnostic findings, an exploratory celiotomy was performed. The lizard was given 0.2 mg butorphanol intramuscularly as a preanesthetic. One hour later she was induced using

Table 23.2. Plasma biochemical results.

		Reference[a]	Reference[b]
Glucose (mg/dL)	222	211–261	149–253
BUN (mg/dL)	2	3–4	1–3
Uric acid (mg/dL)	3.1	2.9–10.0	1.8–7.0
Total protein (biuret) (g/dL)	5.6	2.0–2.7	3.6–6.4
Albumin (g/dL)	3.2	1.3–4.6	1.8–3.4
Globulin (g/dL)	2.4	1.0–4.4	1.4–3.2
Aspartate aminotransferase (IU/L)	22	0–92	4–50
Creatine kinase (IU/L)	1,579	59–7,000	0–2,785
Calcium (mg/dL)	22.2	8–13	5–27.4
Phosphorus (mg/dL)	3.2	2.7–15.1	3.1–8.1
Sodium (mEq/L)	149	137–186	145–167
Potassium (mEq/L)	3.5	1.3–6.3	2.6–5.0
Chloride (mEq/L)	116	107–163	111–141
Bicarbonate (mEq/L)	18.5	—	—
Anion gap (calculated)	19	—	—
Cholesterol (mg/dL)	403	160–900	231–619
Calculated osmolality	297	—	—

[a]Diethelm and Stein (2006).
[b]Carpenter (2005).

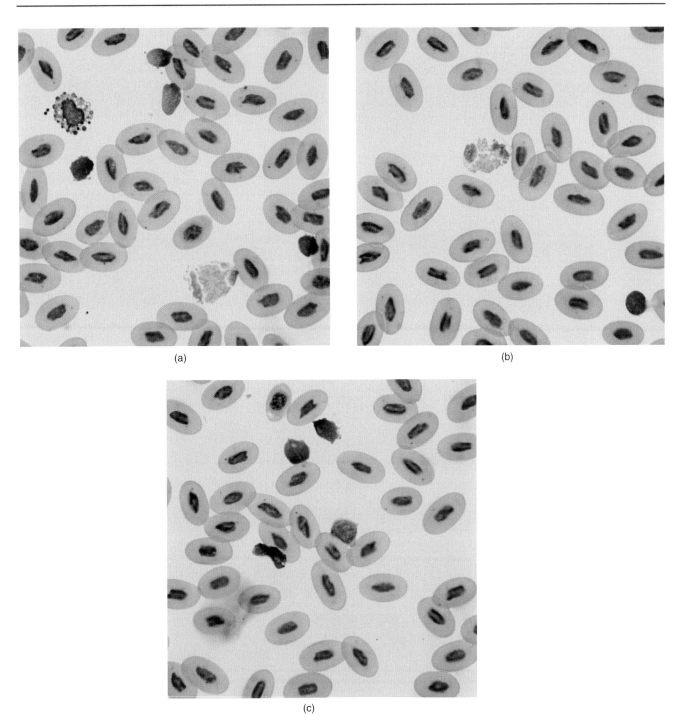

(a)

(b)

(c)

Fig. 23.2. (a–c) Blood films (Wright–Giemsa stain, 100×).

16.4 mg propofol intravenously into the caudal vein. A 2 mm noncuffed endotracheal tube was used to maintain isoflurane anesthesia.

A ventral left-sided paramedian incision was made through the skin and body wall. A cluster of 15 ovarian follicles was identified on the left side. The left ovarian artery and vein were located and ligated using hemoclips, and the left cluster of follicles was removed from the coelomic cavity. The liver was identified and noted to be pale in color. A cluster of 12 ovarian follicles was identified on the right side. The right ovarian artery and vein were located and ligated using hemoclips, and the right cluster of follicles was removed from the coelomic cavity. The coelomic cavity was flushed several times with warm sterile saline before the body wall was closed using a simple continuous pattern with a 4-0

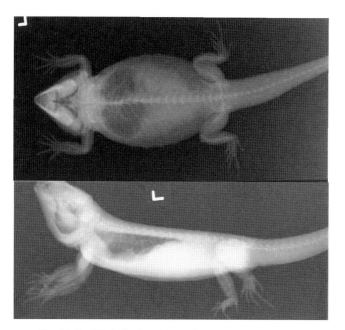

Fig. 23.3. Whole body radiographs.

monofilament glycomer suture. The skin was closed using six interrupted horizontal mattress sutures with 3-0 nylon suture.

The total anesthetic time was 1 hour. She received 0.12 mg meloxicam intramuscularly when the anesthetic was removed. The endotracheal tube was removed 40 minutes later.

A biopsy of the liver was not performed; however, the appearance of the liver associated with prolonged anorexia was indicative of hepatic lipidosis. Postoperatively, the lizard was tube-fed a gruel made from a carnivore critical care diet, which was to be continued as daily feeding as long as the patient remained anorectic. She was also given an oral calcium glubionate solution to be given daily for 30 days to support her apparent negative body calcium balance. Oral meloxicam was also given daily for 5 days for pain management.

One week post-operatively, the lizard was reported to be more active but still relied on tube feeding. By 7 weeks, when the lizard returned for reevaluation and skin suture removal, she was eating well and exhibited normal activity. The skin incision was healed.

An 18-Month-Old Lizard with an Oral Mass

24

Signalment

An 18-month-old female Green iguana (*Iguana iguana*) was presented with difficulty eating owing to an oral mass and swollen jowls (Fig. 24.1).

History

The client noted the swollen jowls 1 month prior to presentation and had taken the iguana to a local veterinary clinic. The lizard was being treated with a combination of antibiotics, cefotaxime and enrofloxacin, for a *Salmonella* infection at the site of the lesion.

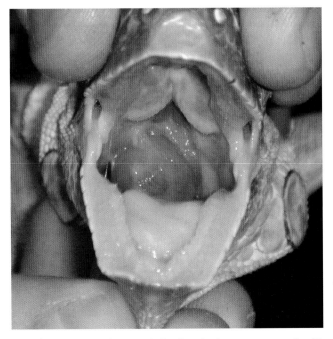

Fig. 24.1. An image of the female iguana presented with swollen jowls.

An esophageal feeding tube was also placed to assist in nutritional support for the iguana because the oral component of the mass appeared to interfere with swallowing. According to the client, the iguana had been doing well at home except for the difficulty in swallowing.

The iguana was obtained from a pet shop and had since been housed in a glass aquarium with reptile carpeting as substrate. The cage temperature ranged between 90 and 100°F, which was provided by a heat lamp and a ceramic heater. The photoperiod provided 14 hours of light and 10 hours of darkness each day. An ultraviolet light source was also provided. The iguana was fed a variety of fruits and vegetables supported by a vitamin and mineral powdered supplement.

Physical Examination Findings

On physical examination, it was determined that the 345 g Green iguana was estimated to be approximately one-half of her predicted size based on age and adequate husbandry. A red rubber esophageal feeding tube was sutured in place. A cystic, cavitating mass was identified on the right side of the oropharynx and the jowls were swollen. Two healed surgical incisions were found on the ventral aspect of the jowls. These were the sites where previous biopsies were obtained, the results of which were pending. The iguana had a respiratory rate of 22 breaths/minute and a heart rate of 48 beats/minute. The lizard was alert and active.

Figure 24.2 is an image of a lateral radiograph of the iguana that accompanied the patient. Blood was obtained via venipuncture of the caudal vein for a blood profile (Tables 24.1 and 24.2 and Figs. 24.3a–24.3c). An ultrasound evaluation was performed to identify any masses within the coelomic cavity.

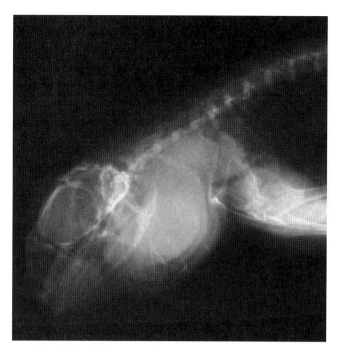

Fig. 24.2. The lateral radiograph (courtesy D. Folland).

a marked leukocytosis and lymphocytosis with an associated anemia. These findings are supportive of lymphoid leukemia with an associated depression anemia.

Figure 24.3a reveals five small, mature lymphocytes. The concentration of lymphocytes in this image would suggest a significant lymphocytosis if the absolute lymphocyte count was not known. Figure 24.3b reveals a normal heterophil, monocyte, and two small, mature lymphocytes. Figure 24.3c reveals a heterophil and four small, mature lymphocytes. The three other cells in this image are thrombocytes, one adjacent to the heterophil and the two small cells in the center of the image.

The chemistry profile is normal based on published reference values. The plasma uric acid concentration appears elevated; however, the degree of increase is not significant as reptiles in general have normal uric acid values less than 10 mg/dL. The apparent elevation in the uric acid concentration could be explained by a postprandial increase if the iguana had been recently fed a meal, especially one containing higher than normal protein, via the feeding tube.

Interpretive Discussion

The lateral radiograph (Fig. 24.2) reveals a large, soft tissue mass in the area of the ventral throat. The mass extends into the back of the oral cavity.

The hemogram reveals a low PCV and high leukocyte and lymphocyte numbers. The hemogram indicates

Summary

On the basis of the hemogram findings supportive of lymphoid leukemia and nonregenerative anemia, a bone marrow aspiration biopsy was obtained from the femur (Figs. 24.4a and 24.4b). The cellularity of the sample was low, and no bony spicules were found. Although

Table 24.1. Hematology findings.

		Reference[a]	Reference[b]
PCV (%)	29	33–44	25–38
Leukocytes			
WBC ($10^3/\mu$L)	38.5	12.0–25.2	3–10
Heterophils ($10^3/\mu$L)	5.8	1.1–5.4	0.35–5.2
Heterophils (%)	15		
Lymphocytes ($10^3/\mu$L)	31.2	4.2–14.6	0.5–5.5
Lymphocytes (%)	81		
Monocytes ($10^3/\mu$L)	1.2	0.3–2.1	0–1.7
Monocytes (%)	3		
Eosinophils ($10^3/\mu$L)	0	0–2	0–0.3
Eosinophils (%)	0		
Basophils ($10^3/\mu$L)	0.4	0–1	0–0.5
Basophils (%)	1		
Thrombocytes			
Estimated number	Adequate	1–5/1,000× field	—
Morphology	Normal, clumped		—
Plasma protein (refractometry) (g/dL)	7.9	—	—

[a]Campbell and Ellis (2007).
[b]Carpenter (2005).

Table 24.2. Plasma biochemical results.

		Reference[a]	Reference[b]
Glucose (mg/dL)	174	105–258	169–288
BUN (mg/dL)	2	—	0–4
Uric acid (mg/dL)	7.1	0.9–6.7	1.2–2.4
Total protein (biuret) (g/dL)	7.3	4.9–7.6	5.0–7.8
Albumin (g/dL)	3.0	1.5–3.0	2.1–2.8
Globulin (g/dL)	4.3	2.8–5.2	2.5–4.3
Aspartate aminotransferase (IU/L)	8	7–102	5–52
Creatine kinase (IU/L)	212	—	0–4,005
Calcium (mg/dL)	13.2	10.8–14.0	8.8–14.0
Phosphorus (mg/dL)	6.5	2.8–9.3	4–6
Sodium (mEq/L)	163	156–172	158–183
Potassium (mEq/L)	3.7	3.7	1.3–3.0
Chloride (mEq/L)	119	113–129	117–122
Bicarbonate (mEq/L)	16.1	—	—
Anion gap (calculated)	31	—	—
Cholesterol (mg/dL)	187	204–347	104–333
Calculated osmolality	320	—	—

[a]Diethelm and Stein (2006).
[b]Carpenter (2005).

the sample appeared to have significant hemodilution, hematopoietic precursors were present, indicating that bone marrow was sampled. Both myeloid and erythroid precursors were present and their maturation appeared orderly and complete; however, the erythroid cell line appeared relatively reduced in numbers. Small and mature lymphocytes comprise 56–71% of the nucleated cell population, supporting a cytodiagnosis of lymphoma with erythroid hypoplasia.

Figure 24.4a reveals a large binucleated cell, representing a rubriblast in the process of dividing, two basophilic rubricytes, and numerous small, mature lymphocytes.

Figure 24.4b shows a progranulocyte (the largest cell with cytoplasmic granules), a heterophil, a prorubricyte, and numerous small, mature lymphocytes.

An ultrasound evaluation of the coelomic cavity failed to reveal an obvious mass or masses elsewhere in the iguana's body. The echogenicity of all internal organs was normal.

Histopathologic examination of the biopsy of the mass obtained from the veterinarian who initially treated the iguana supported the diagnosis of lymphoma. On the basis of these diagnostic findings, the iguana was treated for lymphoma using radiation and chemotherapy.

A subcutaneous vascular access port was placed in the ventral abdominal vein, and the port was anchored subcutaneously on the left thorax. This allowed safe and accurate intravenous delivery of chemotherapeutic agents.

Following radiation therapy using a 1,000 Gy fraction of radiation targeted on the mass in the area of the jowls, the chemotherapy treatment was started using a combination of cyclophosphamide, vincristine sulfate, doxorubicin, and prednisolone for the chronic lymphocytic leukemia. The iguana was started on oral prednisolone at 2 mg/kg for 2 weeks followed by a 1 mg/kg dose for the duration of therapy. Vincristine sulfate (0.003 mg) was given intravenously on days 1, 3, 6, 8, 11, 15, 19, and 23 of the 25-day chemotherapy period. Cyclophosphamide (1.12 mg) was given intravenously on days 2, 7, 13, and 21 of the protocol period. Intravenous doxorubicin (0.1 mg) was given on days 4, 9, 17, and 25 of the protocol period. No intravenous chemotherapy was given on days 5, 10, 12, 14, 16, 18, 20, 22, and 24.

The iguana was also given oral enrofloxacin (5 mg/kg) daily to help with the potentially immunosuppressive action of the chemotherapy. The chemotherapy was to be managed by the initial veterinarian on the case with the instructions that if the heterophil count fell below 1,500 cells/μL, the next treatment should be delayed by 3 days.

The esophageal feeding tube was left in place to provide nutritional support for the iguana during the initial chemotherapy. The feeding tube was removed when the lizard began eating well on her own.

Six months following the initial visit, the iguana was doing well according to the owner. She had doubled her body weight and was not acting sick. During

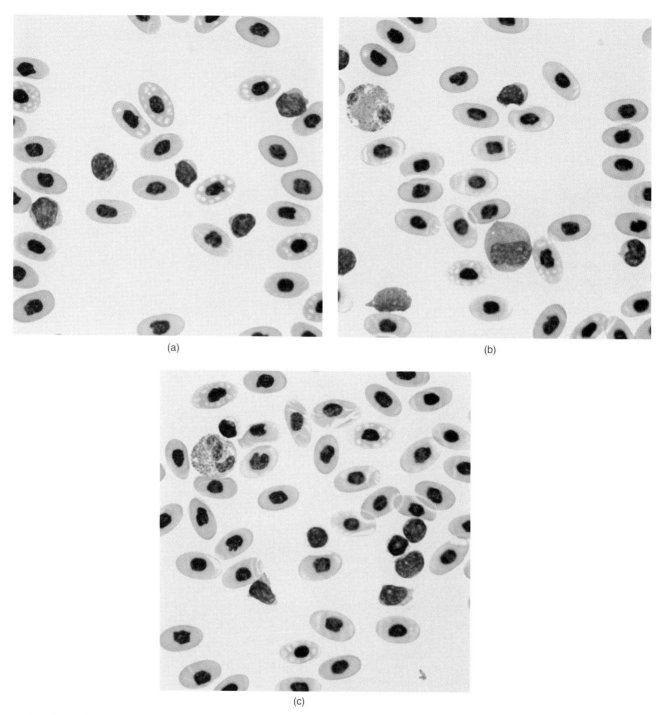

(a)

(b)

(c)

Fig. 24.3. (a–c) Blood films (Wright–Giemsa stain, 100×).

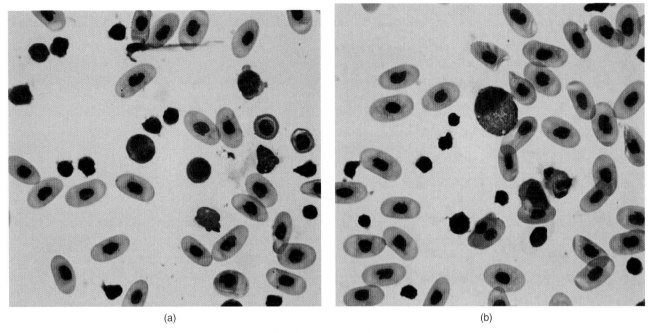

(a)

(b)

Fig. 24.4. (a and b) The bone marrow aspirate (Wright–Giemsa stain, 100×).

that period, the iguana would receive chemotherapy every other week provided by her local veterinarian. During the following year, the iguana continued to do well and would be given chemotherapy every 3 weeks when-ever her total leukocyte and lymphocyte count increased above normal. The client planned to provide such care until the chemotherapy no longer helped.

25

A 35-Year-Old Tortoise with Anorexia, Lethargy, and Constipation

Signalment

A 35-year-old male desert tortoise (*Gopherus agassizii*) was presented with a 3-week history of anorexia, lethargy, and constipation.

History

The client had owned the tortoise for 25 years and reported no previous medical problems. Her veterinarian referred her to an exotic animal veterinary specialist who obtained blood for a complete blood count and diagnostic profile (see day 1 profile results) as well as whole body radiographs (see Figs. 25.1a and 25.1b). It was noted that the captive husbandry had been suboptimal, with a diet rich in vegetable proteins instead of the roughage necessary to maintain urinary and gastrointestinal tract health in a desert tortoise. It was also noted that on physical examination the tortoise had a moderate hyperkeratosis of the dorsal aspect of the nose and malocclusion, which the owner reported had remained unchanged over the past several years. A large (3–4 cm) cystic calculus in the "left outpouching" of the urinary bladder and diffuse distention of bowel loops filled with fecal material was diagnosed based on radiographs; however, the following morning no urinary calculus was found on repeat radiographic evaluation (Fig. 25.2). According to the medical record, it was suspected that "the urinary calculus broke up overnight in the hospital, making it no longer radiographically visible" on the repeat radiograph and a diagnosis of spontaneous resolution of urinary calculus was made. A pharyngostomy tube was inserted and the owner was instructed to feed 55 mL of a commercial critical care formula for herbivores once daily. Cisapride (2 mg/kg given orally daily for 7 days) was also prescribed to potentially increase gastrointestinal motility. At that time, it was suspected that the tortoise's anorexia, lethargy, and constipation were secondary to the urinary calculus that was caused by the owner feeding a large amount of high-protein vegetables that included leafy greens and squash. It was recommended that the owner change the tortoise's diet to a high-fiber, low-protein diet, such as dried grass hay, while reserving leafy greens and other vegetables for occasional "treats." During the following 2 weeks, the tortoise was treated with warm water soaks, physical therapy, mineral oil, enemas, nutritional support, and acupuncture therapy for gastrointestinal hypomotility. During that period, 10 inches of feces was removed during an enema and the tortoise defecated a small amount on his own, 3 days later. The tortoise also appeared more active outside and began to eat grass and dandelions enthusiastically. The pharyngostomy tube was removed because the client felt that it may be interfering with the tortoise's ability to swallow; however, during the following 2 days the tortoise again became anorectic and lethargic.

Physical Examination

On presentation, the 6.0 kg tortoise appeared alert and responsive, but was lethargic and had an extensive history of constipation and partial anorexia. A blood sample was obtained for a complete blood count and diagnostic chemistry panel (see day 21). Whole body radiographs were also obtained (Tables 25.1 and 25.2 and Figs. 25.3–25.5).

Interpretive Discussion

The initial radiographs shown in Figs. 25.1a, 25.1b, and 25.2 reveal a marked amount of particulate matter within the gastrointestinal tract. The ovoid opacity within the lateral mid left side of the coelomic cavity originally identified as a cystic calculus likely represents an end-on intestinal structure based on appearance and location. The remainder of the examination is within normal limits. These findings represent ileus.

111

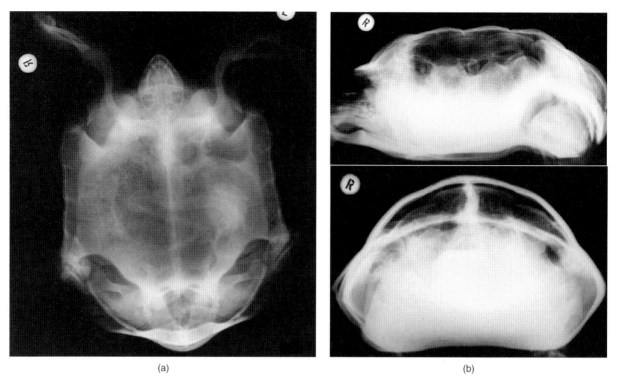

Fig. 25.1. (a) The initial dorsoventral radiograph of the tortoise. (b) The initial lateral radiograph of the tortoise (top). The initial craniocaudal (anterior–posterior) radiograph of the tortoise (bottom).

The dorsoventral view of the radiographs taken the following day (Fig. 25.2) indicated the ovoid opacity overlying the lateral mid left side of the coelomic cavity is no longer identified. The granular material seen throughout the bowel persists and is unchanged. There is slightly less air within the loop of bowel in the cranial left side of the coelomic cavity than on the prior examination. The bowel pattern is otherwise unchanged. The round structure superimposed over the mid left side of the coelomic cavity on the previous study simply may have been due to superimposition of normal soft tissue and bony structures. There is persistent evidence for a generalized adynamic ileus of the bowel.

The radiographs taken on the day of presentation (Figs. 25.3a and 25.3b) revealed similar findings to the previous radiographs. There is granular material seen throughout the bowel. There is more air within the bowel loops than noted previously. This represents persistent evidence for a generalized adynamic ileus of the bowel.

The hemogram on day 1 indicates a leukopenia with a relative heterophilia, lymphopenia, and monocytosis, according to published reference values. The apparent reduced number of thrombocytes on the blood film suggests a thrombocytopenia. These findings are suggestive of either a stress response or mild inflammatory response.

The plasma biochemistry profile on day 1 indicates a mild hyperglycemia, which could be associated with a stress response. There is also a decrease in urea nitrogen, total protein, phosphorus, sodium, chloride, and

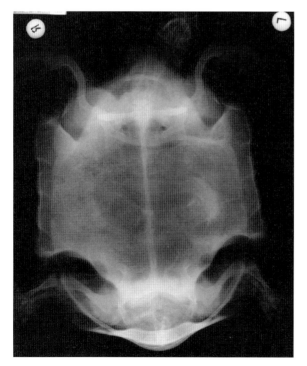

Fig. 25.2. The dorsoventral radiograph of the tortoise the following day.

Table 25.1. Hematology findings.

	Day 1	Day 21	Day 31	Reference[a]
PCV (%)	36	6	25	23–37
Leukocytes				
WBC ($10^3/\mu$L)	4.6	2.0	6.4	6.6–8.9
Heterophils ($10^3/\mu$L)	3.9	1.8	5.6	—
Heterophils (%)	85	88	87	35–60
Lymphocytes ($10^3/\mu$L)	0.1	0.2	0.1	—
Lymphocytes (%)	3	8	2	25–50
Monocytes ($10^3/\mu$L)	0.3	0	0.3	—
Monocytes (%)	7	0	5	0–4
Eosinophils ($10^3/\mu$L)	0	0	0.1	—
Eosinophils (%)	1	0	1	0–4
Basophils ($10^3/\mu$L)	0.2	0.1	0.3	—
Basophils (%)	4	4	5	2–15
Leukocyte morphology				
Thrombocytes				
Estimated number	Reduced	Adequate	Adequate	1–5/1,000× field
Morphology	Normal	Normal, clumped		
Plasma protein (refractometry) (g/dL)	2.1	0.1	1.3	

[a]Carpenter (2005).

cholesterol that are likely a result of the prolonged anorexia. The mild hypercalcemia is unexpected and may not be significant. The hyperkalemia may reflect an acidosis (likely a respiratory acidosis owing to an apparent normal bicarbonate concentration) or decrease urinary excretion of potassium.

The hemogram on day 21 indicates a marked decrease in the hematology parameters. Likewise, the plasma biochemistry profile shows a marked decrease in all analytes except sodium, chloride, bicarbonate, and osmolality. These findings indicated significant lym-phatic fluid contamination of the blood sample. Sodium, chloride, and osmolality are likely not affected owing to the likelihood that these analytes are equivalent in plasma and lymphatic fluid. Lymphatic contamination of blood samples are a common occurrence when sampling blood from chelonians. When this happens, the results of the blood profile should be ignored.

Figure 25.4 reveals six leukocytes in this 50× magnification, suggesting an increase in the total leukocyte count. The four heterophils in the image exhibit increased cytoplasmic basophilia and a reduction in the

Table 25.2. Plasma biochemical findings.

	Day 1	Day 21	Day 31	Reference[a]
Glucose (mg/dL)	97	62	125	69–82
BUN (mg/dL)	10	6	7	30–62
Uric acid (mg/dL)	6.8	0.7	5.3	2.2–9.2
Total protein (biuret) (g/dL)	2.3	0.4	1.5	3.4–3.8
Albumin (g/dL)	1.1	0.1	0.4	1.0–1.2
Globulin (g/dL)	1.2	0.3	1.1	2.3–2.6
Aspartate aminotransferase (IU/L)	65	24	191	47–70
Creatine kinase (IU/L)	1,640	202	9,130	296–3,862
Calcium (mg/dL)	11.9	7.1	11.2	9.6–10.3
Phosphorus (mg/dL)	1.7	0.9	0.9	2.2–4.5
Sodium (mEq/L)	128	133	127	130–157
Potassium (mEq/L)	4.8	2.7	5.6	3.5–3.9
Chloride (mEq/L)	104	114	110	109–112
Bicarbonate (mEq/L)	25.3	22.8	20.4	—
Anion gap (calculated)	3	—	3	—
Cholesterol (mg/dL)	43	9	36	60–89
Calculated osmolality	255	258	257	—

[a]Carpenter (2005).

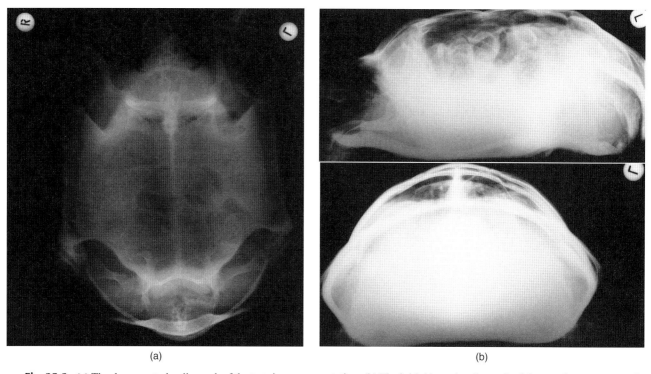

(a)   (b)

Fig. 25.3. (a) The dorsoventral radiograph of the tortoise on presentation. (b) The initial lateral radiograph of the tortoise on presentation (top). The initial craniocaudal (anterior–posterior) radiograph of the tortoise on presentation (bottom).

number of cytoplasmic granules indicating toxicity. The two dark cells are basophils. Two thrombocytes can be found between the heterophil and basophil in the upper right-hand corner of the image.

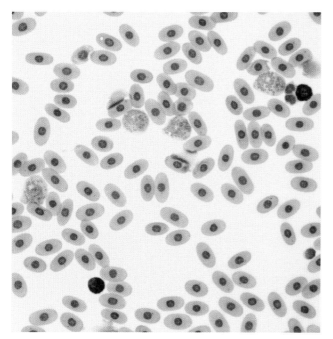

Fig. 25.4. A blood film (Wright–Giemsa stain, 50×).

Figure 25.5a shows clumping of thrombocytes and heterophils. This frequently occurs in blood samples collected in heparin used as an anticoagulant and results in erroneous leukocyte counts. Blood collected from chelonians and exposed to ethylenediaminetetraacetic acid (EDTA) used as an anticoagulant commonly results in hemolysis, therefore, requiring the use of heparin as an anticoagulant in this group of animals.

Figure 25.5b is a higher magnification of the heterophils showing features of toxicity. These include cytoplasmic basophilia and decreased numbers of definitive granules. The apparent inclusions in the cytoplasm of the erythrocytes are generally regarded as artifacts that are commonly found in reptilian red blood cells.

Regardless of the results of the total leukocyte count, the presence of toxic heterophils in the peripheral blood of a reptile is indicative of a severe inflammatory response.

Summary

Because of the radiographic findings indicating a generalized adynamic ileus of the bowel, a leukopenia with the presence of toxic heterophils in the peripheral blood, and the failure of medical management to improve the overall condition of the patient, an exploratory celiotomy was performed on the tortoise in an effort to determine the cause of the diagnostic findings.

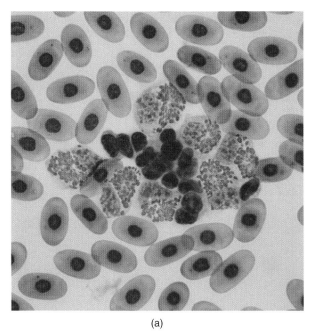
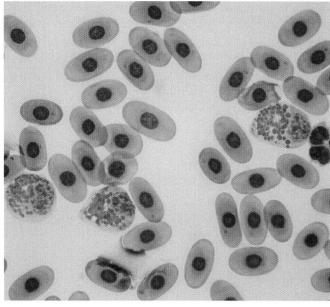

(a)   (b)

Fig. 25.5. (a and b) Blood films (Wright–Giemsa stain, 100×).

Atropine (0.12 mg) and butorphanol (3.0 mg) were given intramuscularly as preanesthetic agents. One hour later, the tortoise was intubated (3.0 mm endotracheal tube) and induced and maintained on isoflurane gas anesthesia (3.5–4.0%). During the anesthesia, the tortoise was given 175 mL of a nonlactated crystalloid solution via jugular catheter.

Surgical exploration of the coelomic cavity began with the removal of a 6 cm × 4 cm block of plastron using a sagittal saw. The muscle below the plastron was dissected using a periosteal elevator. On entering the coelomic cavity, there were fibrinous debris, yellow tinged fluid, and multiple adhesions present. The fluid was evacuated with suction, and a large amount of fibrinous debris was scooped out with a spoon. A culture of the fibrinous material was collected. The liver, stomach, and intestines were all visualized. The liver was enlarged with an accentuated lobular pattern. Fluid was present on the cut surface of the liver when a biopsy and culture were obtained. The stomach contained feed material and multiple loops of intestines were empty on palpation. Motility of the intestines was not visualized. The coelomic cavity was flushed with 2 liters of saline. The coelomic lining was closed using 4-0 nonabsorbable suture in a horizontal mattress continuous pattern. The plastron was replaced in its normal position and a fiberglass mesh sealed with epoxy was used to fix it in place (Fig. 25.6).

The exploratory surgery revealed a severe coelomitis, resulting in a large amount of fibrinous exudate surrounding the internal organs, especially the liver and stomach. No cause of the exudate, such as gastrointestinal leakage, was found during careful examination of the tortoise's organs. Surprisingly, after receiving a large amount of food via the feeding tube and having relatively little fecal output, the stomach and the gastrointestinal tract were found to be relatively empty. The liver appeared diffusely yellow and greasy, suggestive of hepatic lipidosis. A liver biopsy was obtained after the exudate and adhesions were removed. Culture of the exudative material and the liver biopsy were submitted. A pharyngostomy tube was reinserted before the tortoise recovered from anesthesia.

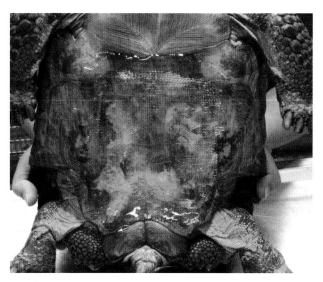

Fig. 25.6. The postoperative appearance of the plastron repair.

The tortoise made an unremarkable recovery from the anesthesia (3.5 hours) and surgery (1 hour and 22 minutes). The fibrinous coelomitis was likely the cause of the gastrointestinal hypomotility. The patient was given a guarded prognosis for recovery owing to the extent of the adhesions in the coelomic cavity, the apparent severe hepatic lipidosis, and the lack of an etiology for his condition. The patient was released to be managed at home with 20 mL of a commercial critical care formula for herbivores to be fed once daily through pharyngostomy tube, ceftazidime (20 mg/kg IM q 72 hours for seven treatments), enrofloxacin (5 mg/kg PO daily for 14 days), metoclopramide (5 mg/kg PO daily for 14 days), lactulose (0.5 mg/kg PO daily for 14 days), and S-adenosyl methionine (90 mg PO daily for 14 days). Daily warm water soaking was also recommended to keep the tortoise hydrated and to encourage gastrointestinal motility. The client was also encouraged to allow the tortoise to be outside along with the other healthy desert tortoise as he normally would be as much as possible.

Histologic examination indicated a suppurative hepatitis, hepatic lipidosis, and severe septic coelomitis. The culture results revealed a heavy growth of *Pasterella*

testudinis from the coelomic cavity sample and *Bacteroides eggerthii* from the coelomic cavity and a light growth from liver. These bacterial isolates were susceptible to all antibiotics tested including enrofloxacin and cephalothin.

The client reported that the tortoise remained lethargic, anorexic, and constipated during the first 2 weeks following the surgery. He passed a large amount of feces on the postoperative day 15, however, and became progressively more bright, alert, and mobile over the next several days. During this time, the tortoise began eating grass on his own and had daily defecations. The tortoise returned for a recheck examination on the postoperative day 21 and was found to be bright, alert, and responsive. Dried grass was present in his mouth, and his pharyngostomy tube was still in place. The plastronotomy site appeared clean and healthy, and several fecal samples provided by the owner appeared grossly normal. A complete blood count and a diagnostic chemistry panel were obtained (see day 31 results). Whole body radiographs revealed no radiographic signs of ileus.

Eight months following surgery, the client reported that the tortoise has remained healthy and the surgery site continues to appear clean and healthy.

26

An Adult Turtle with a Fractured Carapace and Leg Laceration

Signalment

An adult Western box turtle (*Terrapene ornata ornata*) was presented with a fractured carapace and leg laceration.

History

The box turtle was presented to a reptile humane society approximately 1 week prior to presentation at the hospital. It was suspected that the turtle was hit by a car, which consequently fractured the carapace, lacerated the right rear limb, and amputated the tail. The staff at the shelter cleaned the carapace and had been applying silver sulfadiazine to the fractured site. They were also administering ceftazidime (20 mg/kg IM q 72 hours). The staff reported that the turtle would walk; however, it was not using the right rear limb. The turtle appeared to do well during the week it had been at the shelter although it had become anorectic in the last several days.

Physical Examination Findings

On physical examination, the turtle appeared bright, alert, and responsive. The turtle was in good body condition and weighed 360 g. The turtle was ambulating well although it was noted that the distal right rear limb was swollen and nonfunctional. When the limb was gently extended, the turtle was able to retract it back into the shell by moving the proximal portion of the limb. An approximately 1 cm long deep laceration was noticed on the ventral aspect of the limb at the level of the stifle. The tail was missing but the vent was intact, and she defecated during the examination. The carapace had an approximately 3 cm longitudinal fracture deep to the coelomic cavity at the mid caudal aspect. It was noted that granulation had begun and the fracture was stable.

Blood collection was difficult and only a small drop was obtained from the jugular vein. The blood was immediately used to make a blood film.

Radiographs were also taken primarily to assess the extent of the injuries sustained to the right rear limb (Figs. 26.1 and 26.2).

Interpretive Discussion

The radiograph (Fig. 26.1) showed the right rear limb with luxation of the stifle. The long bones of that limb appear to be intact. There was also a small pelvic

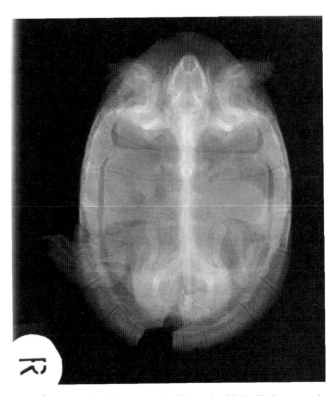

Fig. 26.1. The dorsoventral radiograph with the limb retracted.

117

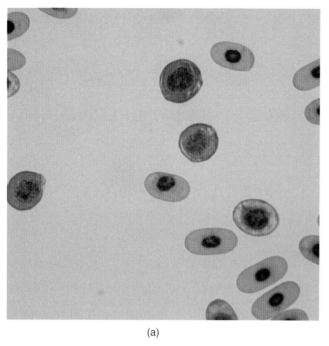

(a)

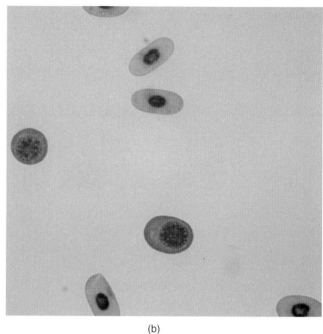

(b)

Fig. 26.2. (a and b) Blood films (Wright–Giemsa stain, 100×).

fracture on the right side noted by the radiologist that is difficult to assess in these images.

Figure 26.2a shows mature elliptical erythrocytes and round immature erythrocytes. The round cells with

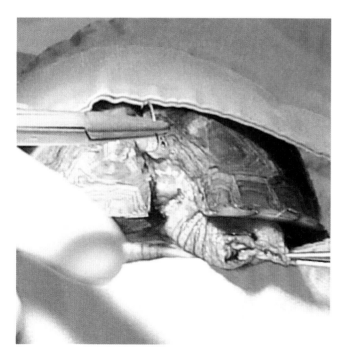

Fig. 26.3. An image of the leg amputation surgery (courtesy A. E. Nash).

the hemoglobin-colored cytoplasm are late polychromatic erythrocytes, whereas the round cell with the gray cytoplasm is a midpolychromatic erythrocyte. Figure 26.2b also reveals immature erythrocytes with the round cell on the left, representing a midpolychromatic erythrocyte and the late polychromatic erythrocyte beginning to take on the flattened ellipsoid shape of a mature cell. These findings likely represent a marked regenerative response involving the erythrocytes possibly associated with blood loss anemia, although a packed cell volume was not obtained.

Summary

A decision was made to amputate the distal portion of the turtle's right rear limb. Dexmedetomidine (0.03 mg/kg IM) and ketamine (3 mg/kg IM) were used for sedation and anesthetic induction. After 20 minutes, the turtle was sedate enough for endotracheal tube placement and she was maintained on 3% isoflurane during surgery.

The right rear limb was prepared for surgery. The laceration was extended using a CO_2 laser to remove the distal portion of the limb (Fig. 26.3). The laser was used in anticipation of controlling hemorrhage; however, there was no extensive bleeding during surgery. The original laceration edges were freshened and the skin was closed over the distal end of the femur. Recovery from anesthesia was uneventful.

A 12-French red rubber tube was placed as a pharyngostomy tube for syringe feedings. The turtle was discharged with instructions to monitor the incision and continue application of the silver sulfadiazine and administration of the ceftazidime.

Two and a half weeks postoperatively, the shelter reported that the turtle had been eating around the pharyngostomy tube and she eventually pulled it out herself. She continued to eat normally and eventually recovered from her injuries.

A 2-Year-Old Lizard with Anorexia and Weight Loss

27

Signalment

A 2-year-old amelanistic spayed female leopard gecko (*Eublepharis macularius*) was presented for anorexia and weight loss.

History

The owner obtained the lizard when it was a hatchling. Beginning at approximately 10 months of age, the gecko developed intermittent diarrhea, anorexia, and weight loss. Approximately 9 months prior to presentation, the gecko was seen by another veterinarian for the reported clinical signs. At that time, it was noted that the lizard was in good body condition and produced normal feces. The only abnormal findings on physical examination in the medical record were an enlarged left ovary observed using transillumination and palpable follicles. The complete blood count at that time was considered normal (see Table 27.1), and the only reported abnormalities on the chemistry profile were an elevated calcium (>20 mg/dL) and phosphorus (11.6 mg/dL). A diagnosis of preovulatory follicular stasis with secondary gastrointestinal involvement was made.

One month later (8 months prior to presentation), the lizard returned to the original veterinarian for a salpingohysterectomy. At that time, the enlarged ovary and follicles could no longer be identified. It was also noted that the distal 1 cm of her tail was necrotic. Aside from her tail necrosis, the owner reported that the lizard was doing well between visits. During the surgery, the liver was tan and friable. The ovary and oviduct were removed and submitted for histopathologic examination along with a biopsy of the liver. The necrotic portion of the tail was also removed during surgery. Histologic evaluation of ovary and liver indicated mild follicular degeneration and hepatic lipidosis, respectively.

The owner reported that the lizard did well postoperatively; however, it was currently exhibiting anorexia

Table 27.1. Hematology findings.

		Reference[a]
Hemacytometer count	30	—
WBC ($10^3/\mu L$)	7.0	5.2–15.6
Band heterophils	0.1	—
Band heterophils (%)	1.0	—
Heterophils ($10^3/\mu L$)	0.7	—
Heterophils (%)	10.0	—
Lymphocytes ($10^3/\mu L$)	4.0	—
Lymphocytes (%)	57.0	—
Monocytes ($10^3/\mu L$)	0.1	—
Monocytes (%)	1.0	—
Eosinophils ($10^3/\mu L$)	0.3	—
Eosinophils (%)	4.0	—
Basophils ($10^3/\mu L$)	1.9	—
Basophils (%)	27.0	—
Plasma protein	8.4	—
PCV	28	27.9–32.7
Adequate thrombocytes	Exist	—

[a]Carpenter (2005).

and weight loss. It was noted that 4 months prior to presentation, a new leopard gecko was introduced into the house, but that gecko died 3 weeks earlier. A necropsy was not performed on the dead gecko.

Currently, the leopard gecko was eating mealworms; however, she was previously syringe-fed high-protein dog and cat food with a commercial pediatric balanced oral electrolyte solution by the owner. According to the owner, the gecko had difficulty hunting and catching crickets. The lizard was housed on a sand substrate and the temperature of the cage was kept between 75 and 80°F. It was also reported that the lizard was consuming large amounts of water and often sat in her water dish for extended periods (Fig. 27.1).

Physical Examination Findings

On physical examination, the leopard gecko was bright, alert, and responsive and weighed 36 g. She had

121

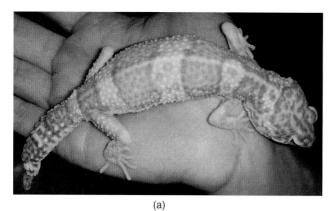

(a)

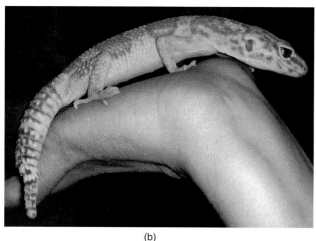

(b)

Fig. 27.1. The leopard gecko at presentation—dorsal and lateral views.

lost 20 g over the last 2 months according to the owner's records. Her body condition was thin at 2/5. Normal regrowth of the distal tail was observed and the area of her surgical site was healed.

The owners had financial concerns due to the monies they had spent on previous examinations and surgery. With the introduction of the recently deceased lizard, it was unknown whether the current condition was a continuation of her previous problem or a new one, although review of the history suggested that the original medical problems of anorexia, intermittent diarrhea, and weight loss had not resolved.

A gastric and cloacal wash was performed for cytologic evaluation. A small amount of blood was obtained via venipuncture of the abdominal vein for preparation of a blood film (Figs. 27.2 and 27.3).

Interpretive Discussion

Figure 27.2a shows two heterophils, epithelial cells, urate crystals, and extracellular bacteria. Figure 27.2b shows two heterophils, urate crystals, and bacteria. The appearance of heterophils in the cloacal wash sample indicates inflammation either in the cloaca or associated with the gastrointestinal tract or possibly the urinary tract. The reproductive tract was removed; therefore, it was not considered unless the inflammation was related to the surgery. Acid-fast stains of both the gastric wash and the cloacal wash for *Cryptosporidia* were negative (not shown).

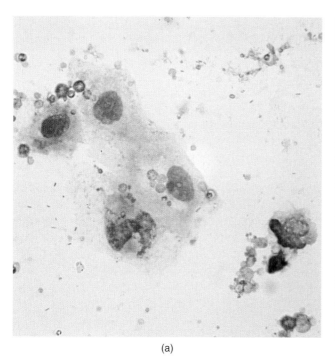

(a)

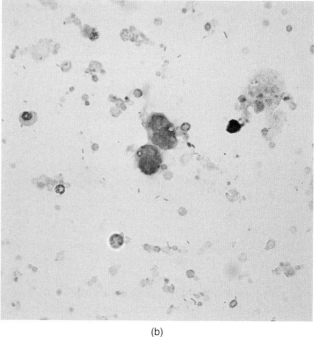

(b)

Fig. 27.2. (a and b) The cloacal wash (Wright–Giemsa stain, 100×).

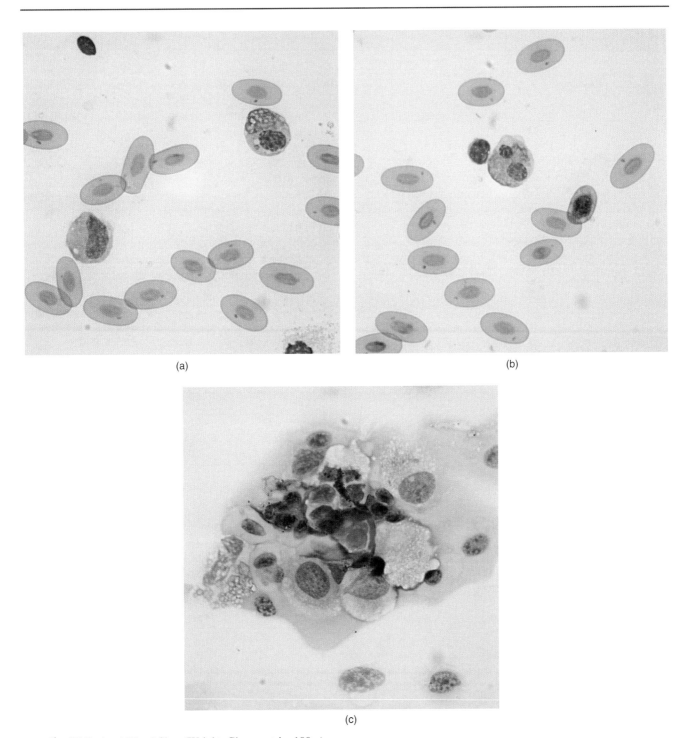

(a)

(b)

(c)

Fig. 27.3. (a–c) Blood films (Wright–Giemsa stain, 100×).

Figure 27.3a shows a heterophil with a nonlobed nucleus exhibiting increased basophilia, vacuolation, and decreased amount of definitive rod-shaped granules in the cytoplasm. This is a young heterophil with features of toxicity. A monocyte is also shown. The erythrocytes contain intracytoplasmic inclusions that are likely an artifact commonly encountered in rep-tilian blood films (Campbell and Ellis, 2007). Figure 27.3b shows a heterophil with a lobed nucleus with a slight increase in cytoplasmic basophilia, a lympho-cyte, and a polychromatic erythrocyte. Figure 27.3c is an image of a different area of the blood film that shows clumping of the cells. The cellular clump con-tains a heterophil, thrombocytes, and macrophages. The blood film indicates an inflammatory response to the hemogram.

Summary

On the basis of the presence of heterophils in the cloacal wash, a presumptive diagnosis of enteritis was made due to a clinical history of intermittent diarrhea. The blood film indicated a severe inflammatory response. Because of the lizard's intermittent eating behavior, she was tube-fed 2% of her body weight (~0.7 mL) a carnivore diet along with fenbendazole (100 mg/kg) and metronidazole (50 mg/kg) partly for treatment of an unknown parasite infestation and as an appetite stimulant. The lizard was treated at home with trimethoprim-sulfa (20 mg/kg PO BID for 10 days)

for the suspected enteritis. The client was given a carnivore diet for syringe feedings as needed. A recommendation of removal of the sand substrate to be replaced with reptile carpet or paper was made as ingested sand may contribute to gastrointestinal irritation and/or partial or complete obstruction. Sand may also irritate the eyes, which may contribute to impaired sight and consequent hunting difficulty. A temperature gradient of 75–95°F in the enclosure was also recommended.

One month following treatment for possible enteritis, the gecko's behavior returned to normal and she was eating insects, including crickets on her own. The gecko had gained weight based on the increased plumpness of the tail, according to the client. The lizard was also observed passing normal fecal material.

Section 4
Fish Hematology Case Studies

An Adult Stingray with Weight Loss and Lethargy

28

Signalment

An adult captive female Southern stingray (*Dasyatis americana*) was presented for weight loss and lethargy.

History

The stingray lived in a touchpool exhibit in a public aquarium. The pool was a marine system with approximately ten other female Southern stingrays and four (two male and two female) Cownose stingrays (*Rhinoptera bonasus*). This was an interactive exhibit where the public may feed and touch the fish.

This stingray was moved into quarantine because she was considered to be very thin and appeared lethargic. She was reportedly one of the more social stingrays and was found laying at the bottom and uninterested in food. She was given an injection of enrofloxacin prior to placement into the quarantine tank.

Physical Examination Findings

She was very thin with a greenish discoloration of her skin (Fig. 28.1a). She also appeared very weak, was not able to move around much, and did not resist handling. The margins of her wings were traumatized (Fig. 28.1b) and her tail was missing skin (Fig. 28.1c). She had multiple abrasions on the ventral aspects of her body (Fig. 28.1d). She had an increased respiratory rate and effort.

A blood sample was collected from the ventral tail vein and submitted for a complete blood count and diagnostic panel (Figs. 28.2a and 28.2b and Tables 28.1 and 28.2).

Interpretive Discussion

The complete blood cell count revealed a leukopenia and anemia. The heterophils show signs of toxicity by the increased cytoplasmic basophilia and cytoplasmic vacuolation (Fig. 28.2a). Figure 28.2b reveals erythrophagocytosis. The hemogram is indicative of severe inflammatory stimulus of the hematopoietic tissue, such as the epigonal organ and consumption of leukocytes, especially heterophils. The erythrophagocytosis suggests a hemolytic cause for the anemia.

The plasma biochemistry profile indicates hypoproteinemia. Little is known about the proteins that make up the total protein of elasmobranchs, except that they normally nearly lack albumin. The hypoproteinemia in this ray could be a result from a decrease in protein synthesis as would result from a decreased intake of amino acids or hepatic failure. A hypoproteinemia could also result from protein loss from the body, such as urinary loss or gastrointestinal loss. The ray exhibits hypocholesterolemia, which is likely associated with decreased synthesis as would occur with hepatic failure; however, decreased absorption from the intestines or lack of a dietary source would also be possible. The plasma creatine kinase (CK) activity is markedly increased, suggesting skeletal muscle injury. The increased plasma aspartate aminotransferase (AST) activity could also relate to skeletal muscle injury or suggest coexisting hepatocellular disease. The hypernatremia in this ray suggests a failure of excess sodium excretion, a function of the rectal gland.

Summary

Antibiotics and force-feeding were started with little to no improvement. Euthanasia was intended, but she died before it could be performed. She died 3 days after presentation and transportation to quarantine. Necropsy findings included external lesions as described on the physical examination. Approximately 20 mL of free fluid was found in the coelomic cavity. The liver was small and dark, presumably lipid depleted. The

127

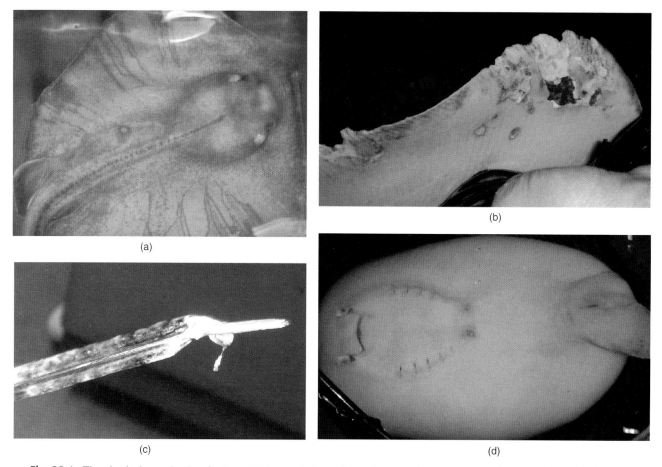

Fig. 28.1. The physical examination findings. (a) A dorsal view of the stingray. (b) The traumatized wing. (c) The skin lesion on the tail tip. (d) A ventral view of the stingray.

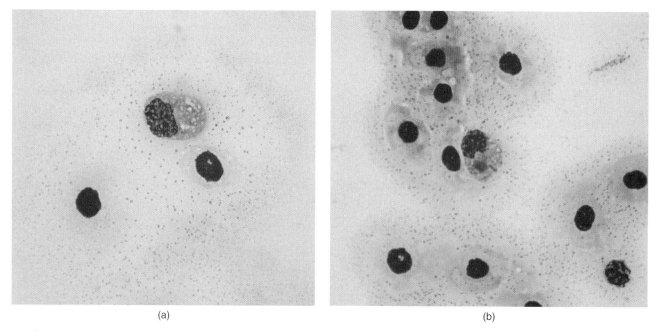

Fig. 28.2. (a and b) Blood films (Wright–Giemsa stain, 100×).

Table 28.1. Hematology Results.

	Results	Normal range Southern stingrays at the aquarium[a]
WBC ($10^3/\mu L$)	2.6	13.6 (3.8–27.9)
G_1 (heterophils) ($10^3/\mu L$)	0.4	4.8 (1.0–8.9)
G_2 (neutrophils) ($10^3/\mu L$)	—	0.3 (0–0.9)
G_3 (eosinophils) ($10^3/\mu L$)	0.4	0.75 (0.1–3.1)
Lymphocytes ($10^3/\mu L$)	1.8	8.25 (1.1–30.1)
Monocytes ($10^3/\mu L$)	0.1	0.2 (0–1.0)
Basophils ($10^3/\mu L$)	0	0.1 (0–0.5)
Plasma protein (g/dL)	4.4	6.1 (5.3–8.6)
PCV (%)	6	26 (21-3-6)
Adequate thrombocytes	Exist	—

[a]Median (min/max) from 20 Southern stingrays during routine physical examination.

epigonal organ was large and hemorrhagic. The large ovary contained numerous yolk-filled follicles. Hemorrhage was seen throughout the skin, muscles, and other organ surfaces (Fig. 28.3). Fluid surrounded the brain and the gills were necrotic.

Table 28.2. Plasma biochemistry results.

	Results	Normal range Southern stingrays at the aquarium[a]
Glucose (mg/dL)	56	36.5 (12–58)
BUN (mg/dL)	1,020	1,052.5 (609–1,330)
Phosphorus (mg/dL)	5.1	4.35 (3.1–7.1)
Calcium (mg/dL)	16.6	16.3 (14.0–18.3)
Uric acid (mg/dL)	<0.2	—
Total protein (g/dL)	1.6	2.7 (2.1–4.9)
Albumin (g/dL)	<1.0	—
Globulin (g/dL)	0.6	1.6 (1.1–3.9)
A/G ratio	1.7	—
Cholesterol (mg/dL)	42	143 (90–291)
CK (IU/L)	4,044	312 (69–1,409)
AST (IU/L)	164	11 (1–55)[b]
Sodium (mg/dL)	313	273.5 (180–292)
Potassium (mg/dL)	5.3	3.5 (1.7–5.8)
Chloride (mg/dL)	267	265.5 (140–313)
Bicarbonate (mg/dL)	4.6	4.4 (3.1–5.7)
Anion gap	46	—
Calculated osmolality	959	—

[a]Median (min/max) from 20 Southern stingrays during routine physical examination.
[b]Collected from 11 stingrays.

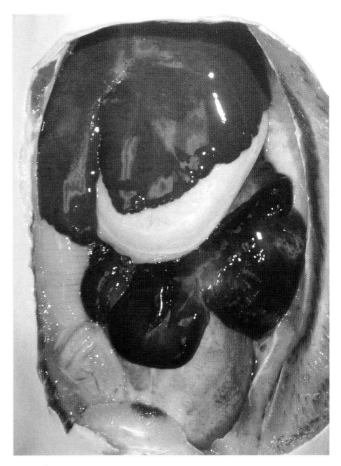

Fig. 28.3. The open coelom during the necropsy. The liver (top of photo) is small and dark brown. The epigonal organ (center of photo) is hemorrhagic.

A kidney culture revealed a mild growth of *Vibrio alginolyticus*. This organism is commonly found in marine environments and can be associated with hemorrhagic septicemia and anemia (Barker, 2001). It is suspected that with such a mild growth this was not the cause of death but more likely the result of an opportunistic pathogen on a compromised animal or an incidental finding.

The diagnosis from histologic examination was a severe chronic active dermatitis and myositis with splenitis, hepatitis, and meningitis. The pathologist also noted that this appeared to be a primary skin and subcutaneous infectious and inflammatory process, which resulted in septicemia. It is possible that this stingray was traumatized (bite wounds) by the other stingrays and was not able to recover.

An Adult Stingray Undergoing a Routine Physical Examination

Signalment

An adult female Southern ray (*Dasyatis americana*) was evaluated as part of an annual wellness examination (Fig. 29.1).

History

This stingray was one of 24 stingrays housed in 12,000-gallon touch pool exhibit in a public aquarium. She was fed a variety of fish supplemented with a commercial elasmobranch vitamin plus shrimp and squid. There had been no health concerns.

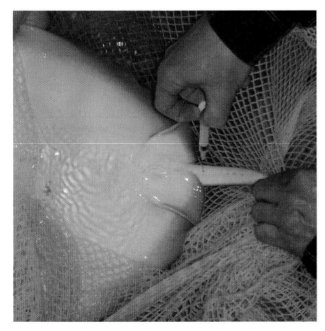

Fig. 29.1. Blood collection from a Southern stingray.

Physical Examination Findings

The stingray was removed from the exhibit for evaluation and blood collection. The ray appeared to be in excellent health, and an ultrasound examination revealed no abnormal findings. A blood sample was obtained via venipuncture of the caudal vein for a blood profile (Tables 29.1 and 29.2 and Figs. 29.2a–29.2c).

Interpretive Discussion

The hemogram appears normal. Figure 29.2a reveals mature erythrocytes, a G_1 granulocyte (heterophil), a G_3 granulocyte (eosinophil), and a thrombocyte. The G_1 granulocyte (the granulocyte on the left of the image) resembles the heterophil of other lower vertebrates and is characterized by having dull eosinophilic staining cytoplasmic granules. The G_3 granulocyte or eosinophil has brightly staining cytoplasmic granules in contrast to those of the G_1 granulocyte. The thrombocyte is the oval cell on the right with a large round nucleus and a basophilic cytoplasm indicating immaturity.

Table 29.1. Hematology results.

		Reference[a]
WBC ($10^3/\mu l$)	12.2	13.6 (3.8–27.9)
G_1 (heterophils) ($10^3/\mu L$)	3.3	4.8 (1.0–8.9)
G_2 (neutrophils) ($10^3/\mu L$)	0	0.3 (0–0.9)
G_3 (eosinophils) ($10^3/\mu L$)	1.5	0.75 (0.1–3.1)
Basophils ($10^3/\mu L$)	0.1	0.1 (0–0.5)
Lymphocytes ($10^3/\mu L$)	7.1	8.25 (1.1–30.1)
Monocytes ($10^3/\mu L$)	0.1	0.2 (0–1.0)
Plasma protein (g/dL)	5.5	6.1 (5.3–8.6)
PCV (%)	24	26 (21–36)
Thrombocytes	Adequate	

[a]Median (min/max) from 20 Southern stingrays during routine physical examination

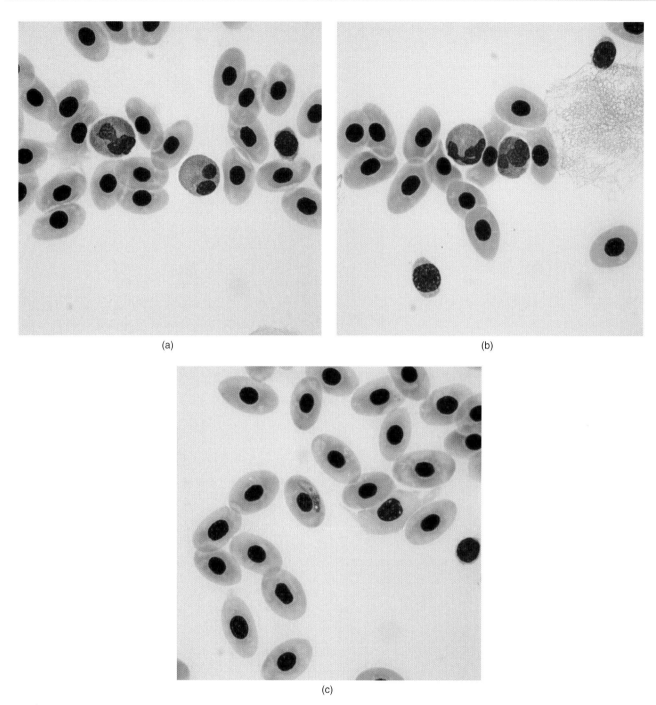

Fig. 29.2. (a–c) A blood film (Wright–Giemsa stain, 100×).

Figure 29.2b shows mature erythrocytes, a G_1 granulocyte or heterophil (the granulocyte on the left with the dull eosinophilic granules), a basophil (the granulocyte on the right), and two thrombocytes. Figure 29.2c shows an erythrocyte with an intracytoplasmic hemogregarine blood parasite. A thrombocyte is also shown in this image.

The plasma chemistry values for this ray are within normal limits. Osmoregulation of marine elasmobranchs is maintained by a high concentration of urea nitrogen and to some extent sodium and chloride in the blood and involves the kidneys, rectal glands, gills, and diet. A high level of urea is maintained by renal tubular reabsorption. The rectal gland of marine elasmobranchs

Table 29.2. Plasma biochemistry results.

		Reference[a]
Glucose (mg/dL)	44	36.5 (12–58)
BUN (mg/dL)	1,070	1,052.5 (609–1,330)
Creatinine (mg/dL)	0	0.35 (0–0.7)
Phosphorus (mg/dL)	4.0	4.35 (3.1–7.1)
Calcium (mg/dL)	17.2	16.3 (14–18.3)
Magnesium (mg/dL)	3.7	3.55 (2.8–5.6)[b]
Total protein (biuret) (g/dL)	4.0	2.7 (2.1–4.9)
Globulin (g/dL)	3.0	1.6 (1.1–3.9)
Alkaline phosphatase (IU/L)	26	21 (1–54)[c]
Aspartate aminotransferase (IU/L)	16	11 (1–55)[c]
Gamma glutamyltransferase (IU/L)	10	7 (0–15)
Creatine kinase (IU/L)	225	312 (69–1,409)
Sodium (mEq/L)	267	273.5 (180–292)
Potassium (mEq/L)	3.0	3.5 (1.7–5.8)
Chloride (mEq/L)	265.5	265.5 (140–313)
Bicarbonate (mEq/L)	4.0	4.4 (3.1–5.7)
Cholesterol (mg/dl)	267	143 (90–291)

[a]Median (min/max) from 20 Southern stingrays during routine physical examination.
[b]Collected from 8 stingrays
[c]Collected from 11 stingrays

is a salt-secreting organ; however, two-thirds of the total sodium and chloride excreted by elasmobranchs occurs in the gills, whereas their gills have low permeability to urea. Metabolic urea is directly related to food availability (Cain et al., 2004).

Summary

The hemogregarine parasite found in the peripheral blood of this ray is considered to be an incidental finding and of no health concern (Saunders, 1958).

Section 5
Mammalian Cytology Case Studies

30

A 6-Year-Old Guinea Pig with Excessive Drinking and Urination, Soft Stools, and Weight Loss

Signalment

A 6-year-old intact male guinea pig (*Cavia porcellius*) was presented with a 6-month history of excessive drinking and urination, soft stools, and weight loss.

History

The guinea pig lived in a cage by himself. He was fed commercial guinea pig pellets and grass hay.

Physical Examination Findings

On physical examination, the guinea pig appeared very thin and weighed 820 g. Palpation of the abdomen revealed intestines that contained excessive amounts of gas. During his initial visit, the guinea pig had multiple episodes of voluminous diarrhea. An enlarged mass was easily palpated in the upper neck region, and an aspirate was obtained for cytologic examination. See Figures 30.1 and 30.2 and Tables 30.1 and 30.2.

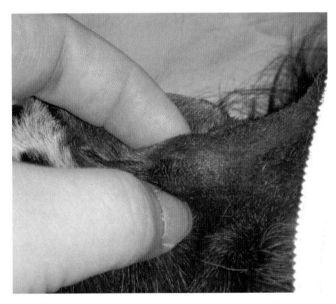

Fig. 30.1. The firm, pea-sized mass that was found in the area of the right thyroid gland.

Interpretive Discussion

The blood profile reveals a hemogram with normal erythrocyte parameters and a stress leukogram. The increased blood glucose also supports a stress response. The slight increase in plasma alanine aminotransferase (ALT) and aspartate aminotransferase (AST) activities associated with a presumed normal creatine kinase (CK) activity suggests hepatocellular disease although these values may not be significantly elevated. The previously (5 years prior) high alkaline phosphatase (ALP) value was likely associated with the osteoblastic activity in a young growing animal.

The fine-needle aspiration biopsy of the mass revealed a highly cellular sample containing primarily epithelial cells that often occurred in adherent groups. Figure 30.2a reveals epithelial cells with round to oval nuclei exhibiting mild nuclear pleomorphism and prominent, multiple nucleoli. Blue–black granules can be seen scattered among the cells. Figure 30.2b reveals a large cluster of tightly adherent epithelial cells with round to oval nuclei that exhibit mild nuclear pleomorphism and prominent nucleoli. Blue–black granules can be found within cells as well as in the noncellular background. Numerous erythrocytes are also present. Figure 30.2c reveals a cluster of epithelial cells with round to oval nuclei with coarse chromatin, mild nuclear pleomorphism, and prominent nucleoli. The cells also contain numerous blue–black granules that are densely packed in areas. Figure 30.2d reveals an isolated cluster of epithelial cells, demonstrating the tendency of these cells to have eccentric nuclei. Two cells contain large perinuclear

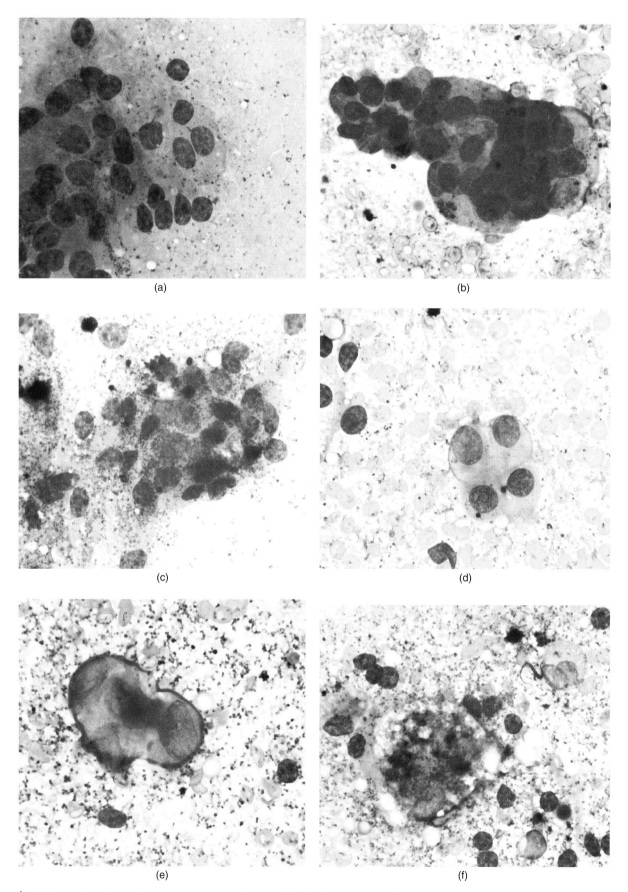

Fig. 30.2. (a–f) A fine-needle aspiration biopsy of mass (Wright–Giemsa stain, 100×).

Table 30.1. Hematology results.

	Day 1	Five years prior	Reference[a]
WBC (10^3/μL)	8.5	10.1	5.5–17.5
Neutrophils (10^3/μL)	4.8	7.0	—
Neutrophils (%)	57	69	22–48
Lymphocytes (10^3/μL)	2.5	2.6	—
Lymphocytes (%)	29	26	39–72
Monocytes (10^3/μL)	0.5	0.5	—
Monocytes (%)	6	5	1–10
Eosinophils (10^3/μL)	0.6	0	—
Eosinophils (%)	7	0	0–7
Basophils (10^3/μL)	0.1	0	—
Basophils (%)	1	0	0–2.7
Plasma protein (g/dL)	—	6.0	—
RBC (10^6/μL)	6.3	5.5	3.2–8.0
Hb (g/dL)	17.2	14.3	10.0–17.2
PCV (%)	49	46	32–50
MCV (fL)	78	83	71–96
MCHC (g/dL)	35	31	26–39
Reticulocytes per microliter	50,480	—	—
Reticulocytes (%)	0.8	—	—
RDW	13.4	15.4	—
Platelets 10^3/μl	285	690	260–740
MPV (fL)	7.7	7.6	—
Clumped platelets	None	Exist	

[a]Quesenberry et al. (2006).

Table 30.2. Plasma biochemical results.

	Day 1	Five years prior	Reference[a]
Glucose (mg/dL)	133	190	60–125
BUN (mg/dL)	14	9	9.0–31.5
Creatinine (mg/dL)	0.3	0.7	0.6–2.2
Phosphorus (mg/dL)	5.8	5.8	3.0–7.6
Calcium (mg/dL)	11.6	11.4	8.2–12.0
Total protein (g/dL)	4.9	5.3	4.2–6.8
Albumin (g/dL)	2.6	2.2	2.1–3.9
Globulin (g/dL)	2.3	3.1	1.7–2.6
A/G ratio	1.1	0.7	—
Cholesterol (mg/dL)	43	22	16–43
Total bilirubin (mg/dL)	0	0.2	0–0.9
CK (IU/L)	275	276	—
ALP (IU/L)	55	294	55–108
ALT (IU/L)	93	33	25–59
AST (IU/L)	94	44	26–68
GGT (IU/L)	7	9	—
Sodium (mg/dL)	136	134	120–152
Potassium (mg/dL)	4.1	5.2	3.8–7.9
Chloride (mg/dL)	97	97	90–115
Bicarbonate (mg/dL)	20.4	20.2	—
Anion gap	22	22	—
Calculated osmolality	272	272	—
Lipemia (mg/dL)	19	19	—
Hemolysis (mg/dL)	40	60	—
Icterus (mg/dL)	0	0	—

[a]Quesenberry et al. (2006).

blue–black cytoplasmic granules. Blue–black granules also appear in the background. Figure 30.2e shows a group of epithelial cells that have failed to divide from each other. The background also contains blue–black granules. Figure 30.2f shows a large epithelial cell with an eccentric nucleus that contains blue–black cytoplasmic granules. The blue–black granules associated with the epithelial cells stained with Wright–Giemsa (Romanowsky) stain are indicative of colloid associated with cells from the thyroid gland. These cells exhibit features of either cellular hyperplasia or benign neoplasia (adenoma) of the thyroid gland.

Summary

On the basis of the guinea pig's clinical signs, location of the mass and cytological findings, a diagnosis of thyroid adenoma was made. This diagnosis was further supported by a blood total T_4 concentration of 6.7 μg/dL. This value is twice the upper limit of the published normal values (2.3–3.5 μg/dL) for males of this species (Depaolo and Masoro, 1989). A thyroid scan was also performed in which 298 microcuries of technetium (Tc) was injected in the cephalic vein of the left forelimb. An immediate marked radiopharmaceutical uptake in the region of the thyroid indicated a large misshapen gland in the center of the neck that was likely unilateral (Figs. 30.3 and 30.4). This finding was indicative of a neoplastic process.

The guinea pig was taken to surgery to remove the abnormal thyroid gland that was contributing to his systemic disease of hyperthyroidism. Hydromorphone (0.47 g/kg), glycopyrrolate (0.009 mg/kg), and midazolam (1 mg/kg) were given subcutaneously as preanesthetic agents 1 hour prior to anesthetic induction and maintenance using 2% isoflurane by face mask and midazolam (0.5 mg/kg) intravenously. The enlarged right thyroid gland was removed following a skin incision and blunt dissection to the glands.

Histopathologic examination of the enlarged right thyroid gland revealed an expansive, compression, and well-demarcated, minimally encapsulated mass composed of sheets, trabeculae, and arborizing cords of neoplastic epithelial cells within a minimal fibrovascular stroma. Neoplastic cells often palisade along the stroma. The neoplastic epithelial cells were columnar with distinct cell borders and abundant eosinophilic cytoplasm that often contained brown intracytoplasmic globular pigment. There was minimal anisocytosis and anisokaryosis. Nuclei were round to oval with coarse clumped chromatin and prominent one to three nucleoli. No mitotic figures were visualized per ten 400× fields. Neoplastic cells often demonstrate intraluminal and associated accumulations of eosinophilic amorphous

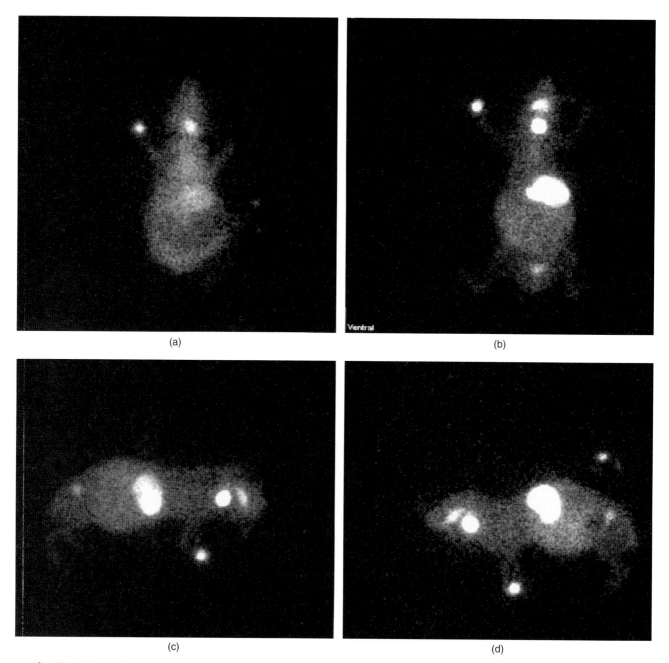

Fig. 30.3. The nuclear scan of the guinea pig with the enlarged thyroid: (a) initial injection, (b) ventral position, (c) right lateral position, and (d) left lateral position.

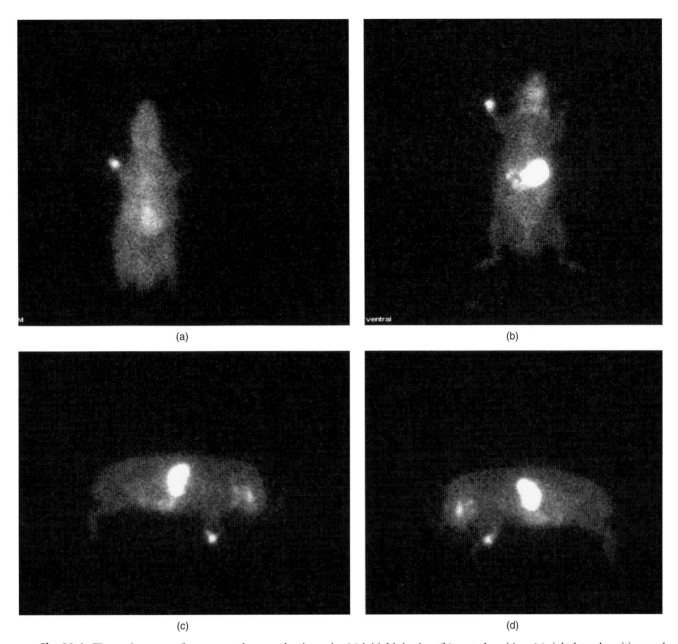

Fig. 30.4. The nuclear scan of an apparently normal guinea pig: (a) initial injection, (b) ventral position, (c) right lateral position, and (d) left lateral position.

material, with occasional associated foamy macrophages. Additionally, neoplastic cells demonstrate apical blebbing. The noninked surgical margin was composed of less than 1 mm of compressed thyroid gland and associated capsules. This supported a histologic diagnosis of a thyroid adenoma.

At the time of suture removal 10 days following surgery, the guinea pig's presenting clinical signs had disappeared and the animal appeared healthy and was gaining weight. The guinea pig lived for another 16 months until he died of left-sided heart failure that resulted in pulmonary edema, as well as right-sided heart failure resulting in hepatic congestion and centrilobular degeneration. There was no evidence of neoplastic metastasis in any organs examined. A leiomyoma within the serosa of the small intestine was also found but was considered to be an incidental finding.

31

A 2-Year-Old Rat with Diarrhea, Dry Skin, and Squinting Eye

Signalment

A 2-year-old intact naked male rat (a variety of fancy rat, *Rattus norvegicus*) was presented with a complaint of a 2-day history of poor appetite, diarrhea, dry skin, and squinting eye (Fig. 31.1).

History

One week prior to presentation, this rat, a member of a colony of 16 naked rats, arrived in the area after a long move from halfway across the country. Since then the colony had lost three rats. An older female and her $1^1/_2$-year-old son suddenly died 2 days after the move and a third adult male died a day later. The surviving rats in the colony became partially anorectic and exhibited diarrhea.

Physical Examination Findings

This male rat was bright, alert, and responsive on physical examination. He tended to hold his left eye closed. The conjunctiva of his left eye was reddened, and a large piece of debris (presumed to be bedding material) was found lodged under the lower lid. The debris was removed and the cornea of the left eye was stained and revealed no evidence of corneal ulceration. This rat was accompanied by two other rats, both of which were also suffering with partial anorexia and diarrhea. A fecal sample was obtained for examination as a wet mount preparation under the microscope (Figs. 31.2–31.5).

Interpretive Discussion

The entire colony of rats is suffering with diarrhea and partial anorexia. Figure 31.2 reveals the appearance

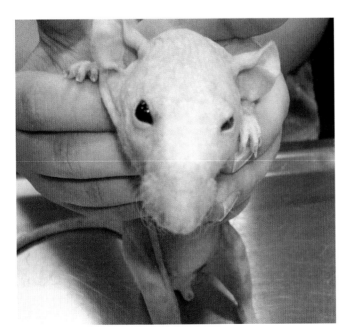

Fig. 31.1. The 2-year-old intact naked male rat that was presented with partial anorexia and diarrhea.

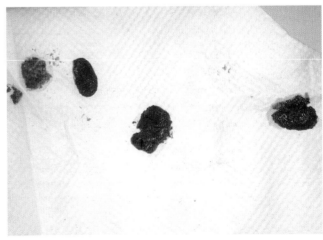

Fig. 31.2. The abnormal feces produced by the rats.

143

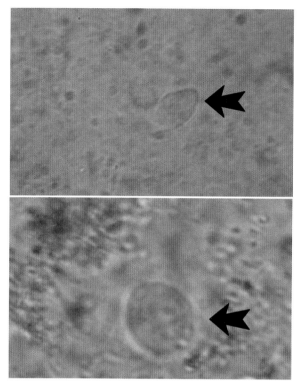

Fig. 31.3. An image from the wet mount preparation of the feces, 100×.

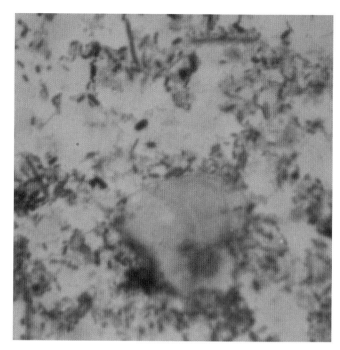

Fig. 31.5. The fecal cytology (Diff-Quik stain, 100×).

of the abnormal feces. A wet mount preparation of the feces revealed numerous highly motile piriform-shaped flagellate protozoa with an undulating membrane (Fig. 31.3). A stained fecal smear (Figs. 31.4 and 31.5) reveals oval to piriform-shaped cells with an eccentric nucleus

and prominent rigid, curved structure seemingly associated with the nucleus in the cytoplasm. This is the typical appearance of trichomonads in stained smears. The drying of the slide and staining process distort the protozoa; however, structures associated with them often provide clues to their identity. For example, they can be identified as poorly staining or lightly staining cells (in most preparations) with a small pyknotic eccentric nucleus,

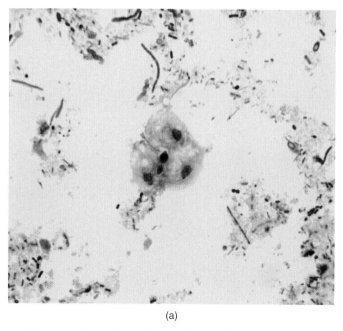

(a)

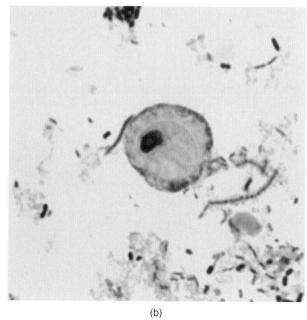

(b)

Fig. 31.4. (a and b) The fecal cytology (Wright–Giemsa stain, 100×).

an axostyle (the pale rigid structure in the figures), an undulating membrane (not seen in the figures), and thin eosinophilic flagella (not seen in Figs. 31.4a and 31.4b, but can be seen in the slightly out of focus image of Fig. 31.5) with Romanowsky-stained specimens.

Summary

This rat along with the entire colony was treated with metronidazole (40 mg/kg PO daily for 5 days) for trichomonad infections. A moisturizing cream was applied daily to the skin of the rat to combat the dry skin that often affects animals that have recently moved from a humid environment to an arid or semiarid one. One drop of a triple antibiotic solution containing a corticosteroid was applied in the left eye twice daily for 10 days to treat the conjunctivitis. After 5 days, the trichomonad infection was completely eliminated in all the rats and they no longer had diarrhea. The male rat's skin and conjunctiva appeared normal after treatment.

A 6-Year-Old Tiger with Two Masses in Her Mouth

32

Signalment

A 6-year-old intact female Bengal tiger (*Panthera tigris tigris*) was presented for two masses in her mouth.

History

This tiger, along with eight other tigers, was traveling across the country as a promotion to save wild tigers. The owners noticed a mass in her mouth when she yawned (Fig. 32.1). Prednisone and antihistamine treat-

ment was started 1 week prior to presentation; however, it was noted that she was having difficulty eating. There were no other abnormalities noted by the owners. She was on the same diet and housed in the same enclosure as the other tigers.

Physical Examination Findings

An estimated 100-kg Bengal tiger appeared normal when viewed in her travel trailer enclosure that

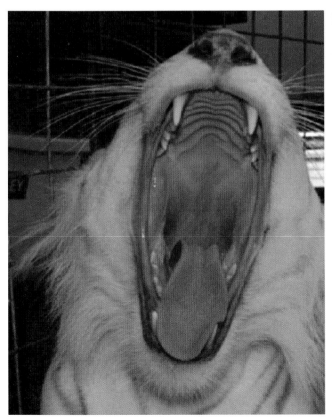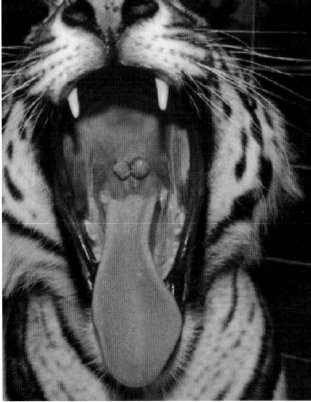

Fig. 32.1. A comparison of normal tiger (on the left) and tiger with lesion when yawning (one the right).

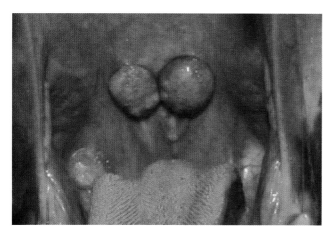

Fig. 32.2. A close-up of lesions in caudal soft palate.

also contained eight other tigers. She was bright, alert, and responsive. In order to perform a more thorough physical examination, injectable anesthetics were necessary. Medetomidine (1 mg), midazolam (10 mg), and ketamine (400 mg) were administered intramuscularly using a spring-loaded pole syringe. Twenty minutes following the delivery of these drugs, the tiger was administered isoflurane via face mask briefly prior to intubation (16 mm endotracheal) and maintenance with isoflurane anesthesia.

Two 2.5–3.0 cm raised, round, well-circumscribed masses were found on the caudal soft palate (Fig. 32.2). There were no other abnormalities noted on physical examination. A fine-needle aspirate of the mass was taken for further evaluation (Figs. 32.3 and 32.4).

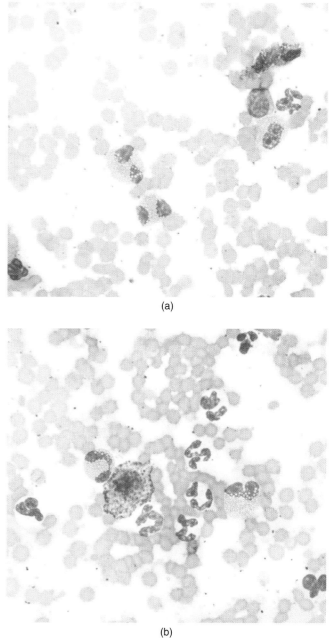

(a)

(b)

Fig. 32.4. (a and b) The aspirate of oral lesion (Wright–Giemsa stain, 100×).

Other Diagnostic Information

A blood sample was obtained for a complete blood count and serum chemistry panel to assess the health status of the tiger (Fig. 32.5 and Tables 32.1 and 32.2).

Interpretive Discussion

Representative examples of the cytologic examination from the fine-needle aspirate are shown (Figs. 32.3 and 32.4). Five eosinophils are seen in Fig. 32.3.

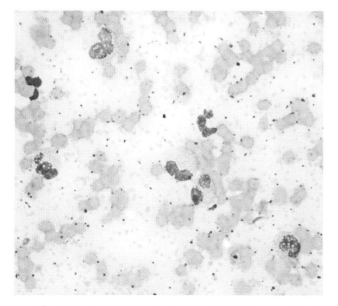

Fig. 32.3. An aspirate of oral lesion (Diff-Quik stain, 100×).

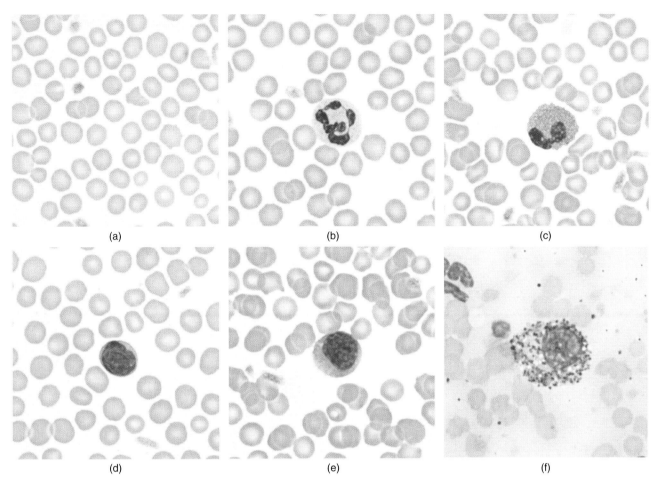

Fig. 32.5. A blood film (Wright–Giemsa stain, 100×): (a) erythrocytes exhibiting mild anisocytosis and poikilocytosis, (b) a normal neutrophil and platelet, (c) a normal eosinophil, (d) a lymphocyte, (e) a monocyte, and (f) a basophil.

Table 32.1. Hematology results.

	Results	Normal range Bengal tigers[a]
WBC ($10^3/\mu$L)	8.5	4.9–17.1
Neutrophils ($10^3/\mu$L)	7.2	0.9–13.9
Lymphocytes ($10^3/\mu$L)	0.7	0–3.5
Monocytes ($10^3/\mu$L)	0.1	0–0.8
Eosinophils ($10^3/\mu$L)	0.5	0–0.6
Basophils ($10^3/\mu$L)	0	0–0.1
Plasma protein (g/dL)	6.8	—
RBC ($10^6/\mu$L)	7.1	4.8–8.3
Hb (g/dL)	14.4	9.6–16.0
PCV (%)	42	29–48
MCV (fL)	59	48.6–69.0
MCHC (g/dL)	34	27.8–38.6
Cell hemoglobin retic	21.8	—
MCV retic	63	—
RDW	15.9	—
Platelets ($10^3/\mu$L)	288	77–389
MPV (fL)	14.6	–

[a]Actual ranges (mean ± 2 standard deviations) for female tiger over 3 years of age. International Species Information System, 2002, Apple Valley, MN.

Erythrocytes and inflammatory cells were present in moderate numbers on the cytology sample. Figure 32.4a shows three eosinophils, a neutrophil, and a lymphocyte. Figure 32.4b shows eight neutrophils, two eosinophils, and a mast cell. The differential of cells on the slide was 46% eosinophils, 38% neutrophils, 10% lymphocytes, 6% large mononuclear cells, and a small number of mast cells. Due to the relatively low number of mast cells, this lesion was more likely a granuloma than a tumor. Owing to a relatively high number of eosinophils, the cytodiagnosis of an eosinophilic inflammation was made.

The hematology and serum chemistry panel appear normal.

Summary

This tiger underwent surgery to remove the masses. Histopathologic examination revealed a mix inflammatory reaction with a predominance of eosinophils and

Table 32.2. Plasma biochemical results.

	Results	Normal range Bengal tigers[a]
Glucose (mg/dL)	154	49.9–213.8
BUN (mg/dL)	36	13–41
Creatinine (mg/dL)	2.8	1.6–4.4
Phosphorus (mg/dL)	4.7	3.6–6.8
Calcium (mg/dL)	9.4	8.9–11.0
Total protein (g/dL)	7.0	6.2–8.2
Albumin (g/dL)	3.5	2.9–4.5
Globulin (g/dL)	3.5	2.7–4.3
A/G ratio	1.0	—
Cholesterol (mg/dL)	151	114.2–342.5
Total bilirubin (mg/dL)	0.2	0–0.4
CK (IU/L)	360	0–1,492
ALP (IU/L)	11	5–41
ALT (IU/L)	42	0–167
AST (IU/L)	22	0–64
GGT (IU/L)	1	0–9
Sodium (mEq/dL)	147	144–156
Potassium (mEq/dL)	3.9	3.5–4.7
Chloride (mEq/dL)	121	112–128
Bicarbonate (mEq/dL)	15.7	11.2–20.4
Anion gap	15	—
Calculated osmolality	303	—
Lipemia (mg/dL)	12	—
Hemolysis (mg/dL)	0	—
Icterus (mg/dL)	0	—

[a]Actual ranges (mean ± 2 standard deviations) for female tiger over 3 years of age. International Species Information System, 2002, Apple Valley, MN.

confirmed the diagnosis of eosinophilic granulomatous stomatitis.

Three weeks after surgery, the mass recurred. The tiger was placed on corticosteroids and antihistamines, which appeared to resolve with this medical treatment.

This condition has been reported in other tigers (Sykes et al., 2007) and is commonly reported in domestic cats (*Felis catus*). The etiology remains unknown. In other cases, clinical signs may or may not be evident and many treatment protocols have been attempted with varying degrees of success, though no case has completely resolved.

A 10-Year-Old Lion with Weight Loss and Lethargy

33

Signalment

A 10-year-old intact female African lion (*Panthera leo*) was presented for weight loss and lethargy (Fig. 33.1).

History

The lioness lived alone in an enclosure at an animal sanctuary where she had lived for many years. She arrived with a 2-week history of vomiting and anorexia and had been constipated for the last 4 days. During the past few months, the sanctuary had been undergoing financial difficulties and as a result had to resort to feeding a variety of meat products to the lioness instead of her

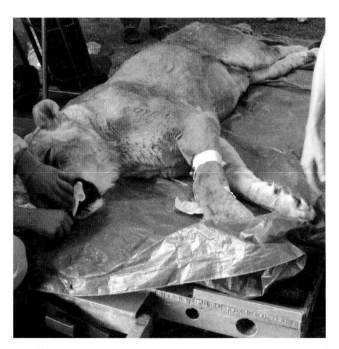

Fig. 33.1. The 10-year-old African lioness that was presented for weight loss and lethargy.

normal steady diet of fortified horsemeat. As a result, she was being fed a varied diet that consisted of whatever was available for the day, such as venison, beef, horsemeat, rabbit, and buffalo. As a result, the lioness began to exhibit signs of lethargy with intermittent bouts of diarrhea and constipation. She had been treated during the past month with trimethoprim-sulfa antibiotic, but showed no improvement.

Physical Examination Findings

The lioness arrived after sedation with a combination of xylazine, tiletamine/zolazepam, and ketamine needed to load her into the transport trailer. She was given yohimbine to reverse the xylazine shortly before her arrival. She appeared thin and dehydrated (at least 10%) with a heart rate of 80 beats/minute, respiratory rate of 10 breaths/minute, and a body temperature of 97°F. On arrival, she was immediately placed under general anesthesia for diagnosis that included a diagnostic panel, complete blood count, abdominal radiographs, and gastrointestinal ultrasound. The 170 kg lioness was given ketamine (4.7 mg/kg) and medetomidine (0.4 mg/kg) intravenously and maintained on isoflurane anesthesia after intubation (size 20 endotracheal tube) (Tables 33.1 and 33.2).

Yellow, hazy urine was obtained by cystocentesis. A urinalysis revealed a pH of 5.0 with a 2+ blood on the test strip. The urine was negative for protein, sulfosalicylic acid protein, glucose, ketones, bilirubin, bacteria, fat, and casts. There were occasional white blood cells, 10–20 red blood cells per high-power field, and few amorphous crystals. The specific gravity was 1.016.

Blood gas evaluation following anesthetic induction revealed a pH of 7.281, pCO_2 of 56, an HCO_3 of 25.5, and an anion gap of 14. The ionized calcium was 1.5.

The lateral abdominal radiograph suggested focal loss of serosal detail within the mid-abdomen. Gastrointestinal structures, kidneys, urinary bladder, and liver

151

Table 33.1. Hematology results.

		Reference[a]
WBC (10^3/μL)	14.7	6.1–26.7
Neutrophils (10^3/μL)	11.8	0.04–22.7
Neutrophils (%)	80	—
Lymphocytes (10^3/μL)	2.2	0.03–6.4
Lymphocytes (%)	15	—
Monocytes (10^3/μL)	0.1	0–1.3
Monocytes (%)	1	—
Eosinophils (10^3/μL)	0.6	0–1.5
Eosinophils (%)	4	—
Basophils (10^3/μL)	0	0–0.3
Basophils (%)	0	—
Plasma protein (g/dl)	7.5	—
RBC (10^6/μL)	8.7	5.2–11.0
Hb (g/dl)	14.6	7.3–18.0
PCV (%)	39	26–53
MCV (fL)	45	33–64
MCHC (g/dL)	37	22.4–49.7
Reticulocytes per microliter	—	0–0.3
Reticulocytes (%)	—	—
RDW	15.5	—
Platelets (10^3/μL)	230	117–734
MPV (fL)	11.6	—
Rouleaux	Increased	—

[a]Actual ranges for female African lions over 10 years of age. International Species Information System, 2002, Apple Valley, MN.

Table 33.2. Plasma biochemical results.

		Reference[a]
Glucose (mg/dL)	117	46–210
BUN (mg/dL)	74	15–47
Creatinine (mg/dL)	8.2	1.5–3.9
Phosphorus (mg/dL)	4.6	3.0–7.4
Calcium (mg/dL)	15.4	7.6–12.0
Total protein (g/dL)	7.4	6.3–8.7
Albumin (g/dL)	3.2	2.6–4.2
Globulin (g/dL)	4.2	2.0–5.4
A/G ratio	0.8	—
Cholesterol (mg/dL)	107	89–269
Total bilirubin (mg/dL)	0.3	0–0.4
CK (IU/L)	1,147	0–1,817
ALP (IU/L)	44	0–48
ALT (IU/L)	42	0–107
AST (IU/L)	50	0–86
GGT (IU/L)	0	0–12
Sodium (mg/dL)	145	130–171
Potassium (mg/dL)	2.8	3.4–5.4
Chloride (mg/dL)	108	109–129
Bicarbonate (mg/dL)	23.5	9.3–20.9
Anion gap	16	—
Calculated osmolality	307	—
Lipemia (mg/dL)	6	—
Hemolysis (mg/dL)	18	—
Icterus (mg/dL)	0	—

[a]Mean ± 2 standard deviations for female African lions over 10 years of age. International Species Information System, 2002, Apple Valley, MN.

appeared within normal limits. The focal loss of serosal detail may be due to superimposition of structures or focal loss of detail as would be seen with small-volume peritoneal effusion or peritonitis.

An ultrasound examination of the gastrointestinal tract of the lioness indicated that the stomach was moderately distended with air, which precluded evaluation of the entire gastric wall; however, the ventral portion of the wall appeared normal. The visualized loops of small bowel were normal, and there was no bowel wall thickening. Normal-appearing peristalsis was observed in several of the small bowel loops. The colon also appeared normal. A lymph node measuring 12 mm in depth and having a normal sonographic appearance was identified in the midline of the caudal abdomen dorsal to the urinary bladder. The mesenteric adipose tissue in the midventral abdomen had variable echogenicity. No obvious mass was identified and there was no free intraperitoneal fluid found. The pancreas was not identified. The variable echogenicity of the mesenteric adipose tissue in the midventral abdomen may represent residual change from previous peritonitis. A mild acute peritonitis could not be ruled out; however, no free fluid was seen. Overall, the gastrointestinal tract sonographically appeared normal.

An abdominal exploratory surgery was performed because of the lack of a diagnosis based on the above-listed diagnostic tests. A 30 cm ventral midline incision was made using a scalpel blade. Cautery was used for controlling soft tissue bleeding and deepening the incision to enter the abdominal cavity. An abdominal explore revealed flaccid, pale, thickened intestines, dilated lymphatics, and cystic ovaries with tortuous vasculature. There was no evidence of a gastrointestinal obstruction. The liver could be palpated, but not visualized. The edges of the liver were sharp, and the liver seemed to be of normal size. Both ovaries were removed at the request of the sanctuary owner. An incisional biopsy was obtained from the jejunum and duodenum, and the biopsy sites were closed with a 3-0 absorbable suture in a simple continuous pattern (Fig. 33.3). A mesenteric lymph node was removed for histopathology using the guillotine method (Fig. 33.2). The abdominal cavity was lavaged with warm saline followed by closure of the body wall using a number 2 absorbable suture in a cruciate pattern. The subcutaneous tissue was closed with a 2-0 absorbable suture in a subcuticular suture pattern, and the skin was closed with the same suture material using an intradermal suture pattern.

Interpretive Discussion

The urinalysis revealed a moderate increase in the amount of erythrocytes in the urine, suggestive of either bleeding somewhere in the urinary tract or red blood

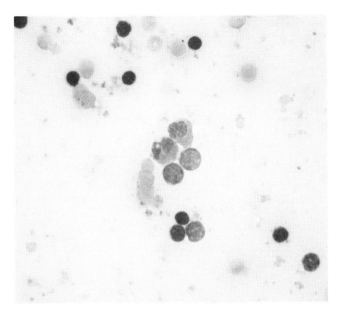

Fig. 33.2. An image of mesenteric lymph node imprint (Wright–Giemsa stain, 100×).

cell contamination of the sample during urine collection via cystocentesis.

The hemogram appeared normal. The significant serum biochemistries indicated an azotemia, hypokalemia, and hypercalcemia. The azotemia was likely to be prerenal in nature because of the urine-specific gravity and serum phosphorus concentration was not low; however, an acute renal failure cannot be completely ruled out due to an unexplained hypercalcemia. Hypercalcemia can also be associated with iatrogenic

causes (such as hypervitaminosis D from oversupplementation of vitamins), malignancy, or endocrine disorders. The low potassium was likely associated with lack of adequate dietary intake due to anorexia and increased loss or inadequate absorption due to vomiting. The increase in serum bicarbonate associated with acidic urine was indicative of metabolic compensation for a systemic acidosis. The blood gas findings indicated a respiratory acidosis with metabolic compensation based on an acid pH (normal should be 7.4), increased pCO_2 (normal should be 40), increased HCO_3 (normal should be 24), and a normal anion gap (normal range of 10–27).

Cytological examination of an imprint from the mesenteric lymph node submitted for histology revealed a moderately cellular sample that consisted of predominantly small normal-appearing lymphocytes. Occasional rare lymphoblasts were present. There were a few eosinophils scattered throughout, and many free eosinophil granules in the background, suggesting the presence of broken eosinophils; therefore, a mild eosinophilic lymphadenitis was reported. Figure 33.2 reveals two eosinophils among the small, mature lymphocytes. No microorganisms were seen.

Cytologic examination of the duodenal imprint revealed a sample with low cellularity. A few lymphocytes and eosinophils were found among normal columnar epithelial cells, suggestive of eosinophilic enteritis. Figure 33.3a reveals normal-appearing columnar epithelial cells arranged in a row. Figure 33.3b reveals lymphocytes and an eosinophil.

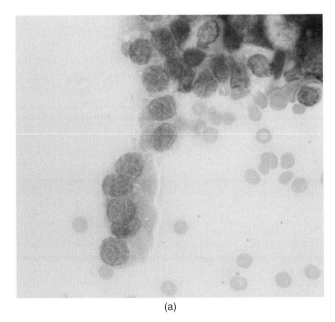

(a)

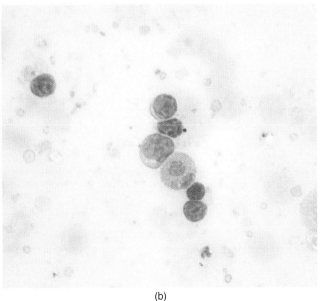

(b)

Fig. 33.3. (a and b) The image of imprint of duodenal biopsy (Wright–Giemsa stain, 100×).

Summary

The lioness made an uneventful recovery from her anesthesia and surgery. She was sent to another wildlife sanctuary for recovery and postoperative convalescence where she was placed on a consistent diet. Although recommended, she was never returned for reevaluation. During the following 2 weeks, her behavior returned to normal and she appeared to be gaining weight although an actual weight was difficult to obtain. In this case, the eosinophilic gastroenteritis and lymphadenitis appeared to be related to the inconsistent diet.

34

A 5^1/$_2$-Year-Old Ferret Presented for a Presurgical Evaluation

Signalment

A 5^1/$_2$-year-old castrated male ferret (*Mustela putorius furo*) was examined for presurgical workup for an exploratory surgery and adrenalectomy.

History

This animal, a blood donor for a veterinary hospital, was housed with one other castrated male ferret. A right adrenalectomy and a partial pancreatectomy were performed 1 year earlier. Alopecia had recurred and was first noted 1 month prior to presentation. There were no other clinical signs, and the ferret appeared healthy with a normal appetite and weight.

Physical Examination Findings

A palpable mass was noted in the cranial abdomen during the physical examination. The ferret was scheduled for an exploratory surgery with the possibility of a left adrenalectomy. Blood was collected for evaluation prior to anesthesia (Tables 34.1 and 34.2).

Table 34.1. Hematology results.

	Pre-op	Reference[a]	Reference[b]	Reference[c]
WBC (10^3/μL)	6.0	4.0–9.0	4.4–19.1	7.7–15.4 (11.3)
Neutrophils (10^3/μL)	4.3	1.5–3.5	—	—
Neutrophils (%)	72	—	11–82	24–78 (40)
Lymphocytes (10^3/μL)	1.2	0.5–5.0	—	—
Lymphocytes (%)	20	—	12–54	28–69 (50)
Monocytes (10^3/μL)	0.2	0–0.5	—	—
Monocytes (%)	3	—	0–9	3.4–8.2 (6.6)
Eosinophils (10^3/μL)	0.2	0–0.5	—	—
Eosinophils (%)	3	—	0–7	0–7 (2)
Basophils (10^3/μL)	0.1	0	—	—
Basophils (%)	2	—	0–2	0–2.7 (0.7)
Plasma protein (g/dL)	8.1	5.0–6.5	—	—
RBC (10^6/μL)	9.0	7.0–11.0	7.3–12.2	—
Hb (g/dL)	16.3	12–18	16.3–18.2	12.0–16.3 (14.3)
PCV (%)	48	35–53	44–61	36–50 (43)
MCV (fL)	53	47–52	—	—
MCHC (g/dL)	34	33–35	—	—
RDW	14.2	—	—	—
Platelets (10^3/μL)	323	297–730 (453)	297–730	—
MPV (fL)	7.6	—	—	—
Clumped platelets	Exist			
Polychromasia	Slight			

[a]Colorado State University reference ranges.
[b]Fox (1988).
[c]Carpenter (2005).

Table 34.2. Plasma biochemical results.

	Pre-op	Reference[a]	Reference[b]	Reference[c]
Glucose (mg/dL)	95	95–140	94–207	63–134 (101)
BUN (mg/dL)	26	10–26	10–45	12–43 (28)
Creatinine (mg/dL)	0.3	0–0.5	0.4–0.9	0.2–0.6 (0.4)
Phosphorus (mg/dL)	5.6	3.0–5.5	4.0–9.1	5.6–8.7 (6.5)
Calcium (mg/dL)	10.1	8.0–9.7	8.0–11.8	8.6–10.5 (9.3)
Total protein (g/dL)	7.6	5.0–6.4	5.1–7.4	5.3–7.2 (5.9)
Albumin (g/dL)	3.5	2.9–4.1	2.6–3.8	3.3–4.1 (3.7)
Globulin (g/dL)	4.1	1.8–3.0	—	2.0–2.9 (2.2)
A/G ratio	0.9	1.0–2.2	—	1.3–2.1 (1.8)
Cholesterol (mg/dL)	119	70–200	64–296	—
Total bilirubin (mg/dL)	0.2	0.0–0.3	<1	—
CK (IU/L)	252	80–400	—	—
ALP (IU/L)	17	10–60	9–84	30–120 (53)
ALT (IU/L)	142	60–270	—	82–289 (170)
AST (IU/L)	33	30–75	28–120	—
GGT (IU/L)	21	1–15	—	5
Sodium (mEq/dL)	147	147–153	137–162	146–160 (152)
Potassium (mEq/dL)	4.0	3.3–4.5	4.5–7.7	4.3–5.3 (4.9)
Chloride (mEq/dL)	115	114–120	106–125	102–121 (115)
Bicarbonate (mEq/dL)	20.0	15–23	—	—
Anion gap	16	14–21	—	—
Calculated osmolality	295	—	—	—
Lipemia (mg/dL)	76	—	—	—
Hemolysis (mg/dL)	55	—	—	—
Icterus (mg/dL)	0	—	—	—

[a]Normal range provided by Colorado State University clinical pathology laboratory (http://www.cvmbs.colostate.edu/pathology/clinpath/2006%20Formulary. htm)
[b]Fox (1988).
[c]Carpenter (2005).

Other Diagnostic Information

During surgery a large mass associated with the greater curvature of the stomach and infiltrating the mucosa was found. There were also several enlarged mesenteric lymph nodes. A lymph node was removed and transected for an impression smear (Fig. 34.1).

Interpretive Discussion

The hemogram revealed a mild neutrophilia. The diagnostic profile indicated a hyperproteinemia with a mild hyperglobulinemia and mild hypercalcemia (according to the first set of reference values).

An imprint of the mesenteric lymph node resulted in a highly cellular sample as demonstrated in Fig. 34.1. This figure shows a predominance of large lymphocytes (compared to adjacent erythrocytes). The nuclei are characterized by a fine granular nuclear chromatin, prominent large and multiple nucleoli, and increased cytoplasmic volume. These findings are consistent with malignancy and supportive of a cytodiagnosis of lymphoma.

Lymphoma is a commonly diagnosed disease in pet ferrets and is the third most occurring neoplasia

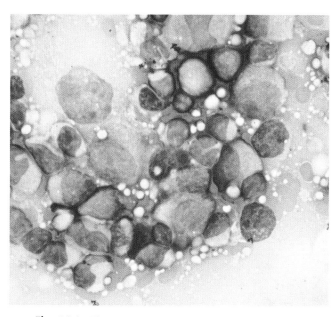

Fig. 34.1. The mesenteric lymph node impression (Wright–Giemsa stain, 100×).

following adrenal neoplasm and pancreatic islet cell tumors (Williams and Weiss, 2004). The mild neutrophilia, hyperglobulinemia, and hypercalcemia may or may not be as a result of the disease. The neutrophilia may be an excitement response and the hyperglobulinemia may be secondary to lymphoma, but it is difficult to assess without knowing which globulins are elevated. Hypercalcemia is a paraneoplastic syndrome rarely seen in ferrets with lymphoma (Hess, 2005).

Summary

On the basis of the strong presumptive diagnosis of lymphoma from the intraoperative cytology, the ferret was euthanized on the surgery table without recovery. A necropsy was performed and lymphoma of the gastrointestinal tract was confirmed. Immunohistochemistry confirmed a T-cell lymphoma.

A 4-Year-Old Ferret with a Tail Mass

35

Signalment

A 4-year-old castrated male ferret (*Mustela putorius furo*) was presented with a tail mass.

History

The ferret was presented for a mass on his tail, which was first noted by the owners less than 2 weeks prior to presentation. The ferret appeared not to be bothered by the lesion, but the owners reported that the mass has significantly increased in size in the last week and had become ulcerated.

Physical Examination Findings

A 2 cm ulcerated mass was found on the ventral mid-tail on an otherwise healthy ferret (Fig. 35.1). A

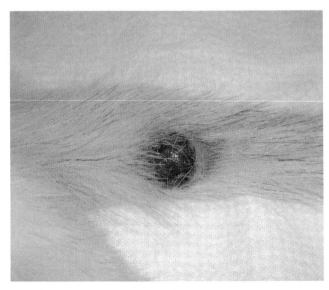

Fig. 35.1. The ferret with a tail mass.

fine-needle aspirate of the mass was obtained for further evaluation (Figs. 35.2a–35.2c).

Other Diagnostic Information

Blood was drawn for preanesthetic hematologic examination and biochemical evaluation (Tables 35.1 and 35.2).

Interpretive Discussion

The cytologic examination of the fine-needle aspirate of the mass revealed a marked inflammatory response characterized by nondegenerate neutrophils and macrophages (Fig. 35.2a). The cytologic examination also reveals several clusters of large epithelial cells (Figs. 35.2b and 35.2c). These cells exhibit a moderate anisocytosis and significant pleomorphism. The cells have an increased nuclear to cytoplasmic (N/C) ratio in most cases. There are also many binucleated and multinucleated cells with large nucleoli and a coarsely granular chromatin pattern. These findings are consistent with malignant neoplasia and more specifically, a carcinoma. It is difficult to determine the tissue of origin based on cytology alone. Inflammatory cells associated with the neoplastic cells indicate a septic inflammatory response (Fig. 35.2c) likely associated with the ulcerative appearance of the lesion.

Neutrophilia, thrombocytopenia, and hyperglobulinemia were noted on the blood profile. Neutrophilia and hyperglobulinemia are likely due to an inflammatory response. The thrombocytopenia may be a result of clumping as noted on the hematology report, therefore, a false decrease.

Summary

On the basis of the history of rapid growth and the cytological interpretation of a presumptive carcinoma, it

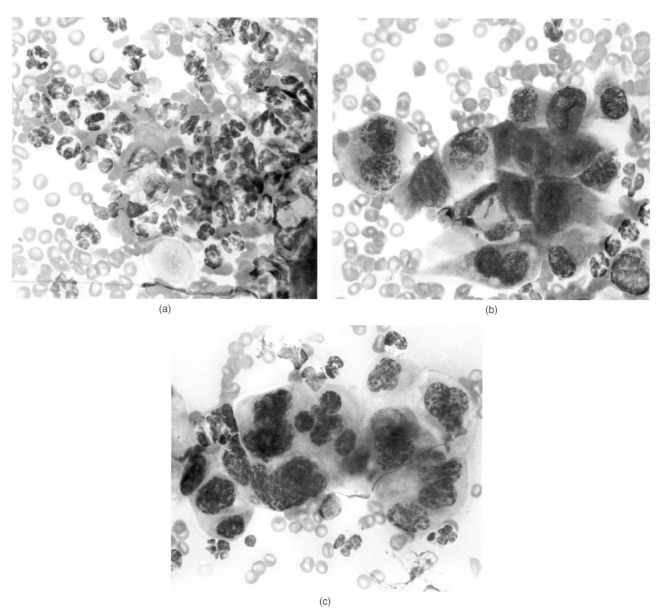

Fig. 35.2. (a–c) The aspirate of the mass (Wright–Giemsa stain, 100×).

Table 35.1. Hematology results.

	Pre-op	Reference[a]	Reference[b]	Reference[c]
WBC ($10^3/\mu$L)	9.3	4.0–9.0	4.4–19.1	7.7–15.4 (11.3)
Neutrophils ($10^3/\mu$L)	7.3	1.5–3.5	—	—
Neutrophils (%)	79	—	11–82	24–78 (40)
Lymphocytes ($10^3/\mu$L)	1.4	0.5–5.0	—	—
Lymphocytes (%)	15	—	12–54	28–69 (50)
Monocytes ($10^3/\mu$L)	0.3	0–0.5	—	—
Monocytes (%)	3	—	0–9	3.4–8.2 (6.6)
Eosinophils ($10^3/\mu$L)	0.2	0–0.5	—	—
Eosinophils (%)	2	—	0–7	0–7 (2)
Basophils ($10^3/\mu$L)	0	0	—	—
Basophils (%)	0	—	0–2	0–2.7 (0.7)
Plasma protein (g/dL)	6.5	5.0–6.5	—	—
RBC ($10^6/\mu$L)	8.5	7.0–11.0	7.3–12.2	—
Hb (g/dL)	14	12–18	16.3–18.2	12.0–16.3 (14.3)
PCV (%)	41	35–53	44–61	36–50 (43)
MCV (fL)	48	47–52	—	—
MCHC (g/dL)	34	33–35	—	—
RDW	12.1	—	—	—
Platelets ($10^3/\mu$L)	192	297–730 (453)	297–730	—
MPV (fL)	8.2	—	—	—
Clumped platelets	Exist			
Polychromasia	Moderate			
Reactive lymphs	Few			

[a]Colorado State University reference ranges.
[b]Fox (1988).
[c]Carpenter (2005).

Table 35.2. Plasma biochemical results.

	Pre-op	Reference[a]	Reference[b]	Reference[c]
Glucose (mg/dL)	128	95–140	94–207	63–134 (101)
BUN (mg/dL)	19	10–26	10–45	12–43 (28)
Creatinine (mg/dL)	0.3	0–0.5	0.4–0.9	0.2–0.6 (0.4)
Phosphorus (mg/dL)	4.8	3.0–5.5	4.0–9.1	5.6–8.7 (6.5)
Calcium (mg/dL)	9.4	8.0–9.7	8.0–11.8	8.6–10.5 (9.3)
Total protein (g/dL)	6.4	5.0–6.4	5.1–7.4	5.3–7.2 (5.9)
Albumin (g/dL)	2.9	2.9–4.1	2.6–3.8	3.3–4.1 (3.7)
Globulin (g/dL)	3.5	1.8–3.0	—	2.0–2.9 (2.2)
A/G ratio	0.8	1.0–2.2	—	1.3–2.1 (1.8)
Cholesterol (mg/dL)	126	70–200	64–296	—
Total bilirubin (mg/dL)	0.1	0.0–0.3	<1	—
CK (IU/L)	240	80–400	—	—
ALP (IU/L)	15	10–60	9–84	30–120 (53)
ALT (IU/L)	66	60–270	—	82–289 (170)
AST (IU/L)	52	30–75	28–120	—
GGT (IU/L)	7	1–15	—	5
Sodium (mEq/dL)	149	147–153	137–162	146–160 (152)
Potassium (mEq/dL)	3.8	3.3–4.5	4.5–7.7	4.3–5.3 (4.9)
Chloride (mEq/dL)	118	114–120	106–125	102–121 (115)
Bicarbonate (mEq/dL)	19.3	15–23	—	—
Anion gap	15	14–21	—	—
Calculated osmolality	298	—	—	—
Lipemia (mg/dL)	0	—	—	—
Hemolysis (mg/dL)	56	—	—	—
Icterus (mg/dL)	0	—	—	—

[a]Normal range provided by Colorado State University clinical pathology laboratory (http://www.cvmbs.colostate.edu/pathology/clinpath/2006%20Formulary.htm)
[b]Fox (1988).
[c]Carpenter (2005).

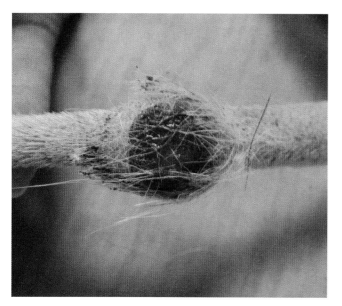

Fig. 35.3. The surgical preparation of the tail.

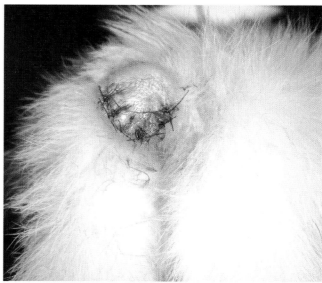

Fig. 35.4. The postoperative tail amputation.

was decided to remove the entire mass instead of obtaining a biopsy for histopathology. The tail was prepared for surgery (Fig. 35.3) and amputated in an effort to obtain 5 cm margins (Fig. 35.4). The amputated part of the tail was submitted for histopathologic examination.

The neoplasm was described as a poorly differentiated carcinoma, presumably an adenocarcinoma. There was vascular invasion, so further assessment for metastatic lesions was recommended. The ferret

returned 2 weeks later for suture removal. He was doing well although he had chewed out two of the sutures. The sutures were removed and silver sulfadiazene cream was applied to the area where he had mutilated the tip. No evidence of metastasis was found on whole body radiographs. Recommendation of further evaluation for metastasis that included regional lymph node assessment or ultrasound was declined by the client.

A 5-Year-Old Rabbit with a Mass Near the Left Nostril

36

Signalment

A 5-year-old castrated male domestic rabbit (*Oryctolagus cuniculus*) was presented with a mass near his left nostril.

History

This rabbit was adopted from a rescue 7 months prior to presentation. The owners first noticed the small growth on the upper left lip 1 month prior to presentation. It had been progressively increasing in size and was now impinging on the left nostril. There were no other problems noted by the owners. A previous biopsy of the mass was inconclusive but thought to be a discrete cell neoplasm.

Physical Examination Findings

The 2.5-kg domestic rabbit was in good body condition. A 1.5–2.0 cm mass was located between the upper left lip and the left nostril (Fig. 36.1). The mass was reddened and ulcerated. Mild lenticular sclerosis was also noted in both eyes.

A fine-needle aspirate of the mass was collected for cytologic examination (Figs. 36.2a and 36.2b).

Other Diagnostic Information

In order to assess the extent and invasiveness of the tumor, a preanesthetic blood profile was obtained. Radiographs and a CT scan were also performed. Blood was submitted for a complete blood count (Table 36.1) and diagnostic panel (Table 36.2).

Other than a mildly elevated alkaline phosphatase (ALP), there were no abnormalities on the blood profile.

Whole body radiographs were taken for metastatic evaluation (Fig. 36.3).

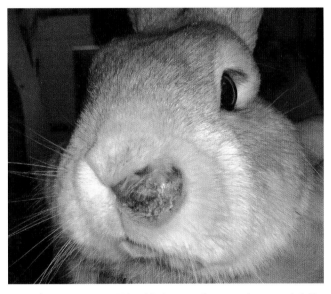

Fig. 36.1. The rabbit with the mass between the upper left lip and the nostril.

The rabbit was placed under general anesthesia for a CT scan. In sternal recumbency, the scan consisted of 1 mm contiguous transverse images of the skull. The images were acquired starting at the first cervical vertebra and extending rostrally to the nasal planum. The mass was described as starting from the left soft tissues of the nasal planum and extending caudally 2.5 cm to the level of the left maxillary incisor roots. Although the mass was adjacent to the maxilla, there were no osseous changes noted.

Interpretive Discussion

The fine-needle aspirate of this mass was poorly cellular. The cells exfoliated individually and did not appear in clusters. The cells exhibited moderate pleo-

163

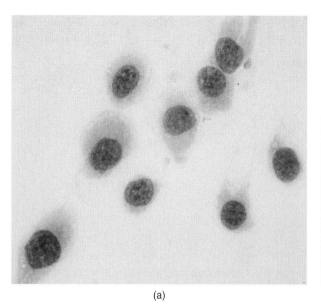
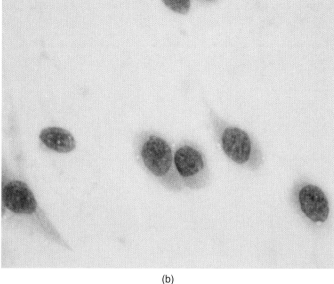

(a)   (b)

Fig. 36.2. (a and b) The fine-needle aspiration biopsy (Wright–Giemsa stain, 100×).

morphism with a tendency toward a spindle shape (Figs. 36.2a and 36.2b), indicating a mesenchymal origin. The nuclei are large, round, and contain a coarse granular pattern. Large irregular nucleoli are occasionally found. The cytology likely represents a soft tissue sarcoma; however, it is difficult to define the tissue origin.

Radiographs showed no evidence of pulmonary metastatic neoplasia. There were multiple mineralized opacities in the cranial abdomen that likely represented saponified fat. Lastly, bridging spondylosis was seen throughout the lumbar and lumbosacral spine.

On the basis of these findings, the history of rapid growth, and the preliminary biopsy results, a malignant neoplasia is very possible. Surgical removal, with possible radiation or chemotherapy, was offered as treatment options.

Table 36.2. Plasma biochemistry results.

	Results	**Reference**[a]
Glucose (mg/dL)	199	75–150
BUN (mg/dL)	16	15–30
Creatinine (mg/dL)	1.0	0.8–2.5
Phosphorus (mg/dL)	3.5	2.3–6.9
Calcium (mg/dL)	15.3	8–14
Total protein (g/dL)	6.4	5.4–7.5
Albumin (g/dL)	3.9	2.5–4.5
Globulin (g/dL)	2.5	1.9–3.5
A/G ratio	1.6	—
Cholesterol (mg/dL)	23	35–60
Total bilirubin (mg/dL)	0	0–0.75
CK (IU/L)	224	0.8–2.5
ALP (IU/L)	66	4–16
ALT (IU/L)	47	14–80
AST (IU/L)	17	14–113
GGT (IU/L)	5	—
Sodium (mEq/dL)	141	138–155
Potassium (mEq/dL)	3.9	3.7–6.8
Chloride (mEq/dL)	103	92–112
Bicarbonate (mEq/dL)	17.8	16.2–31.8
Anion gap	25	—
Calculated osmolality	287	—
Lipemia (mg/dL)	30	—
Hemolysis (mg/dL)	0	—
Icterus (mg/dL)	0	—

Table 36.1. Hematology results.

	Results	**Reference**[a]
WBC (10^3/μL)	3.5	6.3–11.0
Neutrophils (10^3/μL)	1.9	1.5–3.2
Lymphocytes (10^3/μL)	1.4	3.4–7.0
Monocytes (10^3/μL)	0.1	0.1–0.5
Eosinophils (10^3/μL)	0	0–0.2
Basophils (10^3/μL)	0	0.1–0.4
Plasma protein (g/dL)	6.6	—
RBC (10^6/μL)	5.6	4–8
Hb (g/dL)	12.6	8–15
PCV (%)	37	30–50
MCV (fL)	66	58–76.2
MCHC (g/dL)	34	29–34
RDW	12.6	—
Platelets (10^3/μL)	436	290–650
MPV (fL)	6.1	—
Polychromasia	Moderate	—

[a]Campbell and Ellis (2007).

[a]Carpenter (2005).

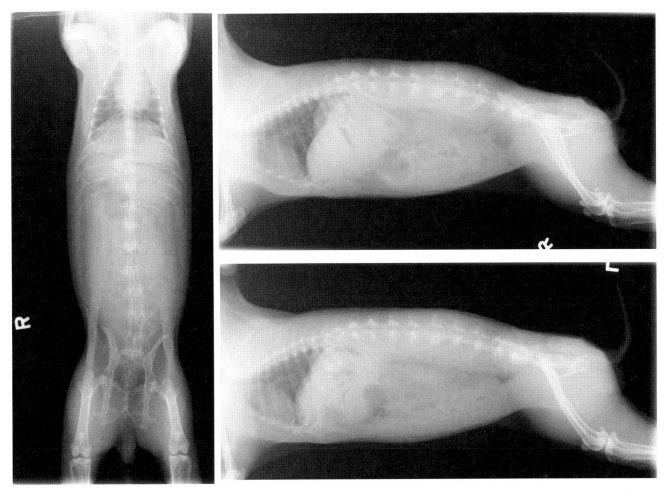

Fig. 36.3. The whole body radiographs.

Summary

With the additional information gained from the diagnostic tests, surgery was scheduled for removal of the mass. Midazolam (1.24 mg), morphine (1.24 mg), and glycopyrolate (0.0247 mg) were given subcutaneously 30 minutes prior to anesthetic induction using midazolam (0.6 mg) and ketamine (13 mg) intravenously. Isoflurane anesthesia was used as maintenance after intubation with a 2.5 mm endotracheal tube.

An incision was made circumferentially around the lip mass and involved the nasal philtrum. The subcutaneous tissues were sharply dissected deep to the mass to the level of the maxillary bone. The mass was excised from the surrounding tissues. A pedicle advancement flap was performed to close the incision. A 4-0 synthetic suture was used to close the subcutaneous tissues with interrupted and continuous patterns. A 4-0 nylon suture was used to close the skin in a simple continuous pattern (Fig. 36.4). The mass was submitted for histopathologic examination.

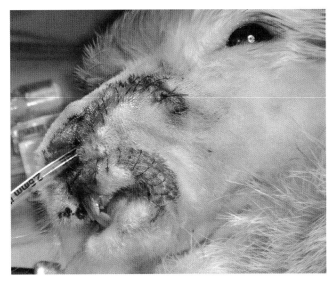

Fig. 36.4. The postoperative appearance of the rabbit.

This rabbit had anesthetic complications, which discouraged further anesthetic procedures. Histopathologic examination confirmed a soft tissue sarcoma with cells along the excisional margin. It was also noted that the atypical mesenchymal proliferation is commonly associated with leporipoxvirus.

The rabbit recovered well from surgery; however, a mass appeared near the right nostril approximately 2 months later. Although samples were not taken, it is presumably a recurrence of the tumor. One month later, several other tumors developed around the rabbit's mouth and eyes. The rabbit was kept comfortable until he passed away approximately 6 months after surgery. No necropsy was performed.

A 1-Year-Old Chinchilla with a Closed Eye

37

Signalment

A 1-year-old intact male chinchilla (*Chinchilla laniger*) was presented with the complaint of an inflamed right eye (Fig. 37.1).

History

The client was a successful chinchilla breeder and provided excellent husbandry for her animals. This chinchilla had been doing fine until yesterday when the client noticed that his eyelids on his right eye were stuck closed until she was able to free them using a commercial artificial tear solution.

Physical Examination Findings

On examination the conjunctivas of the chinchilla's right eye were reddened and inflamed. A conjunctival scraping was performed for cytological examination following application of a topical ophthalmic anesthetic (Figs. 37.2a and 37.2b).

Interpretive Discussion

The conjunctival scraping was poorly cellular as demonstrated in Figs. 37.2a and 37.2b. The few cells present are neutrophils and indicate a neutrophilic inflammation (conjunctivitis). The neutrophils of chinchillas have polymorphic nuclei and faint acidophilic cytoplasmic granules. These should not be confused with eosinophils. Bacteria can be seen in the background, but none were found inside the neutrophils.

Summary

Fluorescent staining of the cornea was negative for the presence of an ulcer. A culture of the lesion identified a pure growth of *Pasteurella multocida* that was susceptible to 11 of the 12 antibiotics tested on the sensitivity screening. The chinchilla was treated at home with one drop of a gentamicin ophthalmic solution given twice daily for 2 weeks. At his 2-week recheck appointment, the chinchilla's conjunctivitis completely resolved.

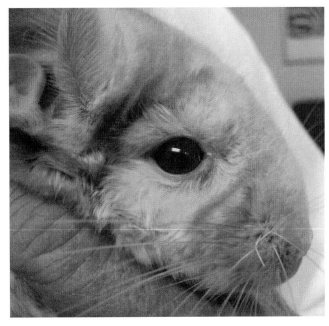

Fig. 37.1. The 1-year-old intact male chinchilla with an inflamed right eye.

167

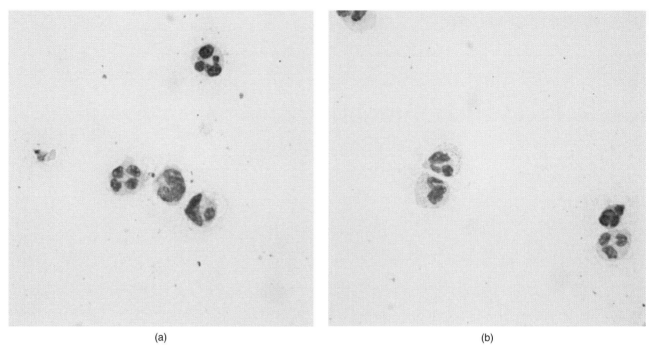

(a)   (b)

Fig. 37.2. (a and b) The conjunctival scraping of the right eye (Wright–Giemsa stain, 100×).

A 5-Year-Old Ferret with a Swollen Head

Signalment

A 5-year-old castrated male ferret (*Mustela putorius furo*) was presented with a nonpainful fluid-filled soft tissue mass located on top of the head just to the right of dorsal midline (Fig. 38.1).

History

During the 1-month duration of this mass, it had been drained weekly by the referring veterinarian. According to the referring veterinarian, the fluid contained within the mass was mucoid in nature. Exophthalmia of the right eye had been noted on one occasion; however, that disappeared following the removal of fluid.

Physical Examination Findings

The 1.1-kg ferret appeared healthy except for the presence of a nonpainful, 3 cm diameter fluctuant mass on top of the head slightly to the right of the dorsal midline. A stainless steel skin staple was found at the caudal aspect of the mass where a Penrose drain had been removed 2 days prior to presentation. The ferret exhibited a mild exophthalmia of the right eye. Blood via jugular venipuncture was collected for a blood profile (Tables 38.1 and 38.2)

Aspiration of the mass revealed a tenacious, honey-colored, blood-tinged fluid (Figs. 38.2–38.4).

Interpretive Discussion

A blood profile revealed a normal hemogram and plasma biochemistries.

Figure 38.3 reveals a highly cellular sample consisting of numerous erythrocytes and inflammatory cells. The inflammatory cells are predominately nondegenerate neutrophils. The linear arrangement of the cells indicates that the sample has high mucin content as

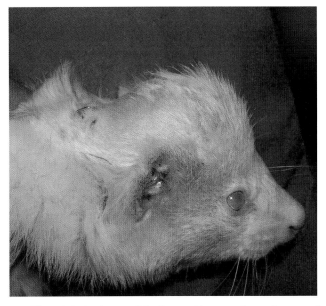

Fig. 38.1. An image of the ferret with a mass located on top of the head.

supported by the gross appearance of the fluid. Higher magnification of the cells (Fig. 38.4) shows the linear arrangement of the cells, nondegenerate neutrophils, and two macrophages. The cytology is indicative of a mixed cell inflammation likely associated with a salivary mucocele based on the location.

Summary

Because of the recurrent nature and the appearance of the fluid provided a presumptive diagnosis of a salivary mucocele. Preoperative radiographs with the possibility of retrograde contrast sialography were offered, but declined by the owner. Examination of the oral cavity revealed a very small and difficult-to-visualize puncta of the zygomatic salivary gland duct, suggesting that if

169

Table 38.1. Hematology results.

		Reference[a]	Reference[b]	Reference[c]
WBC ($10^3/\mu$L)	6.6	4.0–9.0	4.4–19.1	7.7–15.4 (11.3)
Neutrophils ($10^3/\mu$L)	4.0	1.5–3.5	—	—
Neutrophils (%)	61	—	11–82	24–78 (40)
Band cells ($10^3/\mu$L)	0	0	0	—
Band cells (%)	0	—	0	0–2.2 (0.9)
Lymphocytes ($10^3/\mu$L)	2.1	0.5–5.0	—	—
Lymphocytes (%)	32	—	12–54	28–69 (50)
Monocytes ($10^3/\mu$L)	0.33	0–0.5	—	—
Monocytes (%)	5	—	0–9	3.4–8.2 (6.6)
Eosinophils ($10^3/\mu$L)	0.13	0–0.5	—	—
Eosinophils (%)	2	—	0–7	0–7 (2)
Basophils ($10^3/\mu$L)	0	0	—	—
Basophils (%)	0	—	0–2	0–2.7 (0.7)
nRBC ($10^3/\mu$L)	0	—	0	—
nRBC (%)	0	—	0	—
Plasma protein (g/dL)	5.4	5.0–6.5	—	—
RBC ($10^6/\mu$L)	10.2	7.0–11.0	7.3–12.2	—
Hb (g/dL)	17.3	12–18	16.3–18.2	12.0–16.3 (14.3)
PCV (%)	50	35–53	44–61	36–50 (43)
MCV (fL)	49.0	47–52	—	—
MCHC (g/dL)	35.0	33–35	—	—
Reticulocytes ($10^3/\mu$L)	50,950	—	—	—
Reticulocytes (%)	0.5	—	1–12	—
RDW	14.0	—	—	—
Platelets ($10^3/\mu$L)	295.0	—	297–730	—
MPV (fL)	7.5	—	—	—

[a]Colorado State University reference ranges.
[b]Fox (1988).
[c]Carpenter (2005).

Table 38.2. Plasma biochemistry results.

		Reference[a]	Reference[b]	Reference[c]
Glucose (mg/dL)	104	95–140	94–207	63–134 (101)
BUN (mg/dL)	17	10–26	10–45	12–43 (28)
Creatinine (mg/dL)	0	0–0.5	0.4–0.9	0.2–0.6 (0.4)
Phosphorus (mg/dL)	6.0	3.0–5.5	4.0–9.1	5.6–8.7 (6.5)
Calcium (mg/dL)	9.3	8.0–9.7	8.0–11.8	8.6–10.5 (9.3)
Total protein (g/dL)	6.2	5.0–6.4	5.1–7.4	5.3–7.2 (5.9)
Albumin (g/dL)	3.2	2.9–4.1	2.6–3.8	3.3–4.1 (3.7)
Globulin (g/dL)	3.0	1.8–3.0	—	2.0–2.9 (2.2)
A/G ratio	1.1	1.0–2.2	—	1.3–2.1 (1.8)
Cholesterol (mg/dL)	105	70–200	64–296	—
Total bilirubin (mg/dL)	0.3	0.0–0.3	<1	—
CK (IU/L)	144	80–400	—	—
ALP (IU/L)	15	10–60	9–84	30–120 (53)
ALT (IU/L)	54	60–270		82–289 (170)
AST (IU/L)	56	30–75	28–120	—
GGT (IU/L)	1	1–15	—	5
Sodium (mg/dL)	148	147–153	137–162	146–160 (152)
Potassium (mg/dL)	4.9	3.3–4.5	4.5–7.7	4.3–5.3 (4.9)
Chloride (mg/dL)	111	114–120	106–125	102–121 (115)
Bicarbonate (mg/dL)	26.0	15–23	—	—
Calculated osmolality	293	—	—	—
Lipemia (mg/dL)	0	—	—	—
Hemolysis (mg/dL)	13	—	—	—
Icterus (mg/dL)	0	—	—	—

[a]Normal range provided by Colorado State University clinical pathology laboratory (http://www.cvmbs.colostate.edu/pathology/clinpath/2006%20Formulary.htm).
[b]Fox (1988).
[c]Carpenter (2005).

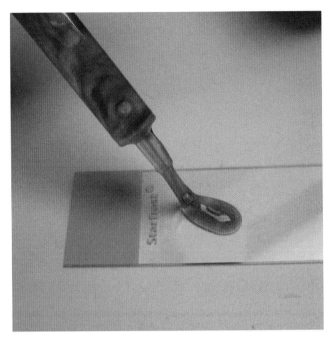

Fig. 38.2. An image of the fluid aspirated from the swelling on top of the head of the ferret.

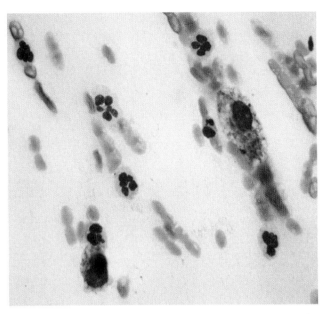

Fig. 38.4. An aspirate of the fluid (Wright–Giemsa stain, 100×).

given permission to perform the contrast sialography, the procedure may have been unsuccessful.

Sixty-two minutes prior to surgery, the ferret was given 0.06 mg hydromorphone and 0.045 mg atropine subcutaneously as preanesthetic treatment. Isoflurane via mask was used to induce anesthesia as well as to maintain anesthesia once the ferret was intubated. The ferret was placed in ventral recumbency, and the dorsal skin on the head was prepared for surgical exploration of the mass. A 3-cm linear skin incision was made over

the mass. Dissection of the fluid-filled mass revealed a well-encapsulated cyst-like structure that extended ventromedially to the right globe and had a visible connection to the right zygomatic salivary gland. Multiple cyst-like structures were noted in the gland. The gland along with the associated sac was removed in its entirety while leaving the zygomatic arch intact. The subcutaneous tissue was closed using 4-0 glycopolymer monofilament synthetic absorbable suture. This was followed by skin closure using 4-0 monofilament nylon suture. A 2 mg

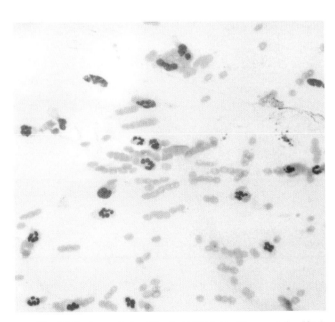

Fig. 38.3. An aspirate of the fluid (Wright–Giemsa stain, 50×).

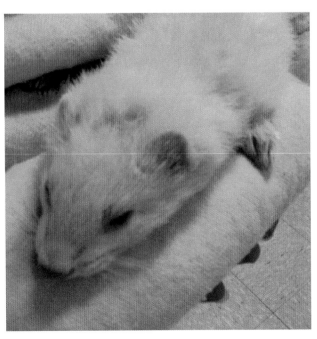

Fig. 38.5. The appearance of the ferret 1 year postoperatively.

bupivacaine line block was peri-incisionally given as a local anesthetic prior to recovery from the inhalant anesthetic. The ferret was given 0.1 mg meloxicam orally daily for 5 days and 0.03 mg buprenorphine orally three times a day for 3 days for pain management.

Histologic results from the biopsy revealed atrophy of the seromucinous salivary gland with sialoadenitis and papillary hyperplasia of the associated ducts. This confirmed the presence of a mucocele associated with the right zygomatic salivary gland.

The right exophthalmia was associated with fluid accumulation above the eye, which resolved once the mucocele was removed. No recurrence of the lesion had been noted 12 months postoperatively (Fig. 38.5).

39

A 2-Year-Old Rat with a Swelling around the Left Inguinal Area

Signalment

A 2-year-old intact female rat (*Rattus norvegicus*) was presented for a swelling around an incision in the left inguinal area (Fig. 39.1).

History

A mass (mammary fibroadenoma) had been surgically removed from the left inguinal area 9 days prior to presentation. The rat was treated with oral pain management (meloxicam) for 5 days postoperatively; however, on day 2, she removed a few of her skin staples. According to the client, multiple attempts at preventing the rat from accessing the incision were unsuccessful until she was fitted with a homemade Elizabethan collar. The rat had not bothered the incision since that day. The client noticed a small swelling near the incision 2 days prior to presentation. Since then the swelling had grown in size.

Physical Examination Findings

The 334 g rat presented with a homemade E-collar around her neck. She appeared healthy on physical examination except for a swelling around an incision in the left inguinal area where she had been shaved for surgery. Four skin staples were found at the cranial end of a healed skin incision in the left inguinal area. The incision had healed in the area where the rat had previously removed the skin staples. Caudal to the healed incision, a 1 cm diameter nonpainful soft swelling was found. A small (<1 mm) red ulcerated area was also found on the right hind footpad. After removal of the skin staples, an aspirate of the swelling was made to obtain a cytological sample (Fig. 39.2). A small amount of clear red fluid was aspirated into the syringe.

Interpretive Discussion

The cytologic examination represented by Figs. 39.2a–39.2c reveals a highly cellular sample containing primarily erythrocytes and inflammatory cells. The mixture of highly vacuolated macrophages and nondegenerate, vacuolated neutrophils indicates a mixed cell inflammation. Note the fine dust-like eosinophilic granules in the cytoplasm of the neutrophils, which is an occasional finding in peripheral blood films of rats. A macrophage in Fig. 39.2b shows evidence of erythrophagocytosis. No infectious agent can be seen; therefore, the cytology likely represents an inflammatory response to a hematoma associated with previous hemorrhage at the site of the swelling.

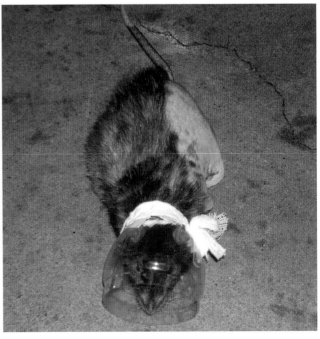

Fig. 39.1. The rat with an Elizabethan collar.

173

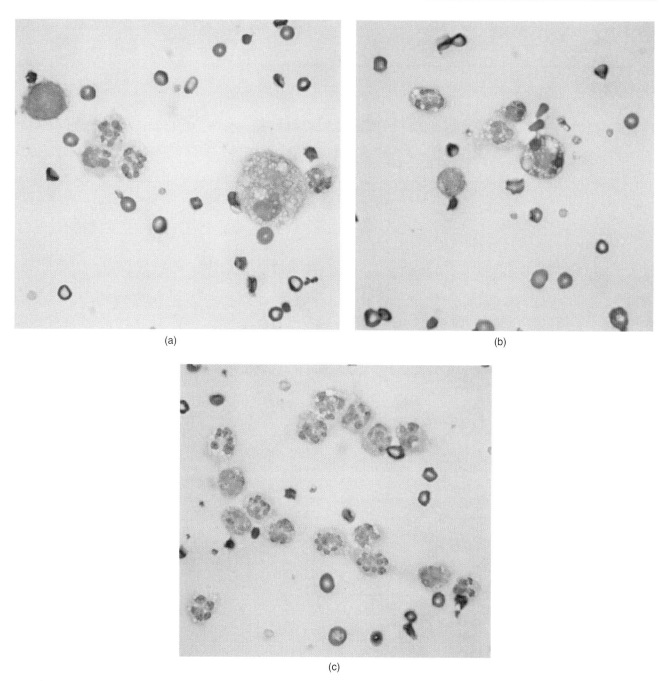

(a)

(b)

(c)

Fig. 39.2. (a–c) The fluid from the subcutaneous swelling on the rat (Wright–Giemsa stain, 100×).

Summary

The rat was treated for 10 days at home with 9.6 mg trimethoprim-sulfa given orally twice daily to help prevent an infection at the site of the swelling. When the rat was reexamined 2 weeks later, the swelling had completely disappeared. According to the owner, the swelling did not recur following the removal of the fluid.

40

A 5-Year-Old Ferret with Lethargy, Dyspnea, Diarrhea, Polyuria, and Polydypsia

Signalment

A 5-year-old castrated male ferret (*Mustela putorius furo*) was presented with lethargy, dyspnea, diarrhea, polyuria, and polydypsia.

History

The ferret had a 2-day history of anorexia. During the past few months, the client was concerned that the ferret was eating and drinking more than normal and as a result had been gaining weight. According to the client, this caused the ferret to develop diarrhea and difficulty in breathing. The client had owned the ferret since he was less than a year old. The ferret lived with a 4-year-old castrated male ferret that appeared healthy. The ferrets were fed a commercial kibbled diet designed for ferrets. According to the owner, this was the first time any of the ferrets had been sick. The ferret was currently being treated with amoxicillin for cystitis as prescribed by another veterinarian who had examined the ferret a week earlier.

Physical Examination Findings

The ferret was obtunded on presentation and weighed 1.7 kg. He appeared dehydrated based on the tenting of the skin. An abdominal mass could easily be palpated on the left side near kidney.

Blood was drawn via jugular venipuncture for hematology and biochemical evaluation. Whole body radiographs were also obtained to evaluate the abdominal cavity (Fig. 40.1 and Tables 40.1 and 40.2).

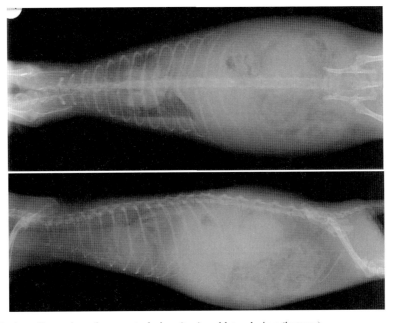

Fig. 40.1. The whole body radiographs—dorsoventral view (top) and lateral view (bottom).

Table 40.1. Hematology results.

		Reference[a]	Reference[b]	Reference[c]
WBC (10^3/μL)	7.4	4.0–9.0	4.4–19.1	7.7–15.4 (11.3)
Neutrophils (10^3/μL)	4.1	1.5–3.5	—	—
Neutrophils (%)	—	—	11–82	24–78 (40)
Lymphocytes (10^3/μL)	2.4	0.5–5.0	—	—
Lymphocytes (%)	—	—	12–54	28–69 (50)
Monocytes (10^3/μL)	0.3	0–0.5	—	—
Monocytes (%)	—	—	0–9	3.4–8.2 (6.6)
Eosinophils (10^3/μL)	0.6	0–0.5	—	—
Eosinophils (%)	—	—	0–7	0–7 (2)
Basophils (10^3/μL)	0	0	—	—
Basophils (%)	—	—	0–2	0–2.7 (0.7)
Plasma protein (g/dL)	7.7	5.0–6.5	—	—
RBC (10^6/μL)	11.7	7.0–11.0	7.3–12.2	—
Hb (g/dL)	19.7	12–18	16.3–18.2	12.0–16.3 (14.3)
PCV (%)	58	35–53	44–61	36–50 (43)
MCV (fL)	50	47–52	—	—
MCHC (g/dL)	34	33–35	—	—
RDW	14.5	—	—	—
Platelets (10^3/μL)	733	297–730 (453)	1–12	—
MPV (fL)	7.9	—	—	—
Clumped platelets	Exist	—	297–730	—
Polychromasia	Slight	—	—	—

[a]Colorado State University reference ranges.
[b]Fox (1988).
[c]Carpenter (2005).

Table 40.2. Plasma biochemical results.

		Reference[a]	Reference[b]	Reference[c]
Glucose (mg/dL)	120	95–140	94–207	63–134 (101)
BUN (mg/dL)	34	10–26	10–45	12–43 (28)
Creatinine (mg/dL)	0.6	0–0.5	0.4–0.9	0.2–0.6 (0.4)
Phosphorus (mg/dL)	5.2	3.0–5.5	4.0–9.1	5.6–8.7 (6.5)
Calcium (mg/dL)	9.9	8.0–9.7	8.0–11.8	8.6–10.5 (9.3)
Total protein (g/dL)	6.7	5.0–6.4	5.1–7.4	5.3–7.2 (5.9)
Albumin (g/dL)	3.6	2.9–4.1	2.6–3.8	3.3–4.1 (3.7)
Globulin (g/dL)	3.1	1.8–3.0	—	2.0–2.9 (2.2)
A/G ratio	1.2	1.0–2.2	—	1.3–2.1 (1.8)
Cholesterol (mg/dL)	193	70–200	64–296	—
Total bilirubin (mg/dL)	0.1	0.0–0.3	<1	—
CK (IU/L)	241	80–400	—	—
ALP (IU/L)	28	10–60	9–84	30–120 (53)
ALT (IU/L)	133	60–270		82–289 (170)
AST (IU/L)	46	30–75	28–120	—
GGT (IU/L)	12	1–15	—	5
Sodium (mEq/dL)	150	147–153	137–162	146–160 (152)
Potassium (mEq/dL)	4.2	3.3–4.5	4.5–7.7	4.3–5.3 (4.9)
Chloride (mEq/dL)	119	114–120	106–125	102–121 (115)
Bicarbonate (mEq/dL)	18.5	15–23	—	—
Anion gap	17	14–21	—	—
Calculated osmolality	306	—	—	—
Lipemia (mg/dL)	5	—	—	—
Hemolysis (mg/dL)	33	—	—	—
Icterus (mg/dL)	0	—	—	—

[a]Normal range provided by Colorado State University clinical pathology laboratory (http://www.cvmbs.colostate.edu/pathology/clinpath/2006%20Formulary.htm).
[b]Fox (1988).
[c]Carpenter (2005).

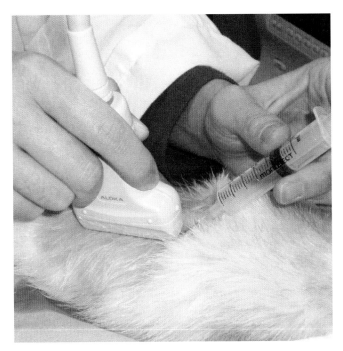

Fig. 40.2. The ultrasound-guided fine-needle aspiration biopsy of the abdominal mass.

Other Diagnostic Information

An ultrasound-guided fine-needle aspirate of the abdominal mass was obtained for cytologic interpretation (Figs. 40.2–40.3).

Interpretive Discussion

The radiographs reveal bilateral pleural effusions. The caudal aspect of the cranial mediastinum is widened. A focal alveolar pattern is seen in the medial aspect of the caudal left lung on the ventral–dorsal (VD) image. Portions of the margins of the cardiac silhouette are not well seen. The heart may be mildly enlarged. There is loss of serosal detail within the abdomen. The liver is enlarged causing caudal displacement of the stomach. On the VD image, a lobulated soft tissue opacity causing displacement of the surrounding bowel is seen within the medial caudal mid left side of the abdomen, L3 through L5. The right kidney is faintly visualized on the VD image. On the lateral view, both kidneys can be seen and each looks of normal size. There is some indistinctness of the dorsal cranial aspect of the abdomen on the lateral image. There is an ill-defined soft tissue mass with associated mass effect in the region of the right kidney on the VD image. This could be related to the mesentery or possibly a neoplasia involving one of the adrenal glands. Enlargement of the liver can be seen secondary to congestion, metabolic disease, or neoplasia. The bilateral pleural effusions could be secondary to right-sided heart failure. Cardiomyopathy cannot be ruled out. The increased opacity and enlargement of the caudal aspect of the cranial mediastinum may be related to fluid within the mediastinum. An echocardiogram and an abdominal ultrasound examination were recommended for further evaluation.

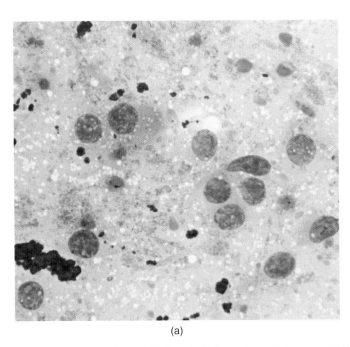
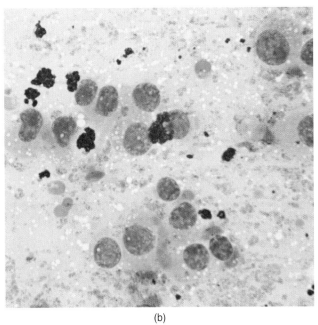

(a)　　　　　　　　　　　　　　　　　　　　(b)

Fig. 40.3. (a and b) The aspirate of the mass (Diff-Quik stain, 100×).

The significant blood profile findings indicate an increase in the packed cell volume (PCV), hemoglobin concentration, hyperproteinemia, and azotemia. This is likely associated with dehydration as noted on the physical examination findings.

The cytologic examination of the fine-needle aspirate of the mass revealed a homogeneous population of mononuclear cells. These cells have an eccentric nucleus and abundant basophilic cytoplasm that often contains small vacuoles. Some cells have prominent large nucleoli, a feature of malignant neoplasia. These mononuclear cells are neuroendocrine in origin and likely represent an adrenal adenocarcinoma based on the anatomical location of the mass.

Summary

Plasma was also submitted for a ferret adrenal panel to the University of Tennessee Diagnostic Lab. The results obtained 1 week later indicated an estradiol of 363.0 pmol/L (normal range 30–180), 17-OH-progesterone of 0.48 nmol/L (normal range 0–0.80), and two androstenedione of 7.1 nmol/L (normal range 0–15). These results support clinical signs for the presence of adrenal disease.

Adrenal disease in ferrets is often associated with an endocrine-patterned hair loss that typically begins with alopecia of the tail. This did not occur in this case; therefore, the abdominal mass could have been related to a granuloma or other type of neoplasia, such as lymphoma, another common neoplasia of ferrets. On the basis of the size of the adrenal mass as well as the age and condition of the ferret, the client decided on euthanasia rather than exploratory surgery to remove the adrenal mass.

The gross necropsy revealed the left adrenal gland effaced with a large 5.5 cm × 5.5 cm × 2.0 cm mass. The mass was multinodular with areas of necrosis and hemorrhage. There were approximately 40 mL of serosanguineous fluid in the peritoneal cavity and 70 mL of serosanguineous pleural effusion. The liver had severe diffuse acute congestion and was moderately friable. The hepatic surface was cobblestone. The diagnoses were a left adrenocortical carcinoma with secondary peritoneal effusion, moderate chronic lymphocytic portal hepatitis, and moderate to marked acute pulmonary congestion and edema. The spleen exhibited diffuse moderate reactive hyperplasia.

A 3-Year-Old Guinea Pig with Anorexia and Decreased Water Intake

41

Signalment

A 3-year-old intact male guinea pig (*Cavia porcellius*) was presented with a 4-day history of partial anorexia and decreased water intake (Fig. 41.1).

History

The guinea pig was housed alone in a commercial guinea pig cage that was kept in a bedroom. He was fed commercial guinea pig pellets, grass hay, carrots, and spinach. He had been eating and drinking less and producing fewer normal-appearing feces during the past 4 days. One week prior to the onset of the clinical signs, the guinea pig was left overnight in an unheated house where the temperature dropped to 40°F. According to the owner, the guinea pig was less active and vocal than normal. The pig was treated for a louse infestation 1 year earlier.

Physical Examination Findings

On physical examination, the 995 g guinea pig was lethargic and moderately dehydrated as determined by tenting of the skin and slight sinking of the eyes into the orbits. He had a pulse rate of 324 beats/minute and exhibited tachypnea. His temperature was 100°F. A pea-sized mass was palpable in the intermandiblar space. A second almond-sized mass was found in the left prescapular region. The guinea pig appeared to be blind and exhibited no papillary light reflex in either eye. Cataracts were found in each eye. A fine-needle aspiration biopsy was obtained from each mass for cytodiagnosis (Figs. 41.2 and 41.3). The guinea pig was given 20 mL of lactated Ringer's solution and 50 mg ascorbic acid subcutaneously along with 5 mL of a commercial critical care diet for herbivores as supportive care.

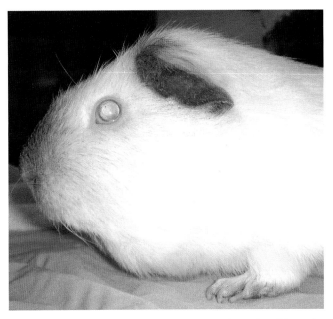

Fig. 41.1. An image of the 3-year-old guinea pig with a submandibular and left prescapular mass.

Interpretive Discussion

Figures 41.2a and 41.2b show a highly cellular sample consisting of a heterogeneous population of lymphoid cells in which the intermediate cells (>90%) predominate. The cells are 1.0–1.25 times the size of a heterophil (neutrophil), have a small amount of deeply basophilic cytoplasm, and a round to oval nucleus with coarse chromatin. Some cells have a prominent nucleolus. Small mature lymphocytes are fewer in number. The background contains a small number of erythrocytes and rare heterophils. The increased population of intermediate-sized lymphocytes exhibiting

179

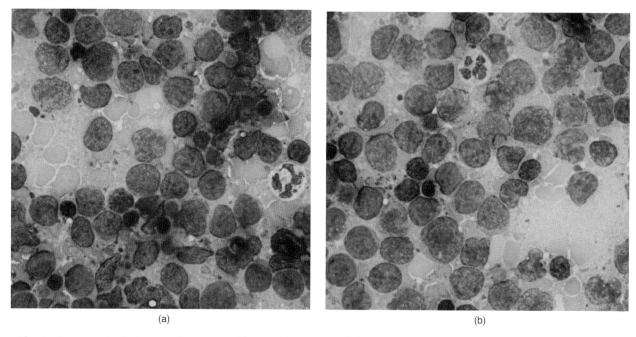

(a)   (b)

Fig. 41.2. (a and b) The fine-needle aspiration biopsy of the submandibular mass (Wright–Giemsa stain, 100×).

a few features of malignancy is indicative of lymphoma.

Figures 41.3a and 41.3b reveal a highly cellular sample that contains primarily a population of lymphocytes, exhibiting features of malignancy as shown in the submandibular sample. The lymphocytes in this sample tend to be slightly larger and exhibit more cytoplasm in comparison to those in the other sample.

Summary

Because of the poor prognosis of lymphoma, the client elected not to pursue further diagnostic testing and treatment. The client was also unaware of the bilateral cataracts causing the guinea pig to be blind. The guinea pig was considered to be older than the age reported by the client. The guinea pig was euthanized; however, no necropsy was performed.

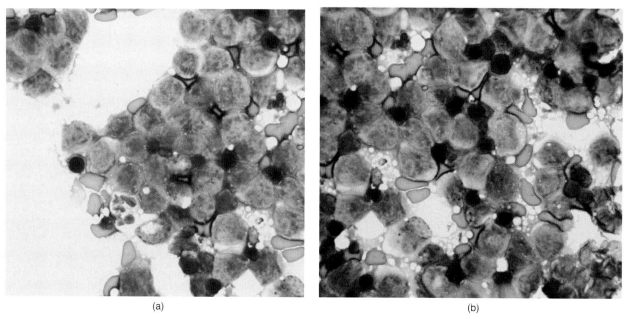

(a)   (b)

Fig. 41.3. (a and b) The fine-needle aspiration biopsy of the prescapular mass (Wright–Giemsa stain, 100×).

A 9-Year-Old Ferret with a Mass on the Ear

Signalment

A 9-year-old spayed female ferret (*Mustela putorius furo*) was presented with a nonpainful soft tissue mass located on the right ear (Fig. 42.1).

History

The mass on the ear had been noticed 3 weeks prior to presentation, according to the client. It appeared to be growing rapidly. The ferret was the only pet in the household. She was fed a commercial kibbled diet made for kittens and ferret treats. The ferret was housed in a commercially made wire ferret cage. The ferret had been eating and drinking normally and there were no other concerns.

Physical Examination Findings

The 530 g ferret appeared healthy except for the presence of a nonpainful, multipedunculated mass on the right pinna. Blood was collected for a blood profile, which proved to be normal. A fine-needle aspiration biopsy of the mass was obtained for cytodiagnosis (Figs. 42.2a and 42.2b).

Interpretive Discussion

Figures 42.2a and 42.2b reveal a highly cellular sample consisting of discrete, round cells with distinct cell margins that exhibit moderate anisocytosis and anisokaryosis. The nuclei are round to oval with no apparent nucleoli or one or multiple prominent nucleoli that vary in size and shape. The cytoplasm is finely granular and basophilic. The background surrounding the cells is a heavy basophilic material. These cells are compatible with a histiocytoma.

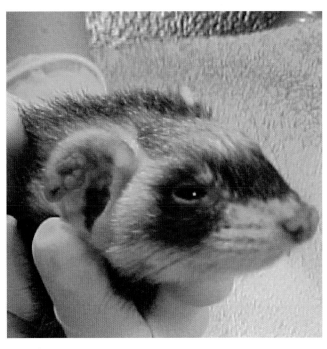

Fig. 42.1. An image of the ferret with a mass located on the right ear.

181

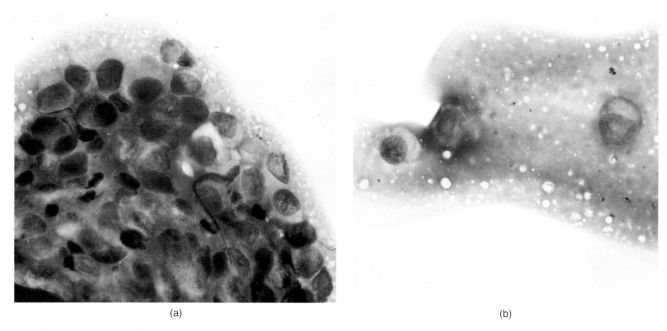

(a)   (b)

Fig. 42.2. (a and b) The aspirate of the mass (Wright–Giemsa stain, 100×).

Summary

Buprenorphine (0.012 mg) was given intramuscularly as a preanesthetic 20 minutes prior to anesthetic induction using isoflurane. A CO_2 laser (0.8 mm ceramic tip, 5 W, continuous pulse) was used to remove the mass. The ferret made an uneventful recovery.

Histopathologic finding of the mass revealed an expansile, neoplastic population of spindloid and histiocytic cells. The neoplastic cells were 20–40 μm in diameter with large ovoid nuclei, clumped chromatin, and abundant, eosinophilic, finely vacuolated cytoplasm. These cells were interspersed with abundant, loose collagen bundles. Numerous multinucleated giant cells were also present. Superficial dermal aggregates of lymphocytes and plasma cells were also found. Neoplastic cells extended to, but did not cross, auricular cartilage. The histopathologic diagnosis was malignant fibrous histiocytoma.

A 3-Year-Old Ferret with Lethargy and Weight Loss

Signalment

A 3-year-old intact male ferret (*Mustela putorius furo*) was presented for lethargy and weight loss.

History

The ferret had a 1-week history of lethargy and weight loss. The clients obtained him from a friend in California approximately 1 year earlier with no known medical problems. It was also noted that the client does body piercing for a living.

Physical Examination Findings

On physical examination, the ferret was obtunded and minimally responsive. Due to his deteriorating condition, blood was collected immediately and an intravenous catheter was placed in his right cephalic vein (Fig. 43.1).

Other findings on physical examination included a body weight of 710 g, body condition score of 3/9, increased respiratory rate and effort, and perianal pasting with melena (Fig. 43.1). Abdominal palpation revealed an irregular splenic surface with multiple small masses.

Ultrasound-guided aspirates of the nodules in the spleen and liver were performed (Figs. 43.2a–43.2d and Tables 43.1 and 43.2).

Interpretive Discussion

The complete blood count (CBC) revealed a leukocytosis with neutrophilia and monocytosis and an elevated plasma protein (refractometric), an indication of an inflammatory leukogram that is possibly associated with an infectious etiology. The presence of band cells indicates an accelerated demand for neutrophils (left shift) associated with an inflammatory stimulus.

The plasma biochemical profile revealed a severe hypoglycemia, a finding commonly associated with an insulinoma in domestic ferrets; however, other possible causes for this include decreased glucose absorption associated with starvation or malabsorption, hepatic failure, sepsis, and neoplasia other than beta cell tumors. The biochemistry profile also revealed an azotemia as indicated by an elevated blood urea nitrogen (BUN) and creatinine and a hyperphosphatemia. This is an indication of a likely loss of 85% of the glomerular filtration rate. The plasma total protein obtained by spectrophotometry on the biochemistry profile does not support a hyperproteinemia as indicated on the CBC. It does,

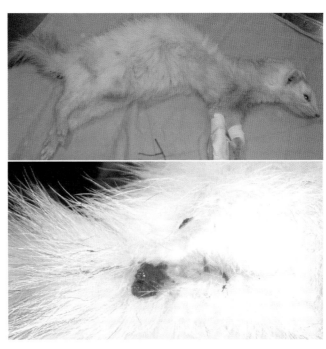

Fig. 43.1. The obtunded ferret on presentation (top) with perianal melena (bottom).

183

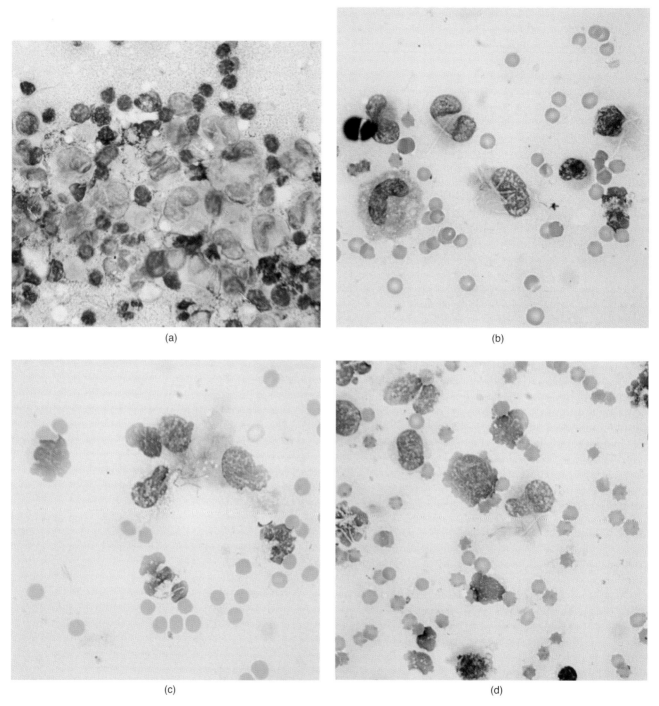

(a)

(b)

(c)

(d)

Fig. 43.2. (a–d) The fine-needle aspiration biopsy of mass (Wright–Giemsa stain, 100×).

however, reveal an alteration in albumin and globulin concentrations (hypoalbuminemia and hyperglobulinemia). A hypoalbuminemia associated with a normal or increased globulin concentration can be an additional indication of hepatic failure. The blood profile supports hepatobiliary disease along with electrolyte imbalances that includes an increased anion gap acidosis. These re-

sults indicate multiple organ involvement, such as hepatic and renal failure.

The physical examination findings of splenic masses were suggestive of lymphoma, a common neoplasia of ferrets and a disease that could result in multiple organ involvement. A lymphocytosis or abnormal lymphocytes, however, were not found on the hemogram.

185

Table 43.1. Hematology results.

	Results	Reference[a]	Reference[b]	Reference[c]
WBC (10^3/μL)	12.6	4.0–9.0	4.4–19.1	7.7–15.4 (11.3)
Segmented neutrophils (10^3/μL)	9.3	1.5–3.5	—	—
Segmented neutrophils (%)	74	—	11–82	24–78 (40)
Band neutrophils (10^3/μL)	1.5	0	0	—
Band neutrophils (%)	12	—	0	0–2.2 (0.9)
Lymphocytes (10^3/μL(	0.6	0.5–5.0	—	—
Lymphocytes (%)	5	—	12–54	28–69 (50)
Monocytes (10^3/μL)	1.1	0–0.5	—	—
Monocytes (%)	9	—	0–9	3.4–8.2 (6.6)
Eosinophils (10^3/μL)	0	0–0.5	—	—
Monocytes (%)	0	—	0–7	0–7 (2)
Basophils (10^3/μL)	0	0	—	—
Basophils (%)	0	—	0–2	0–2.7 (0.7)
Plasma protein (g/dL)	8.3	5.0–6.5	0	—
RBC (10^6/μL)	8.0	7.0–11.0	0	—
Hb (g/dL)	12.6	12–18	—	—
PCV (%)	41	35–53	7.3–12.2	—
MCV (fL)	52	47–52	16.3–18.2	12.0–16.3 (14.3)
MCHC (g/dL)	30	33–35	44–61	36–50 (43)
RDW	11.9	—	—	—
Platelets (10^3/μL)	114	—	1–12	—
MPV (fL)	5.4	—	—	—
Clumped platelets	Exist	—	297–730	—
Adequate platelets	Exist	—	—	—
Echinocytes	Few			
Moderate rouleaux	Noted			

[a]Colorado State University reference ranges.
[b]Fox (1988).
[c]Carpenter (2005).

Table 43.2. Plasma biochemical results.

	Pre-op	Reference[a]	Reference[b]	Reference[c]
Glucose (mg/dL)	30	95–140	94–207	63–134 (101)
BUN (mg/dL)	105	10–26	10–45	12–43 (28)
Creatinine (mg/dL)	1.2	0–0.5	0.4–0.9	0.2–0.6 (0.4)
Phosphorus (mg/dL)	13.2	3.0–5.5	4.0–9.1	5.6–8.7 (6.5)
Calcium (mg/dL)	8.2	8.0–9.7	8.0–11.8	8.6–10.5 (9.3)
Total protein (g/dL)	5.6	5.0–6.4	5.1–7.4	5.3–7.2 (5.9)
Albumin (g/dL)	2.0	2.9–4.1	2.6–3.8	3.3–4.1 (3.7)
Globulin (g/dL)	3.6	1.8–3.0	—	2.0–2.9 (2.2)
A/G ratio	0.6	1.0–2.2	—	1.3–2.1 (1.8)
Cholesterol (mg/dL)	266	70–200	64–296	—
Total bilirubin (mg/dL)	1.5	0–0.3	<1	—
CK (IU/L)	388	80–400	—	—
ALP (IU/L)	127	10–60	9–84	30–120 (53)
ALT (IU/L)	341	60–270		82–289 (170)
AST (IU/L)	227	30–75	28–120	—
GGT (IU/L)	205	1–15	—	5
Sodium (mEq/dL)	143	147–153	137–162	146–160 (152)
Potassium (mEq/dL)	5.0	3.3–4.5	4.5–7.7	4.3–5.3 (4.9)
Chloride (mEq/dL)	109	114–120	106–125	102–121 (115)
Bicarbonate (mEq/dL)	5.9	15–23	—	—
Anion gap	33	14–21	—	—
Calculated osmolality	314	—	—	—
Lipemia (mg/dL)	70	—	—	—
Hemolysis (mg/dL)	17	—	—	—
Icterus (mg/dL)	2	—	—	—

[a]Normal range provided by Colorado State University clinical pathology laboratory (http://www.cvmbs.colostate.edu/pathology/clinpath/2006%20Formulary.htm).
[b]Fox (1988).
[c]Carpenter (2005).

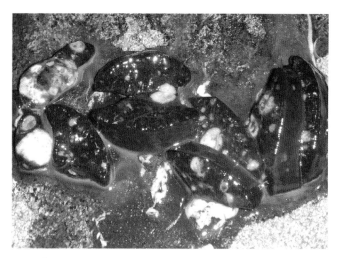

Fig. 43.3. The gross image of the sliced spleen during necropsy.

Multiple ultrasound-guided aspirates were obtained from the nodules palpated on the spleen as well as those found on the liver. Figure 43.2a reveals a macrophagic inflammation with a predominance of macrophages and lymphocytes. Figures 43.2b–43.2d show additional images of macrophages that contain negative staining filamentous inclusions suggestive of mycobacteriosis.

Summary

The ferret was euthanized because of a poor prognosis for survival. The necropsy revealed multiple granulomatous lesions throughout the spleen and liver (Figs. 43.3 and 43.4). The nodules were white, firm, and ranged in size from pinpoint to 5 mm. The mediastinal and

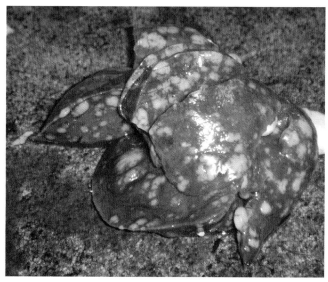

Fig. 43.4. The gross image of the sliced liver during necropsy.

mesenteric lymph nodes were four times and twice normal size, respectively. The lung lobes were bilaterally mottled and firm.

Histopathologic examination revealed multiple granulomas with extracellular and intracellular acid-fast filamentous bacteria in the lungs, liver, spleen, mesenteric, and mediastinal lymph nodes. Histologic finding also revealed a chronic, moderate interstitial nephritis and myocardial degeneration with interstitial fibrosis.

Bacterial culture confirmed a *Mycobacterium* sp. that was identified as *Mycobacterium goodii* using 16S rDNA sequencing. This species of mycobacterium has not been reported in ferrets but has been reported in dogs (Bryden et al., 2004).

A 3-Month-Old Ferret with a Prolapsed Rectum

Signalment

A 3-month-old neutered female ferret (*Mustela putorius furo*) was presented with a prolapsed rectum (Fig. 44.1).

History

The owner obtained the ferret when she was 5 weeks old. According to the owner, the ferret's rectum had been prolapsed during the past 18 hours. The ferret had a history of intermediate episodes of a rectal prolapse since she was 5 weeks of age. Lately, the ferret had been normal except for bouts of small yellow feces during the past 2 days. During the past few weeks, the owner had been offering multiple diets in an effort to change what the ferret eats with the thought that the cause for the rectal prolapse was dietary.

Physical Examination Findings

On physical examination, the ferret was bright, alert, and responsive and her activity level was normal. Her temperature was 101.3°F, her heart rate was 312 beats/minute, and her respiratory rate was 38 breaths/minute. She weighed 545 g with a body condition score of 5/9. Approximately 1–2 mm of her rectum was prolapsed. Abdominal palpation revealed a large mass in the right cranial abdomen. The ferret's feces were soft, yellow, and had a "bird seed" appearance (Fig. 44.2). The feces were sampled for cytologic examination (Figs. 44.3a and 44.3b).

A blood sample was obtained via jugular venipuncture for a complete blood count and plasma biochemical profile. An ultrasound evaluation of the abdomen was also performed (Tables 44.1 and 44.2).

Interpretive Discussion

The complete blood count revealed only a mild neutrophilia and has limited significance as it likely represents a stress leukogram or physiological response associated with excitement.

The hypoalbuminemia associated with normal globulin concentration on the plasma biochemistry profile could result from either a decrease in albumin production or an increase in albumin loss from the body. Decreased albumin production results from liver failure, starvation, intestinal malabsorption of amino acids, gastrointestinal parasitism, or exocrine pancreatic insufficiency. Loss of albumin from the body can occur with glomerular disease and gastrointestinal parasitism. In this case, intestinal malabsorption is likely because of the abnormal appearance of the feces (Fig. 44.2).

Figures 44.3a and 44.3b show the presence of eosinophils in the fecal sample and support a diagnosis of eosinophilic gastroenteritis. This is a common disease of ferrets and is considered to be associated with an immune-mediated or hypersensitivity reaction related to the diet. Affected ferrets often produce feces with a "bird seed" appearance that is considered to be the result of a malabsorption disorder.

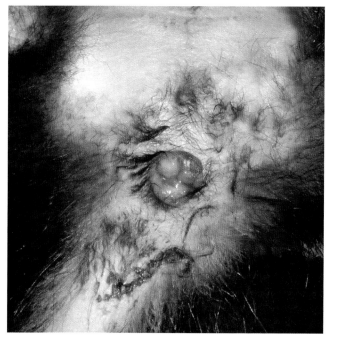

Fig. 44.1. The 3-month-old spayed female ferret with a pro-lapsed rectum.

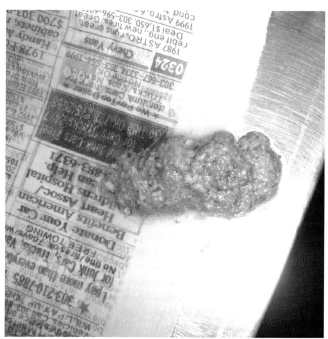

Fig. 44.2. A gross image of the feces.

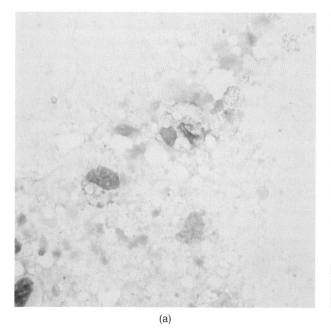

(a)

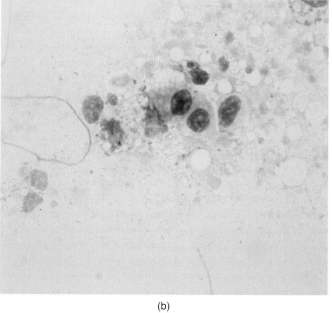

(b)

Fig. 44.3. (a and b) The fecal cytology (Wright–Giemsa stain, 100 ×).

Table 44.1. Hematology results.

	Results	Reference[a]	Reference[b]	Reference[c]
WBC ($10^3/\mu L$)	7.7	4.0–9.0	4.4–19.1	2.5–8.6 (5.9)
Segmented neutrophils ($10^3/\mu L$)	5.2	1.5–3.5	—	—
Segmented neutrophils (%)	68	—	11–82	12–41 (31)
Lymphocytes ($10^3/\mu L$)	2.1	0.5–5.0	—	—
Lymphocytes (%)	27	—	12–54	25–95 (58)
Monocytes ($10^3/\mu L$)	0.4	0–0.5	—	—
Monocytes (%)	5	—	0–9	1.7–6.3 (4.5)
Eosinophils ($10^3/\mu L$)	0.1	0–0.5	—	—
Eosinophils (%)	1	—	0–7	1–9 (4)
Basophils ($10^3/\mu L$)	0	0	—	—
Basophils (%)	0	—	0–2	0–2.9 (0.8)
Plasma protein (g/dL)	6.3	5.0–6.5	—	—
RBC ($10^6/\mu L$)	8.2	7.0–11.0	7.3–12.2	—
Hb (g/dL)	14.3	12–18	16.3–18.2	15.2–17.4 (15.9)
PCV (%)	43	35–53	44–61	47–51 (48)
MCV (fL)	52	47–52	—	—
MCHC (g/dL)	34	33–35	—	—
RDW	13.8	—	—	—
Platelets ($10^3/\mu L$)	693	—	297–730	—
MPV (fL)	7.3	—	—	—
Clumped platelets	Exist			
Echinocytes	Few			
Polychromasia	Moderate			

[a]Colorado State University reference ranges.
[b]Fox (1988).
[c]Carpenter (2005).

Table 44.2. Plasma biochemical results.

	Pre-op	Reference[a]	Reference[b]	Reference[c]
Glucose (mg/dL)	123	95–140	94–207	63–134 (101)
BUN (mg/dL)	20	10–26	10–45	12–43 (28)
Creatinine (mg/dL)	0.3	0–0.5	0.4–0.9	0.2–0.6 (0.4)
Phosphorus (mg/dL)	5.2	3.0–5.5	4.0–9.1	5.6–8.7 (6.5)
Calcium (mg/dL)	9.3	8.0–9.7	8.0–11.8	8.6–10.5 (9.3)
Total protein (g/dL)	5.1	5.0–6.4	5.1–7.4	5.3–7.2 (5.9)
Albumin (g/dL)	2.6	2.9–4.1	2.6–3.8	3.3–4.1 (3.7)
Globulin (g/dL)	2.5	1.8–3.0	—	2.0–2.9 (2.2)
A/G ratio	1.0	1.0-2.2	—	1.3–2.1 (1.8)
Cholesterol (mg/dL)	235	70–200	64–296	—
Total bilirubin (mg/dL)	0.1	0–0.3	<1	—
CK (IU/L)	326	80–400	—	—
ALP (IU/L)	114	10–60	9–84	30–120 (53)
ALT (IU/L)	122	60–270		82–289 (170)
AST (IU/L)	64	30–75	28–120	—
GGT (IU/L)	2	1–15	—	5
Sodium (mEq/dL)	142	147–153	137–162	146–160 (152)
Potassium (mEq/dL)	3.7	3.3–4.5	4.5–7.7	4.3–5.3 (4.9)
Chloride (mEq/dL)	114	114–120	106–125	102–121 (115)
Bicarbonate (mEq/dL)	18.4	15–23	—	—
Anion gap	13	14–21	—	—
Calculated osmolality	284	—	—	—
Lipemia (mg/dL)	15	—	—	—
Hemolysis (mg/dL)	15	—	—	—
Icterus (mg/dL)	0	—	—	—

[a]Normal range provided by Colorado State University clinical pathology laboratory (http://www.cvmbs.colostate.edu/pathology/clinpath/2006%20Formulary.htm).
[b]Fox (1988).
[c]Carpenter (2005).

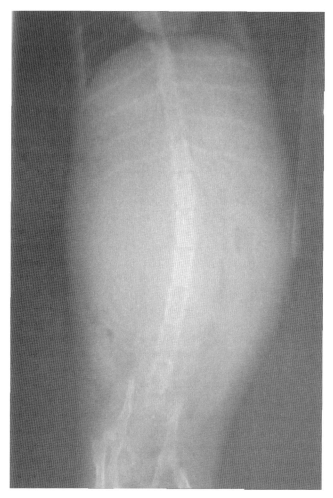

Fig. 44.4. The whole body dorsoventral radiograph of the 3-month-old ferret.

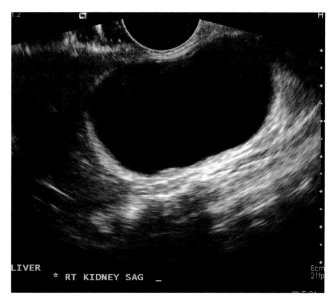

Fig. 44.5. An ultrasound image in the region of the right kidney.

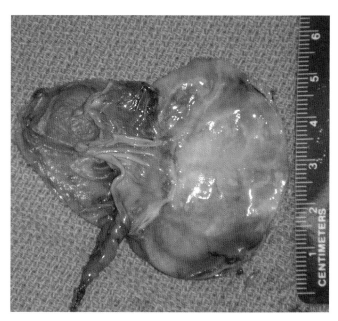

Fig. 44.6. The hydronephrotic right kidney removed from the 3-month-old ferret.

Summary

Whole body dorsoventral radiograph (Fig. 44.4) revealed a large soft tissue mass in the right side of the abdomen. The mass is displacing the gastrointestinal tract.

The abdominal ultrasound revealed a normal liver and gallbladder. Numerous, small, hypoechoic foci were scattered throughout the splenic parenchyma. These foci were not vessels as indicated by a color Doppler examination. The left kidney appeared normal. A 5.2 cm × 2.9 cm anechoic structure with a well-defined wall filled the right side of the abdomen and extended across midline. The mass distorted the abdominal anatomy. The right kidney was not identified. Neither the adrenal gland nor the pancreas could be identified during the ultrasound examination. A multilobulated soft tissue structure with a mildly heterogenous echo pattern was seen in the caudal left side of the abdomen. This structure measured 8 mm × 18.4 mm × 9.4 mm. Several normal-appearing segments of small bowel were identified in the caudal abdomen. The urinary bladder appeared normal, contained a small volume of urine, and was separate from the anechoic mass in the right side of the abdomen. The large, well-delineated anechoic mass in the right side of the abdomen was in the normal anatomic region for the right kidney and likely represented a markedly hydronephrotic right kidney and a congenital anomaly (Fig. 44.5). The lobulated soft tissue structure in the caudal left abdomen likely represented a lymph node. The lobulated lymph node and presence of numerous hypoechoic foci in the spleen provided concern for neoplasia, specifically lymphoma.

The ferret was admitted for exploratory surgery. She was given the preanesthetic agents—0.02 mg atropine, 0.2 mg hydromorphone, and 0.1 mg midazolam—subcutaneously 1 hour prior to induction of anesthesia. Intravenous propofol (5 mg) and midazolam (0.1 mg) were used to induce anesthesia. Anesthesia was maintained using 1% isoflurane after the ferret was intubated with a 3.0 mm endotracheal tube. The total anesthetic time was 106 minutes during which the ferret received 11.37 mL of intravenous lactated Ringer's solution.

Following aseptic preparation, an 8 cm skin incision was made from 1 inch caudal to the xyphoid to the pubis using a #15 scalpel blade. Once the linea alba was located, a stab incision was made into it just below the xyphoid and the linea alba incision was extended using Mayo scissors. A 4 cm kidney was visualized on the right side of the abdomen. An abdominal exploration was performed, and all other organs appeared normal. A syringe and needle were used to aspirate 40 mL of urine from the right kidney in an effort to better visualize the renal artery and vein. An incision was made into the retroperitoneal area, and the peritoneum was bluntly dissected from the kidney capsule using sterile cotton-tipped applicator. The renal artery and vein were isolated, and two encircling ligatures and one transfixing between the encircling ligatures were placed around the vessels using a 4-0 polytrimethylene carbonate suture. The vessels were transected between the transfixing and distal-encircling ligatures. The ureter was located and an attempt was made to follow it to its attachment at the urinary bladder; however, abundant retroperitoneal fat surrounded the middle portion and prevented visualization of the ureter. A stay suture was placed in the bladder with a 4-0 polytrimethylene carbonate suture to aid visualization of the ureter attachment. The ureter was located and ligated with two encircling ligatures using a 4-0 polytrimethylene carbonate suture before transection of the ureter (Fig. 44.6). The abdomen was flushed with copious amounts of sterile saline before the body wall was closed using a 4-0 polytrimethylene carbonate suture in a simple continuous pattern. The skin was closed using a 4-0 nylon suture in a simple continuous pattern. A line block using bupivocaine (2 mg/kg) was administered while the skin was being closed.

The rectal prolapse was likely associated with the pressure placed on the gastrointestinal tract from the large cystic mass that was a hydronephrotic kidney. The prolapsed rectum was manually reduced, and the ferret was treated postoperatively with meloxicam (0.5 mg/kg PO daily) as an analgesic for 5 days and chloramphenicol (50 mg/kg PO BID) for 14 days for the inflammatory bowel disease. It was possible that the inflammatory bowel disease was related to the pressure on the intestines from the cystic kidney and not the diet. The ferret made an uneventful recovery and there was no recurrence of the rectal prolapse.

45

A 2^1/$_2$-Year-Old Gerbil with Lethargy and Anorexia

Signalment

A 2^1/$_2$-year-old intact male gerbil (*Meriones unguiculatus*) was presented for lethargy and anorexia (Fig. 45.1).

History

The gerbil had not been opening his eyes for the past 4 days. He had not been eating for the past 2 days. The gerbil would move around when aroused; otherwise, he remained inactive. This was the only pet in the house. He was housed in a commercial pet cage designed for gerbils with a recycled paper product as bedding. He was fed a commercial diet designed for gerbils supplemented with eggs and a mixture of fruits and vegetables. According to the owner, the gerbil's feces and urine had been normal. The client noted a thin line of blood on the ventral abdomen prior to presentation.

Physical Examination Findings

The 140 g intact male gerbil was weak and responded slowly when handled. The eyelids remained closed when being handled owing to a green discharge and slight amount of blood located at the margins. Matted hair containing a small amount of blood was noted on the ventral part of the mid-abdomen. Further investigation revealed an ulcerated skin mass encrusted with dried exudate and blood. This lesion was associated with two masses. The largest mass measured 1 cm in diameter and was hairless and irregular in shape. A smaller (4 mm) mass was located adjacent to the larger mass. A fine-needle aspiration biopsy of the large mass was performed for cytodiagnosis (Figs. 45.2a–45.2c).

Interpretive Discussion

Figures 45.2a and 45.2b show cohesive clusters of epithelial cells. The cells have a high nucleus–cytoplasm ratio with a small amount of deeply basophilic cytoplasm. The cells have a round to oval nucleus with coarse nuclear chromatin and multiple, often large, nucleoli. Figure 45.2c reveals a cluster of these cells exhibiting cytoplasmic vacuolation, suggestive of secretory tissue origin. The background contains round, fat-like droplets.

The cytologic examination reveals epithelial cells with features of malignancy. The location of the mass and the appearance of vacuolated cells suggest that the tumor is an adenocarcinoma, likely originating from the scent gland.

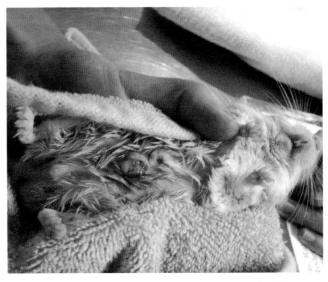

Fig. 45.1. The gerbil with a cutaneous mass on the abdomen.

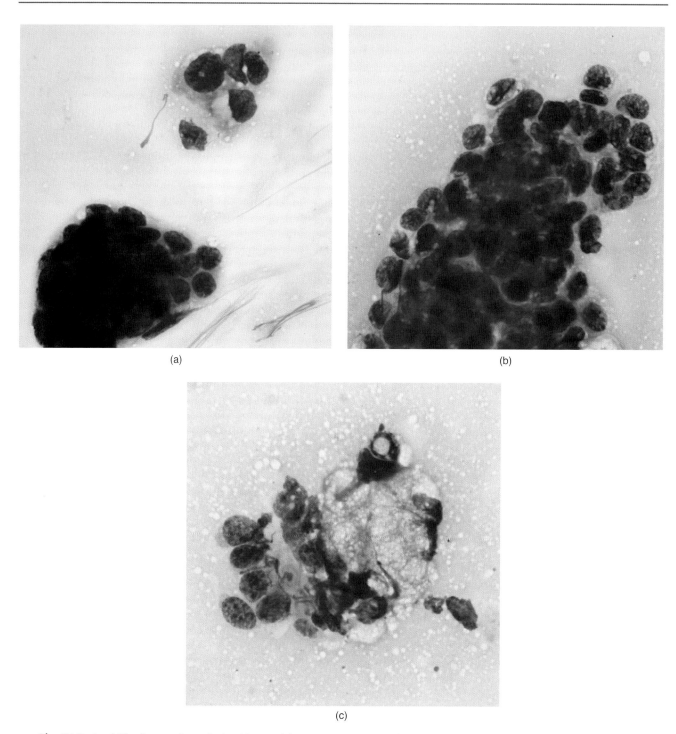

(a)

(b)

(c)

Fig. 45.2. (a–c) The fine-needle aspiration biopsy of the cutaneous mass (Wright–Giemsa stain, 100×).

Summary

The gerbil died during abdominal palpation that revealed several irregular internal masses. The client elected to submit the body for a private cremation; however, permission to obtain a biopsy sample for histopathologic examination was granted.

The histopathologic examination revealed a tumor that consisted of epithelial cells that formed into clumps, masses, and glandular structures. The round nuclei were pleomorphic and contained prominent nucleoli. Mitotic figures were moderate in number. The tumor was invasive into the surrounding tissue. The tumor appeared to be an adenocarcinoma of the scent gland, an aprocrine gland.

A 5-Year-Old Guinea Pig with an Ulcerated Swelling in the Abdominal Area

46

Signalment

A 5-year-old intact male guinea pig (*Cavia porcellius*) was presented with an ulcerated swelling in the left caudal abdominal area (Fig. 46.1).

History

The client noticed that a mass was developing on the skin of the abdominal area of her guinea pig 3 weeks prior to presentation. The skin overlying the mass began to ulcerate and bleed 2 weeks prior to presentation. The guinea pig was the only pet in the household. He was fed a diet of timothy hay, commercial guinea pig pellets, and a variety of vegetables as treats. The guinea pig had been doing fine except for the mass.

Physical Examination Findings

The 1.1-kg intact male guinea pig appeared generally healthy except for a 2.5 cm × 2.5 cm firm mass in the area of the left mammary gland. The associated teat was enlarged and a 1-cm area of skin overlying the mass was ulcerated. The physical examination also revealed an enlarged left testicle. The left testicle was three times the size of the right testicle. The client declined an offer for radiographic evaluation and a blood profile. A fine-needle aspiration biopsy was performed for cytodiagnosis (Figs. 46.2–46.5).

Interpretive Discussion

The cytologic results represented by Fig. 46.2 reveal numerous erythrocytes and a cohesive group of epithe-

lial cells with oval nuclei exhibiting mild anisokaryosis arranged in an acinar configuration (cells arranged around a clear space likely representing a lumen). Figures 46.3a and 46.3b reveal numerous erythrocytes and a cohesive raft of epithelial cells arranged in an acinar configuration. The oval nuclei contain coarse nuclear chromatin and one or more distinct nucleoli. The light blue homogenous cytoplasm varies from scant to

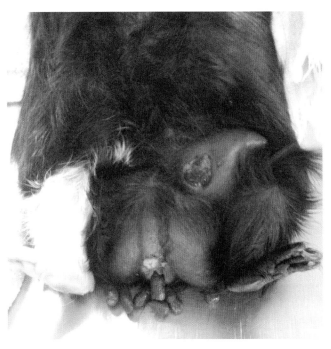

Fig. 46.1. A close-up view of the ulcerated mass on the 5-year-old male guinea pig.

195

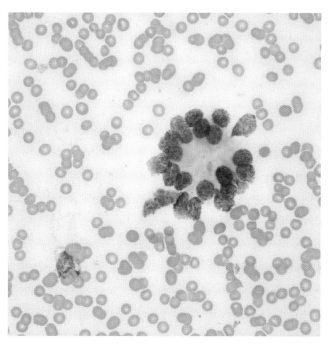

Fig. 46.2. A fine-needle aspiration of the mass (Wright–Giemsa stain, 50×).

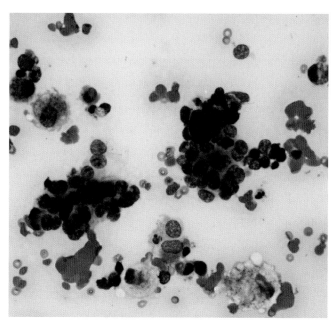

Fig. 46.4. A Fine-needle aspiration of the mass (Wright–Giemsa stain, 50×).

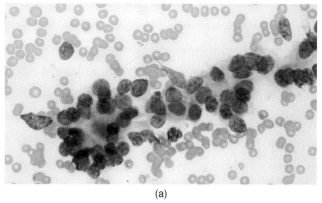

(a)

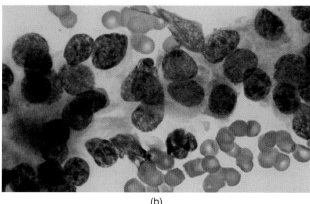

(b)

Fig. 46.3. (a) A fine-needle aspiration of the mass (Wright–Giemsa stain, 50×). (b) A fine-needle aspiration of the mass (Wright–Giemsa stain, 100×).

moderate. Figure 46.4 reveals numerous erythrocytes and two cohesive groupings of epithelial cells exhibiting features of malignancy. These features include cells with high nuclear to cytoplasmic ratios, basophilic cytoplasm, slight to moderate anisokaryosis, anisocytosis, one or more distinct nucleoli, and coarsely clumped nuclear chromatin. This figure also reveals cells that resemble foamy macrophages containing eosinophilic granules that likely represent phagocytized secretions. It is also possible that these cells represent vacuolated epithelial cells from secretory tissue. Figure 46.5a is a higher magnification of a group of epithelial cells exhibiting features of malignancy that include distinct nucleoli, coarse nuclear chromatin, high nucleus/cytoplasm ratios, and moderate anisocytosis and anisokaryosis. Figure 46.5b reveals numerous erythrocytes. Five heterophils (cells with dull eosinophilic granules) and one eosinophil (cell with brightly colored eosinophilic granules) embedded in a dense clump of platelets.

The cytologic examination supports a cytodiagnosis of malignant epithelial cells, such as an adenocarcinoma. On the basis of the location of the mass involving the area of the mammary gland, these likely represent a mammary adenocarcinoma. The inflammatory cells present likely, in part, come from peripheral blood contamination of the sample and associated inflammation (mastitis) owing to the ulcerative nature of the lesion.

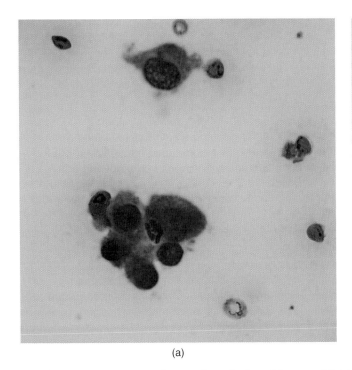

(a)

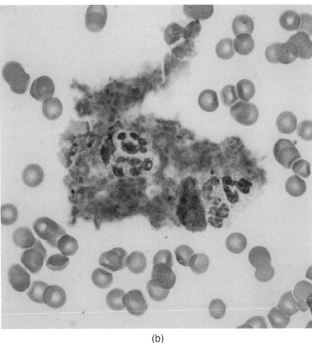

(b)

Fig. 46.5. (a and b) The fine-needle aspiration of the mass (Wright–Giemsa stain, 100×).

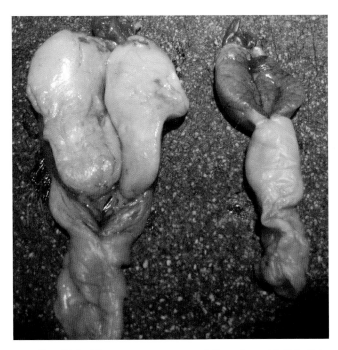

Fig. 46.6. The gross appearance of the enlarged left testicle compared to the normal right testicle.

Summary

The client was offered evaluation of the guinea pig for metastases followed by surgical removal of the mass and regional lymph node, if negative. After being informed of the highly malignant nature of mammary gland neoplasms of male guinea pigs, the client elected euthanasia both from a humane point of view and financial constraints.

The gross necropsy revealed a 2 cm × 1.5 cm exophytic dermal and subcuticular mass within the left inguinal area. The mass is firm on palpation and consists of homogeneous, tan tissue with a thin, pseudocapsule on cut section. The left testicle is enlarged approximately twice the size of the right (Fig. 46.6). The testicle is enlarged by a poorly demarcated, off-white to yellow homogeneous mass, which resembles normal adipose tissue on cut section. Present within the caudal aspect of the left caudal lung lobe is a well-demarcated, 2 mm in diameter mass, which appears as off-white, homogeneous tissue on cut section. The remaining organs and structures of the thoracic cavity are properly formed and within normal limits. The remaining organs and structures of the abdominal cavity are within normal limits.

Histopathologic examination of the subcuticular lesion from the inguinal region revealed a multilobulated, pseudo-encapsulated, cellular mass composed of polygonal to cuboidal cells, which are arranged in acini and frequently having variable amounts of arborizing fibrous stroma. This tissue expanded the deep dermis and subcutis. The cells are moderately sized and contain a moderate amount of light eosinophilic cytoplasm. Nuclei are oval with finely clumped, chromatin and variably distinct nucleoli. Mitotic figures are approximately two to three per 400× field. There is a mild degree of anisocytosis and anisokaryosis. Frequently present within the acini is homogeneous, eosinophilic material. There is extensive invasion of the cellular mass through the fibrous pseudocapsule. There is regionally extensive ulceration of the overlying epithelium, which is replaced by a serocellular crust, composed of numerous degenerating neutrophils admixed with homogeneous, finely fibrillar material (fibrin) and colonies of bacterial cocci. Within one area, there is irregular refractile material embedded in the serocellular crust. The histology indicates an apocrine gland carcinoma, likely mammary gland in origin.

Histopathologic findings of the left testicle revealed an unencapsulated mass composed of sheets of well-differentiated adipocytes admixed with more cellular areas and a compressing remnant of seminiferous tubules completely lacking in mature spermatogonia and spermatids. The cells are frequently large with a single large, clear, discrete vacuole, which peripheralizes the nucleus. Other cells admixed within the stroma contain numerous, variably sized discrete vacuoles within the light eosinophilic cytoplasm. The nuclei of these cells are large with finely stippled chromatin and variably distinct nucleoli. Mitotic figures are uncommonly encountered. There is a marked degree of anisocytosis and anisokaryosis. Multifocally, there are areas of coagulative necrosis with retention of architecture and nuclear absence. The peritesticular tissue is a liposarcoma based on histologic findings.

Histopathologic examination also revealed an unencapsulated, well-demarcated cellular mass composed of trabeculae and occasional acini-like structures focally expanding the pulmonary parenchyma. The cells composing these structures have distinct cell borders and are polygonal with abundant, finely vacuolated cytoplasm. The nuclei are oval with finely stippled to peripheralized chromatin and variably distinct nucleoli. Mitotic figures are approximately $0-1/400\times$ field. There is a mild degree of cellular atypia within this population. There is local invasion into the adjacent alveolar spaces. Within the adjacent parenchyma, alveolar spaces are occasionally filled by alveolar histiocytes, which are multifocally aggregated and contain refractile, coarsely granular, greenish/brown pigment. These findings indicate a bronchoalveolar adenoma.

A 6-Year-Old Ferret with Pawing at the Mouth

47

Signalment

A 6-year-old castrated male ferret (*Mustela putorius furo*) was presented with a 1-day history of pawing at his mouth.

History

The ferret was housed with a female ferret of the same age that presented 5 days earlier showing similar clinical signs of pawing at the mouth. That ferret was diagnosed with having an insulinoma and hepatocellular disease of unknown etiology. At the age of 4 years, this patient had an adrenalectomy to remove a left adrenal mass (adenoma) and a partial pancreatectomy as treatment for an insulinoma. At the same time the ferret was medically treated for *Helicobacter* gastritis. During the past 9 months, the ferret began to exhibit bilaterally symmetrical alopecia, signaling recurrence of adrenal disease. The client elected not to perform a second surgery or pursue medical treatment at that time owing to financial reasons. The ferret was being treated with flutamide, an antiandrogen, to reduce the chance of prostate hyperplasia. There had been no husbandry change except for a new bag of ferret food (same brand) that was obtained 3 weeks earlier.

Physical Examination Findings

The 1.4-kg castrated male ferret was alert and active on physical examination. A 1 cm diameter cutaneous mass was found on the left flank area (Fig. 47.1). The skin mass was a well-delineated, reddened, lesion partially devoid of hair with a central white area. According to the client, the mass had been present for several months. During the examination, the ferret produced loose, semiformed feces. A sample was collected for cytodiagnosis.

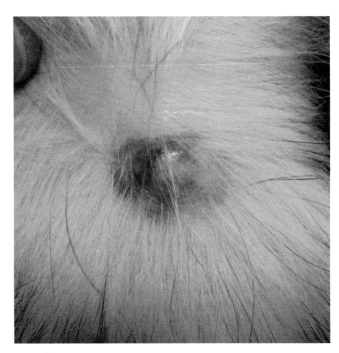

Fig. 47.1. A close-up view of a cutaneous lesion on the 6-year-old male ferret.

A blood sample was obtained via jugular venipuncture for a blood profile. A fine-needle aspiration biopsy of the cutaneous lesion was performed for cytodiagnosis (Tables 47.1 and 47.2 and Figs. 47.2–47.4).

Interpretive Discussion

The significant findings in the hemogram include an increased mean cell volume (MCV) and decreased mean cell hemoglobin concentration (MCHC), indicating the presence of macrocytic, hypochromic erythrocytes in a nonanemic ferret. Macrocytic erythrocytes are commonly associated with immature erythrocytes reported as polychromatic cells on Wright-stained blood films

199

Table 47.1. Hematology results.

		Reference[a]	Reference[b]	Reference[c]
WBC (10^3/μL)	7.4	4.0–9.0	4.4–19.1	7.7–15.4 (11.3)
Neutrophils (10^3/μL)	3.6	1.5–3.5	—	—
Neutrophils (%)	49	—	11–82	24–78 (40)
Lymphocytes (10^3/μL)	3.0	0.5–5.0	—	—
Lymphocytes (%)	41	—	12–54	28–69 (50)
Monocytes (10^3/μL)	0.4	0–0.5	—	—
Monocytes (%)	5	—	0–9	3.4–8.2 (6.6)
Eosinophils (10^3/μL)	0.4	0–0.5	—	—
Eosinophils (%)	5	—	0–7	0–7 (2)
Basophils (10^3/μL)	0	0	—	—
Basophils (%)	0	—	0–2	0–2.7 (0.7)
Plasma protein (g/dL)	6.7	5.0–6.5	—	—
RBC (10^6/μL)	9.1	7.0–11.0	7.3–12.2	—
Hb (g/dL)	15.6	12–18	16.3–18.2	12.0–16.3 (14.3)
PCV (%)	49	35–53	44–61	36–50 (43)
MCV (fL)	54	47–52	—	—
MCHC (g/dL)	32	33–35	—	—
RDW	11.9	—	—	—
Platelets (10^3/μL)	175	—	297–730	—
MPV (fL)	8.9	—	—	—
Clumped platelets	Exist	—	—	—

[a]Colorado State University reference ranges.
[b]Fox (1988).
[c]Carpenter (2005).

Table 47.2. Plasma biochemical results.

		Reference[a]	Reference[b]	Reference[c]
Glucose (mg/dL)	65	95–140	94–207	63–134 (101)
BUN (mg/dL)	11	10–26	10–45	12–43 (28)
Creatininc (mg/dL)	0	0–0.5	0.4–0.9	0.2–0.6 (0.4)
Phosphorus (mg/dL)	3.5	3.0–5.5	4.0–9.1	5.6–8.7 (6.5)
Calcium (mg/dL)	9.4	8.0–9.7	8.0–11.8	8.6–10.5 (9.3)
Total protein (g/dL)	6.1	5.0–6.4	5.1–7.4	5.3–7.2 (5.9)
Albumin (g/dL)	3.5	2.9–4.1	2.6–3.8	3.3–4.1 (3.7)
Globulin (g/dL)	2.6	1.8–3.0	—	2.0–2.9 (2.2)
A/G ratio	1.3	1.0–2.2	—	1.3–2.1 (1.8)
Cholesterol (mg/dL)	99	70–200	64–296	—
Total bilirubin (mg/dL)	0.2	0–0.3	<1	—
CK (IU/L)	154	80–400	—	—
ALP (IU/L)	13	10–60	9–84	30–120 (53)
ALT (IU/L)	76	60–270	—	82–289 (170)
AST (IU/L)	42	30–75	28–120	—
GGT (IU/L)	1	1–15	—	5
Sodium (mEq/dL)	146	147–153	137–162	146–160 (152)
Potassium (mEq/dL)	4.1	3.3–4.5	4.5–7.7	4.3–5.3 (4.9)
Chloride (mEq/dL)	114	114–120	106–125	102–121 (115)
Bicarbonate (mEq/dL)	23.7	15–23	—	—
Anion gap	13	14–21	—	—
Calculated osmolality	287	—	—	—
Lipemia (mg/dL)	25	—	—	—
Hemolysis (mg/dL)	13	—	—	—
Icterus (mg/dL)	0	—	—	—

[a]Normal range provided by Colorado State University clinical pathology laboratory (http://www.cvmbs.colostate.edu/pathology/clinpath/2006%20Formulary.htm).
[b]Fox (1988).
[c]Carpenter (2005).

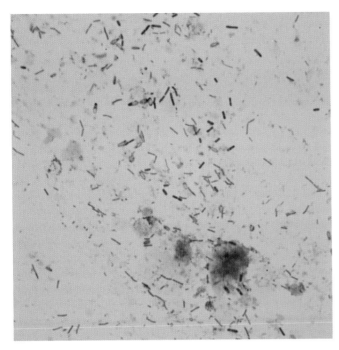

Fig. 47.2. The fecal cytology (Diff-Quik stain, 100×).

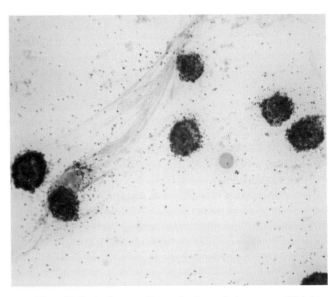

Fig. 47.4. A fine-needle aspiration of the mass (Wright–Giemsa stain, 100×).

and are an indication of a regenerative response. Macrocytosis without evidence of an appropriate regenerative response, such as increased polychromasia, in an anemic animal is indicative of a myeloproliferative disorder; however, this ferret is not anemic. Hypochromasia is also associated with immature polychromatic erythro-

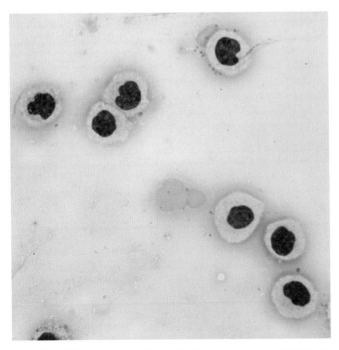

Fig. 47.3. A fine-needle aspiration of the mass (Diff-Quik stain, 100×).

cytes because their hemoglobin content is less than mature cells owing to an increased volume. Some drugs may cause macrocytosis. The only medication the ferret had been taking was flutamide, which has been reported to cause methemoglobinemia in humans (Jackson et al., 1994).

The platelet count is decreased; however, platelet clumping found on the blood film suggests that this is an artifact.

The only significant finding on the plasma chemistry profile was hypoglycemia. This likely indicates a recurrence of hypoglycemia associated with an insulinoma that was treated 2 years ago. In general, the fasting blood glucose of a normal ferret is greater than 90 mg/dL. Ferrets exhibiting values less than 70 mg/dL are likely to have an insulinoma. Those with a fasting glucose between 70 and 90 mg/dL may be hypoglycemic for other reasons; however, an insulinoma cannot be ruled out.

Figure 47.2 represents the fecal cytologic finding that reveals a mixed population of bacteria represented by a variety of morphological types. There are numerous rod-shaped bacteria, with a lighter area likely representing spore formation. These bacteria that take on a safety pin-like appearance are considered to represent a Clostridium sp. of bacteria. In general, such bacteria represent less than three per oil-immersion field in the fecal cytology from a normal ferret. Confirmation of clostridial enteritis requires a positive culture and/or endotoxin assay.

Figure 47.3 reveals round cells with distinct cell margins with slight anisocytosis and anisokaryosis. The medium-sized oval nucleus of the cells frequently has irregular margins, can be eccentrically positioned, contains granular chromatin, and has poorly defined nucleoli. The cytological features are consistent with a discrete cell or round cell tumor, which include a histiocytoma, mast cell tumor, and lymphoma. If this were a canine patient, a transmissible venereal tumor would also be included in the list.

Figure 47.4 reveals many fully granulated, well-differentiated mast cells. These cells have the same characteristics as those described in Fig. 47.3 except for the presence of the basophilic granules in the cytoplasm and the background (freed from ruptured cells). Diff-Quik and Wright–Giemsa are both Romanowsky stains; however, Diff-Quik may not stain the granules in some subsets of mast cells as demonstrated by this example.

Summary

Mast cell tumors of ferrets are considered to be benign and are often self-limiting; however, owing to the chronicity and unusual appearance of the mast cell tumor on this patient, a decision for surgical removal was made. The ferret was given subcutaneous buprenorphine (0.03 mg/kg) as a preanesthetic agent. This was followed by providing general anesthesia using isoflurane. A lidocaine block (2 mg/kg) around the mass was made prior to surgical removal. The mass along with 2 mm skin margins was removed in its entirety. The subcutaneous tissue was closed using 4-0 glycopolymer monofilament synthetic absorbable suture. This was followed by skin closure using 4-0 monofilament nylon suture. The ferret was provided with meloxicam (0.3 mg/kg PO BID) postoperatively for 3 days.

The ferret was treated with amoxicillin (11 mg/kg PO BID) for 10 days for a potential clostridial overgrowth. The ferret was also treated medically for the recurrence of clinical signs of an insulinoma using prednisolone (0.25 mg/kg PO BID) to be started 24 hours after the meloxicam treatment.

Reevaluation of the ferret 10 days later indicated that the treatment for the insulinoma was controlling his hypoglycemia. At that time, the skin incision had healed and the sutures were removed. The appearance of the ferret's feces had returned to normal and no longer contained the clostridial-like organisms.

A 7-Year-Old Ferret with Bilateral Alopecia

48

Signalment

A 7-year-old castrated male ferret (*Mustela putorius furo*) was presented with bilateral alopecia.

History

According to the owner, the ferret had been sleeping a lot lately and was not as active as he normally would be. The ferret had been losing his hair during the past few months as well. The ferret was the only pet in the household and was kept in a commercial ferret cage. He was fed a commercial kibbled ferret diet.

Physical Examination Findings

On physical examination, the ferret appeared alert and responsive, but was not as active as would be expected from a healthy ferret in a new environment. He also appeared thin and weighed 620 g. His body temperature was 101.2°F, his heart rate was 240 beats/minute, and his respiratory rate was 36 breaths/minute. A palpable mass in the mid-abdomen was found on abdominal palpation.

A blood sample via jugular venipuncture was obtained for a complete blood count and plasma biochemical profile.

An ultrasound evaluation of the abdomen was also performed. The palpable mass on the physical examination was an enlarged lymph node according to the ultrasound evaluation. A round mass measuring 15 mm × 17 mm was found between the cranial aspect of the left kidney and the spleen and just left of the aorta. That mass had small areas of mineralization within the dorsal aspect. A normal-appearing adrenal gland (left or right) could not be identified during the ultrasound study. The ultrasound conclusions were a mild lymphadenopathy in the abdomen and a neoplastic left adrenal gland. An ultrasound-guided fine-needle aspiration biopsy of

the enlarged abdominal lymph node was obtained for cytology (Tables 48.1 and 48.2 and Figs. 48.1 and 48.2).

Interpretive Discussion

The complete blood count was normal except for an insignificant slight increase in neutrophils and the appearance of a few nucleated erythrocytes. These could be associated with increased levels of corticosteroids.

The significant finding on the plasma biochemistry panel is a marked hypoglycemia. This is likely associated with increased insulin levels because of an

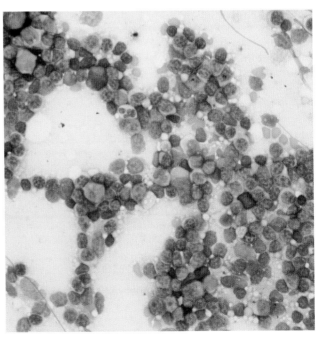

Fig. 48.1. A fine-needle aspirate of an abdominal lymph node (Wright–Giemsa stain, 50×).

203

Table 48.1. Hematology results.

		Reference[a]	Reference[b]	Reference[c]
WBC ($10^3/\mu L$)	5.9	4.0–9.0	4.4–19.1	7.7–15.4 (11.3)
Neutrophils ($10^3/\mu L$)	4.2	1.5–3.5	—	—
Neutrophils (%)	71	—	11–82	24–78 (40)
Lymphocytes ($10^3/\mu L$)	1.4	0.5–5.0	—	—
Lymphocytes (%)	24	—	12–54	28–69 (50)
Monocytes ($10^3/\mu L$)	0.2	0–0.5	—	—
Monocytes (%)	3	—	0–9	3.4–8.2 (6.6)
Eosinophils ($10^3/\mu L$)	0	0–0.5	—	—
Eosinophils (%)	0	—	0–7	0–7 (2)
Basophils ($10^3/\mu L$)	0.1	0	—	—
Basophils (%)	2	—	0–2	0–2.7 (0.7)
nRBCs ($10^3/\mu L$)	0.1	0	—	—
Plasma protein (g/dL)	5.8	5.0–6.5	—	—
RBC ($10^6/\mu L$)	8.0	7.0–11.0	7.3–12.2	—
Hb (g/dL)	14.2	12–18	16.3–18.2	12.0–16.3 (14.3)
PCV (%)	42	35–53	44–61	36–50 (43)
MCV (fL)	52	47–52	—	—
MCHC (g/dL)	34	33–35	—	—
RDW	19.2	—	—	—
Platelets ($10^3/\mu L$)	490	—	297–730	—

[a]Colorado State University reference ranges.
[b]Fox (1988).
[c]Carpenter (2005).

Table 48.2. Plasma biochemical results.

		Reference[a]	Reference[b]	Reference[c]
Glucose (mg/dL)	46	95–140	94–207	63–134 (101)
BUN (mg/dL)	24	10–26	10–45	12–43 (28)
Creatinine (mg/dL)	0.2	0–0.5	0.4–0.9	0.2–0.6 (0.4)
Phosphorus (mg/dL)	3.7	3.0–5.5	4.0–9.1	5.6–8.7 (6.5)
Calcium (mg/dL)	8.0	8.0–9.7	8.0–11.8	8.6–10.5 (9.3)
Total protein (g/dL)	5.2	5.0–6.4	5.1–7.4	5.3–7.2 (5.9)
Albumin (g/dL)	3.0	2.9–4.1	2.6–3.8	3.3–4.1 (3.7)
Globulin (g/dL)	2.2	1.8–3.0	—	2.0–2.9 (2.2)
A/G ratio	1.4	1.0–2.2	—	1.3–2.1 (1.8)
Cholesterol (mg/dL)	140	70–200	64–296	—
Total bilirubin (mg/dL)	0.1	0–0.3	<1	—
CK (IU/L)	139	80–400	—	—
ALP (IU/L)	24	10–60	9–84	30–120 (53)
ALT (IU/L)	73	60–270	—	82–289 (170)
AST (IU/L)	45	30–75	28–120	—
GGT (IU/L)	8	1–15	—	5
Sodium (mEq/dL)	152	147–153	137–162	146–160 (152)
Potassium (mEq/dL)	4.5	3.3–4.5	4.5–7.7	4.3–5.3 (4.9)
Chloride (mEq/dL)	118	114–120	106–125	102–121 (115)
Bicarbonate (mEq/dL)	23.6	15–23	—	—
Anion gap	15	14–21	—	—
Calculated osmolality	302	—	—	—
Lipemia (mg/dL)	0	—	—	—
Hemolysis (mg/dL)	0	—	—	—
Icterus (mg/dL)	0	—	—	—

[a]Normal range provided by Colorado State University clinical pathology laboratory (http://www.cvmbs.colostate.edu/pathology/clinpath/2006%20Formulary.htm).
[b]Fox (1988).
[c]Carpenter (2005).

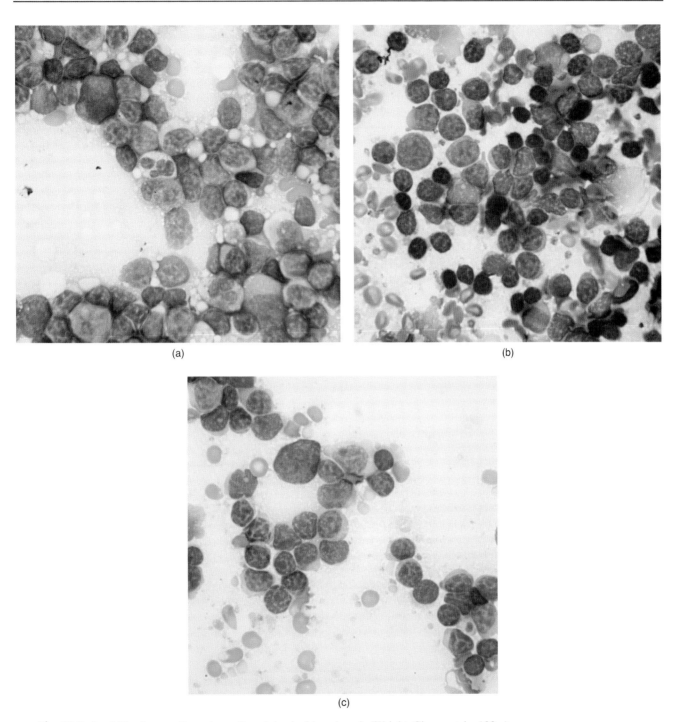

(a)

(b)

(c)

Fig. 48.2. (a–c) The fine-needle aspirate of an abdominal lymph node (Wright–Giemsa stain, 100×).

insulinoma, a common disorder of geriatric ferrets fed a diet high in carbohydrates, such as the kibbled diet.

Figures 48.1 and 48.2a show a highly cellular sample consisting primarily of lymphocytes. The majority of the cells are small and intermediate lymphocytes (the actual percentage was 79%) with an increase in the number of lymphoblasts (19%). An occasional neutrophil and eosinophil could be seen. A moderate number of erythrocytes are also seen. Figure 48.2a is a higher magnification of these cells. Figures 48.2b and 48.2c also reveal a similar cytological finding. Note the lymphoglandular bodies, cytoplasmic fragments, which are common in lymphoid tissue in the background of these two images. A cytodiagnosis of a reactive lymph node was made.

Summary

The ferret underwent exploratory surgery for a left adrenal mass and pancreatic insulinoma (based on the low blood glucose concentration). The ferret was given 0.012 mg butorphanol subcutaneously 50 minutes prior to face mask induction with isoflurane anesthesia. Isoflurane anesthesia was maintained after intubation using a 3.0 mm tube for 1 hour during the surgical procedure.

A ventral midline incision was made between the xyphoid and pubis to approach the abdominal cavity. Multiple nodules were seen throughout the pancreas. Many of the large nodules were removed by blunt dissection and submitted for histopathologic examination. (This was an older case as the current method of dealing with insulinomas of the pancreas in the ferret is to perform a partial pancreatectomy by removing the left lobe after removing visible nodules in the main body of the pancreas.) An enlarged abdominal lymph node was removed and submitted for histologic examination. A 2 cm diameter adrenal mass was also removed and submitted for histopathologic examination. A saline lavage of the abdominal cavity was performed prior to closing the abdominal wall using a 2-0 polydioxanone suture in a simple continuous pattern. The skin was closed using a 3-0 nylon suture in a Ford interlocking pattern. Recovery from anesthesia and surgery was uneventful.

Histopathologic results showed that the left adrenal mass was an adrenocortical carcinoma. Histology of the pancreas confirmed an insulinoma. The lymph node was histologically normal.

Section 6
Avian Cytology Case Studies

A 20-Year-Old Parrot with Dyspnea, Weight Loss, and Persistent Ascites

Signalment

A 20-year-old African grey parrot (*Psittacus erithacus*) of unknown gender was presented with a 3-week history of dyspnea, weight loss, and persistent ascites (Fig. 49.1).

History

The parrot had been the only bird in the household for the past 20 years with no exposure to other birds. Multiple therapeutic abdominocentesis had been performed by the referring veterinarian over the past 3 weeks to maintain the patient's comfort.

Physical Examination Findings

On presentation, the parrot appeared thin with a body weight of 490 g. The keel was moderately prominent, suggestive of pectoral muscle atrophy. The patient had a markedly distended coelomic region and exhibited signs of tachypnea and dyspnea. The respiratory effort significantly worsened when the patient was tilted backward anywhere from 45° to complete dorsal recumbency. Cardiac auscultation revealed a regular rhythm with a grade III/VI holosystolic heart murmur.

Other Diagnostic Testing

A blood sample was obtained via jugular venipuncture and submitted for a complete blood cell count and plasma biochemical profile (Tables 49.1 and 49.2). Whole body radiographs were also taken. Analysis of the clear coelomic fluid revealed a total protein of 2.6 g/dL, 80 nucleated cells/μL, and red blood cells more than 100,000/μL. A cell differential revealed 25% heterophils, 64% large mononuclear cells, and 11% lymphocytes. No microorganisms were seen (Figs. 49.2–49.4).

Interpretive Discussion

The increased packed cell volume (PCV) is possibly associated with dehydration. The low refractometric total protein suggests hypoproteinemia. This finding in association with an elevated PCV indicates that the hypoproteinemia may be worse than it appears and likely to become critical when the bird becomes better hydrated. It is also possible that the bird has polycythemia associated with chronic hypoxia. The leukogram is unremarkable.

The plasma biochemistries confirmed the severe hypoproteinemia and hypoalbuminemia, indicating severe protein loss or lack of production. The low potassium was associated with either poor dietary intake or excessive loss. The low plasma cholesterol concentration indicates either decreased synthesis by the liver,

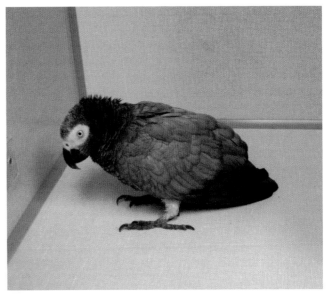

Fig. 49.1. The 20-year-old African grey parrot with weight loss and dyspnea.

Table 49.1. Hematology results.

		Reference[a]
PCV (%)	61	38–48
Leukocytes		
WBC ($10^3/\mu$L)	6.1	5–11
Heterophils ($10^3/\mu$L)	4.8	—
Heterophils (%)	78	55–75
Bands ($10^3/\mu$L)	0	0
Bands (%)	0	0
Lymphocytes ($10^3/\mu$L)	1.1	—
Lymphocytes (%)	18	25–45
Monocytes ($10^3/\mu$L)	0.1	—
Monocytes (%)	2	0–3
Eosinophils ($10^3/\mu$L)	0	—
Eosinophils (%)	0	0–2
Basophils ($10^3/\mu$L)	0.1	—
Basophils (%)	2	0–1
Thrombocytes		
Estimated number	Adequate	1–5/1,000× field
Morphology	Normal, clumped	
Plasma protein (refractometry) (g/dL)	1.5	3–5

[a]Johnston-Delaney and Harrison (1996).

increased catabolism, or decreased dietary absorption. The increased bile acid concentration was indicative of hepatobiliary disease resulting in abnormal hepatic uptake, bile acid storage, excretion, or hepatic perfusion.

The whole body referral radiographs (Figs. 49.2 and 49.3) indicate severe generalized cardiomegaly based on a cardiac silhouette width to thorax width of 70%. The normal should be 51–61% (Straub et al., 2002). The

Table 49.2. Plasma biochemical results.

		Reference[a]
Glucose (mg/dL)	259	190–350
BUN (mg/dL)	2	3.0–5.4
Uric acid (mg/dL)	7.4	4.5–9.5
Total protein (biuret) (g/dL)	1.0	3.0–4.6
Albumin (g/dL)	0.4	1.6–3.2
Globulin (g/dL)	0.6	0.4–1.9
Aspartate aminotransferase (IU/L)	90	100–365
Creatine kinase (IU/L)	380	165–412
Calcium (mg/dL)	8.5	8.5–13.0
Phosphorus (mg/dL)	4.5	3.2–5.4
Sodium (mEq/L)	150	157–165
Potassium (mEq/L)	2.6	2.9–4.6
Chloride (mEq/L)	116	—
Bicarbonate (mEq/L)	20.3	13—25
Anion gap (calculated)	17	—
Cholesterol (mg/dL)	64	160–425
Bile acids (mol/L)	99	20—85
Calculated osmolality	299	—

[a]Johnston-Delaney and Harrison (1996).

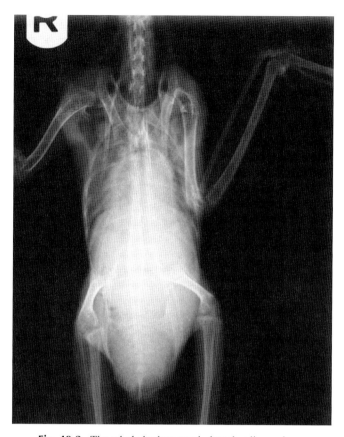

Fig. 49.2. The whole body ventral–dorsal radiograph.

cardiac silhouette width to coracoid width of 745% is also indicative of cardiomegaly. The normal should be 545–672% (Straub et al., 2002). The radiographs also reveal a marked hepatomegaly. Although the pulmonary parenchyma appears normal, the air sacs are only minimally visible owing to severe compression from the distended coelomic cavity. The coelomic cavity has a

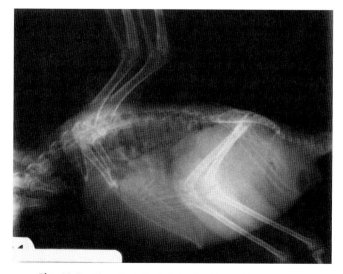

Fig. 49.3. The whole body lateral radiograph.

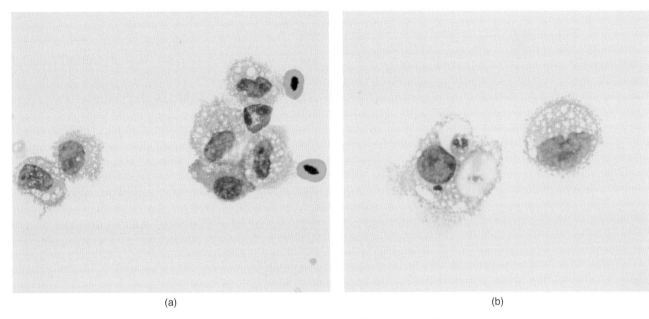

(a)   (b)

Fig. 49.4. (a and b) Images of concentrated fluid (cytospin) (Wright–Giemsa stain, 100×).

generalized loss of serosal detail. Exposed human fingers were noted on the lateral radiograph.

Figure 49.4a indicates a normal-appearing heterophil and vacuolated macrophages. Figure 49.4b shows two foamy macrophages and one that has phagocytized other cells. The low cellularity with a predominance of mononuclear leukocytes and slightly increased protein indicates a modified transudative effusion. Removal of this fluid with its protein content likely contributed to the systemic hypoproteinemia.

Summary

An echocardiogram found severe right ventricular hypertrophy and dilation with systolic dysfunction, moderate right atrioventricular valve insufficiency, a significantly elevated estimated pulmonary arterial pressure, hepatic venous congestion, and coelomic effusion. The clinical diagnosis of chronic cor pulmonale was established (Sedacca et al., 2009).

A therapeutic abdominocentesis was performed to indirectly improve respiratory function by giving the air sacs more room to expand. Careful attention was made to remove a minimal amount of fluid as possible to not only make the patient more comfortable but also minimize potential worsening of the hypoproteinemia. After successful stabilization, the parrot was discharged with instructions to start the following cardiac therapies: furosemide (1 mg/kg PO q 12 hours), benazepril (0.5 mg/kg PO q 24 hours), and pimobendan (0.25 mg/kg PO q 12 hours). A high-protein diet was also recommended.

One week following the initial examination, the patient returned for reevaluation. The owner reported that the parrot was doing better, with an improved attitude and appetite. Although less coelomic distension was appreciated on physical examination and the respiratory effort was improved, the keel was more prominent than it had been the week prior and the bird had lost more weight (5 g). The plasma albumin concentration had decreased even further from 0.4 to 0.3 g/dL. Although the degree of coelomic effusion appeared subjectively less on echocardiogram, a significant amount of fluid was present and had reformed over the past week. Specific chamber measurements were not evaluated at that time. The combination of diuretic spironolactone/hydrochlorothiazide 1 mg/kg PO q 12 hours, was started with recommendations to keep all other medications the same as previously prescribed.

Three weeks later the parrot was found dead in its cage by the owner. A postmortem examination revealed marked dilation and hypertrophy of the right ventricle with a dilated and thin-walled right atrium. The interventricular septum and outer wall of the right ventricle were as thick as the left ventricular free wall. No gross abnormalities to the right AV valve, or remainder of the heart, were appreciated. Although the large elastic arteries of both the systemic and pulmonary circulations were grossly normal, histologic findings confirmed significant evidence of circumferential atherosclerosis. Histologic findings also confirmed moderate to severe hepatic hemosiderosis most likely secondary to chronic passive congestion.

The clinical, echocardiography, and necropsy findings of the African grey parrot are consistent with chronic cor pulmonale and right-sided congestive heart failure secondary to significant pulmonary arterial hypertension, right AV valve insufficiency, and right ventricular systolic dysfunction. Although atherosclerosis most commonly affects the systemic and coronary arteries of parrots, pulmonary hypertension secondary to severe pulmonary atherosclerosis was strongly speculated in this case. The incidence of atherosclerosis in the African grey species has been reported to be as high as 92.4% (Bavelaar and Beynen, 2003).

An 11-Year-Old Cockatiel with a Mass in the Ear

50

Signalment

An 11-year-old male cockatiel (*Nymphicus hollandicus*) was presented with a soft tissue mass protruding from the right ear (Fig. 50.1).

History

According to the client, the mass had doubled in size in just 2 days. The client had recently been away from the house for 3$^1/_2$ weeks and noticed a mass in the bird's ear when she returned. She has owned the bird since it was 6–8 weeks old and since then there had been no other birds in the household. There were two dogs, but they had never bothered the bird. The bird lived in a 3 ft × 2 ft nonpainted metal cage that contained two wooden dowel perches and ceramic food and water bowls. The bird was fed a seed mixture purchased from a feed store and vegetables. The bird had no other medical problems until now. He was still behaving normally.

Physical Examination Findings

The 101 g bird appeared normal in all respects except for a 1 cm diameter, round, raised, pink soft tissue mass protruding from his right ear (Fig. 50.1). An attempt to aspirate the mass for cytological examination resulted in the rapid withdrawal of approximately 0.5 mL of blood into the syringe. More blood would have been drawn if the procedure had not been stopped. The bird was anesthetized using isoflurane via face mask for radiographic evaluation of the head to determine the extent of the mass. The radiographs revealed a 5 mm × 10 mm soft tissue mass in the region of the right ear, and there was no evidence of osseous involvement of this mass. The ear canal appeared to be open and free of tissue. Rule-outs for the mass included neoplasia, abscess, or hematoma. While the bird was under anesthesia, an attempt to remove the mass by strangulation using a 3-0

synthetic suture was made. The removed tissue was imprinted on a microscope slide for cytology and submitted for histopathologic examination (Figs. 50.2a–50.2d).

Interpretive Discussion

Figures 50.2a–50.2d reveal a cytology that is highly cellular and contains numerous erythrocytes. Pleomorphic mesenchymal cells are present. The cytoplasm is moderate, wispy to fusiform, and basophilic with margins that are indistinct or appear as if the cell has been ripped apart. The cells have an oval nucleus that contains coarse chromatin and prominent multiple nucleoli. These are supportive of a cytological diagnosis of a sarcoma, possibly a hemangiosarcoma because of the amount of associated blood.

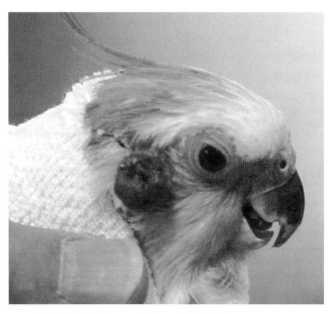

Fig. 50.1. An image of the cockatiel with an ear mass.

213

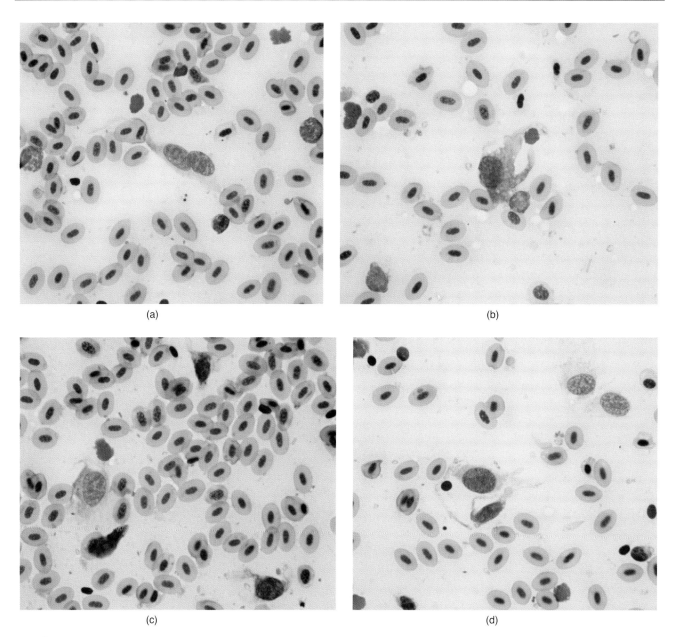

Fig. 50.2. (a–d) The images of the imprint of the mass (Wright–Giemsa stain, 100×).

Summary

Histologic examination revealed an expansile dermal mass characterized by abundant, variably sized, irregular blood-filled vessels, sinusoids, and clefts surrounded by mature fibrous connective tissue. The vessels and sinusoids were lined by plump endothelial cells overlying arborizing collagenous stroma. The tumor extended to the edge of the surgical margin submitted. Special stains using immunohistochemistry for Factor 8 proved to be inconclusive. The special stains utilized were nonspecific for both the normal and neoplastic tissues, which may be attributable to differences in avian cell markers. The mass was diagnosed as a hemangiosarcoma.

The client was informed of these findings and told that the lesion is likely to recur because of its location and difficulty to remove in its entirety.

A 4-Year-Old Cockatiel with a Swollen Head

Signalment

A 4-year-old intact female cockatiel (*Nymphicus hollandicus*) was presented with a swollen head.

History

The cockatiel was presented with a complaint of having a swollen head for a 2-week duration. She had been slightly more lethargic lately but continued to eat, drink, and produce normal droppings. She lived with another female cockatiel that appeared healthy to the owners.

Physical Examination Findings

The cockatiel weighed 110 g. She was quiet, alert, and responsive and in good body condition. The periocular tissue was swollen bilaterally, and there was a large, approximately 1 cm diameter, ulcerated mass below the left eye near the neck (Figs. 51.1a and 51.1b).

A fine-needle aspirate of the mass was performed for cytologic evaluation (Figs. 51.2–51.4).

Other Diagnostic Information

A drop of blood was taken to prepare a blood film for an examination of the hemic cytology (Fig. 51.5).

A bone marrow aspiration biopsy was obtained using a 22-gauge spinal needle inserted into the proximal tibiotarsus (Figs. 51.6a and 51.6b).

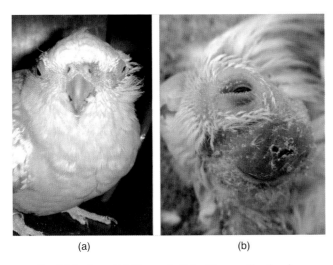

(a)   (b)

Fig. 51.1. (a and b) The cockatiel with a swollen head.

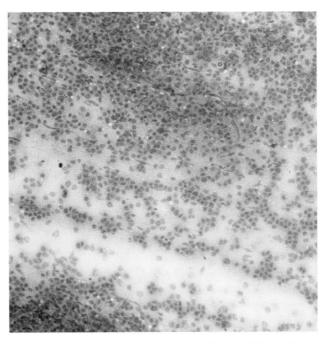

Fig. 51.2. A fine-needle aspiration biopsy (Wright–Giemsa stain, 20×).

215

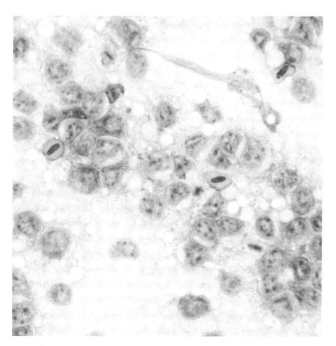

Fig. 51.3. A fine-needle aspiration biopsy (Diff-Quik stain, 100×).

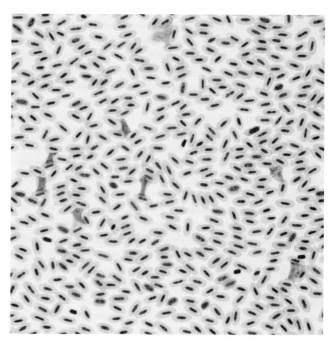

Fig. 51.5. A blood film (Wright–Giemsa stain, 50×).

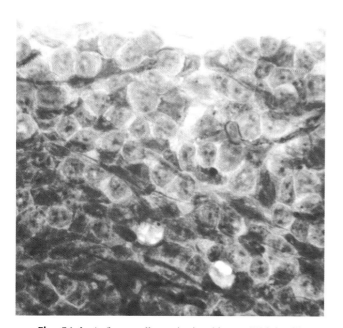

Fig. 51.4. A fine-needle aspiration biopsy (Wright–Giemsa stain, 100×).

Interpretive Discussion

Figure 51.2 is a low-magnification image of the fine-needle aspirate of the mass. It reveals a highly cellular population of discrete round cells. Figure 51.3 represents a higher magnification of the cellular sample and reveals many large "round cells" (when compared to erythrocytes) with light blue cytoplasm and large round nuclei, many of which have clumped chromatin. Figure 51.4 shows a dense population of the round cells that are staining darker but have identical features to those in the other two images. These round cells are atypical lymphocytes and considered suspicious for lymphosarcoma as the majority of cells are large and small lymphocytes are rare.

Figure 51.5 reveals a blood film with a high cellularity when viewed with a 50× objective. All the leukocytes were small mature lymphocytes that tend to mold around adjacent cells. This finding represents the leukocyte differential of 95% lymphocytes and supports a marked lymphocytosis indicative of lymphoid leukemia.

The cytologic examination of the bone marrow demonstrated in Figs. 51.6a and 51.6b reveals a highly cellular sample that contains numerous mature erythrocytes. The only other cell type is the lymphocyte, the

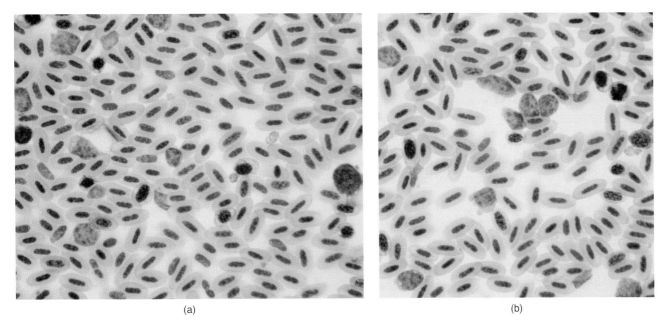

Fig. 51.6. (a and b) The bone marrow aspirate (Wright–Giemsa stain, 100×).

majority of which appear large. This finding supports a lymphocytic leukemia.

Summary

On the basis of the clinical diagnosis of the large cell lymphoma and likely associated lymphoid leukemia, the bird was euthanized. Necropsy revealed that nearly all major organs that were examined contained a neoplastic population of lymphocytes including the facial mass. Affected organs included liver, spleen, lung, kidney, bone marrow, skin, bursa, ovary, meninges, esophagus, trachea, proventriculus, and conjunctiva. The presence of neoplastic lymphocytes within vascular lumina suggests that this bird was likely leukemic. A final diagnosis of disseminated lymphosarcoma was made.

An Adult Owl with a Swollen Elbow

52

Signalment

An adult Barn owl (*Tyto alba*) was presented with a swollen right elbow.

History

The owl presented to a raptor rehabilitation facility, and there was little information available concerning the owl's history. The owl appeared to be in good condition, according to the rehabilitators except for a swelling on the right elbow.

Physical Examination Findings

The owl was in good condition. A fluid-filled swelling was found on the ventral aspect of the right elbow. The elbow exhibited normal range of motion and the owl showed no pain response when it was manipulated. An aspirate of the swelling revealed a small volume of clear, viscous fluid (Figs. 52.1–52.2).

Interpretive Discussion

The cytologic examination revealed in Figs. 52.2a and 52.2b indicates a moderately cellular sample with a heavy eosinophilic granular background. The cells are large mononuclear cells with eccentric nuclei and

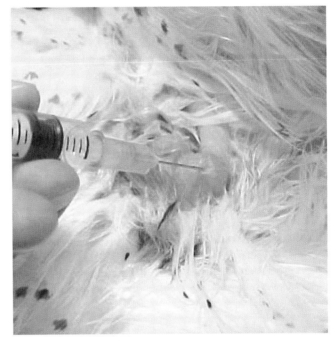

Fig. 52.1. An aspiration of the fluid-filled swelling on the elbow of the Barn owl.

abundant cytoplasm containing pink-staining granules. These cells are synovial lining cells or synoviocytes. The presence of synoviocytes and the heavy granular

219

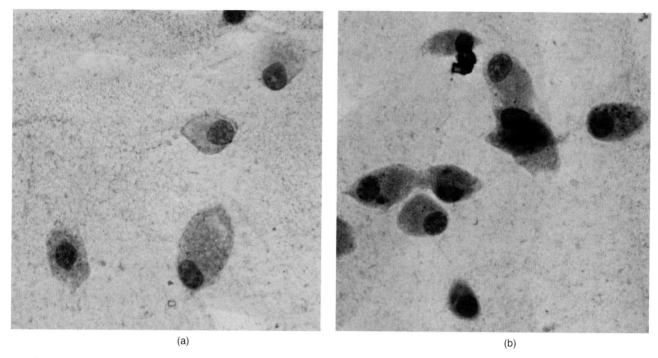

(a)   (b)

Fig. 52.2. (a and b) The cytology of fluid removed from a cystic lesion on the elbow (Wright–Giemsa stain, 100×).

background indicative of the presence of mucin supports the cytodiagnosis of synovial fluid. Because this sample was not obtained by aspiration of a joint, but rather a cystic lesion adjacent to a joint, a diagnosis of a synovial cyst was made.

Summary

After the cyst was drained during aspiration, a bandage was applied to the wing to provide gentle pressure to the area of the lesion. The bandage was removed 3 days later after which the lesion did not recur.

53

A 2-Year-Old Macaw with Left Leg Lameness

Signalment

A 2-year-old male Military macaw (*Ara militaris*) was presented with left leg lameness.

History

The macaw was presented with the chief complaint of left leg lameness. A complete blood count and a plasma biochemistry profile performed at another veterinary hospital were normal.

Physical Examination Findings

On physical examination, the macaw was bright, alert, and responsive and weighed 896 g. He was reluctant to bear weight on his left leg, which was markedly swollen in the region of the proximal tibiotarsus.

The diagnostic plan included radiographic evaluation of the left leg and an aspiration biopsy of the swollen area of the bone for cytodiagnosis (Figs. 53.1–53.4).

Interpretive Discussion

The radiographs (Figs. 53.1–53.3) reveal that the proximal one-third of the left tibiatarsus is nearly completely lytic where small amounts of the cortex remain visible. There is soft tissue swelling around the proximal tibiotarsus with areas of mineralization. There is a pathologic fracture of the proximal tibiotarsus. The tibiotarsus appears malaligned on the lateral view. The distal left femur is normal. No other soft tissue or bony abnormalities are detected. The radiographic differential diagnoses included bacterial or fungal osteomyelitis or primary bone neoplasia.

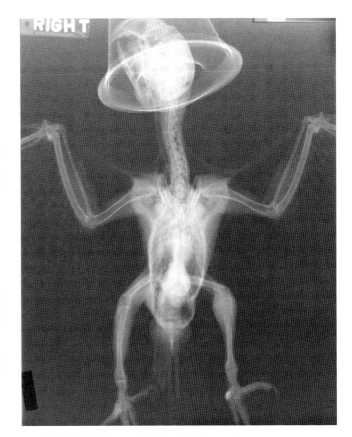

Fig. 53.1. The ventral–dorsal radiograph.

The aspiration biopsy of the lesion revealed a highly cellular sample with numerous erythrocytes. The sample also contains numerous large mesenchymal cells.

Figure 53.4a shows a highly cellular sample that contains numerous erythrocytes and many pleomorphic spindle-shaped cells (mesenchymal cells) with high and variable nucleus–cytoplasm (N/C) ratios, anisocytosis, anisokaryosis, and nuclear pleomorphism. The nuclei have coarse, granular chromatin and are often lobed.

221

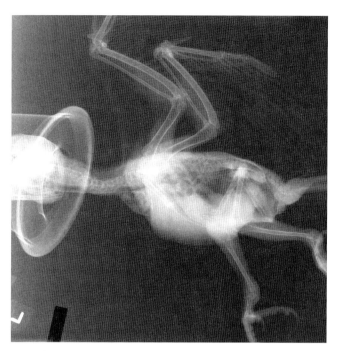

Fig. 53.2. The lateral radiograph.

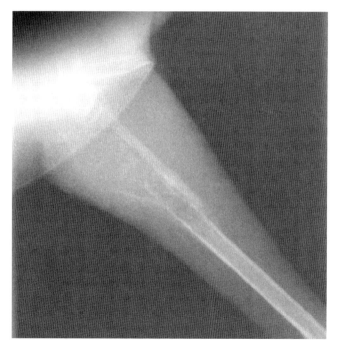

Fig. 53.3. An enlarged view of the swollen left leg.

The cytoplasm of these cells stains light blue and some cells have cytoplasmic vacuolation. Two mitotic figures can be seen.

Figure 53.4b is a higher magnification of Fig. 53.4a. At the bottom of the image, there is a mitotic figure. The two spindle-shaped cells in the center of the image have large nuclei with prominent large and multiple nucleoli and pale blue cytoplasm. Vacuoles can be seen in the cytoplasm of the cell on the left.

Figure 53.4c shows large, pleomorphic spindle-shaped cells with large, sometimes binucleated, pleomorphic nuclei. The nuclei have coarse, granular chromatin with large prominent nucleoli. The cytoplasm of these cells is dark blue and often vacuolated.

Figure 53.4d shows an extremely large, multinucleated, spindle-shaped cell with coarse, nuclear chromatin, multiple large nucleoli with anisonucleoliosis, and dark cytoplasmic basophilia.

Figure 53.4e shows a large cell on the right with an abnormal mitotic figure. The cell on the left has a high N/C ratio with a large, angular nucleolus.

Figure 53.4f shows a multinucleated, spindle-shaped giant cell with a blue cytoplasm that contains numerous pink-staining inclusions that stain similar to the nucleus. These inclusions could represent numerous satellite nuclei or a secretory product.

The cytologic examination represents a mesenchymal cell neoplasm, and a cytodiagnosis of a sarcoma involving the bone was made.

Summary

On the basis of the cytologic interpretation of a sarcoma and the extent of the lytic bone lesion, the left leg was amputated at the hip. The bird was given butorphanol (0.67 mg) intramuscularly 35 minutes prior to anesthesia induction with sevoflurane anesthesia via face mask. The butorphanol provided poor sedation. The macaw had an uneventful recovery from the anesthesia and surgery.

Histopathologic examination revealed a poorly differentiated sarcoma, which was consistent with the cytological findings. Histology of the tumor had some features that made fibrosarcoma a likely diagnosis. The tumor extended to the edge of soft tissue surgical margins and the distal femur was free of tumor.

The macaw died 2 months later owing to metastasis to the liver.

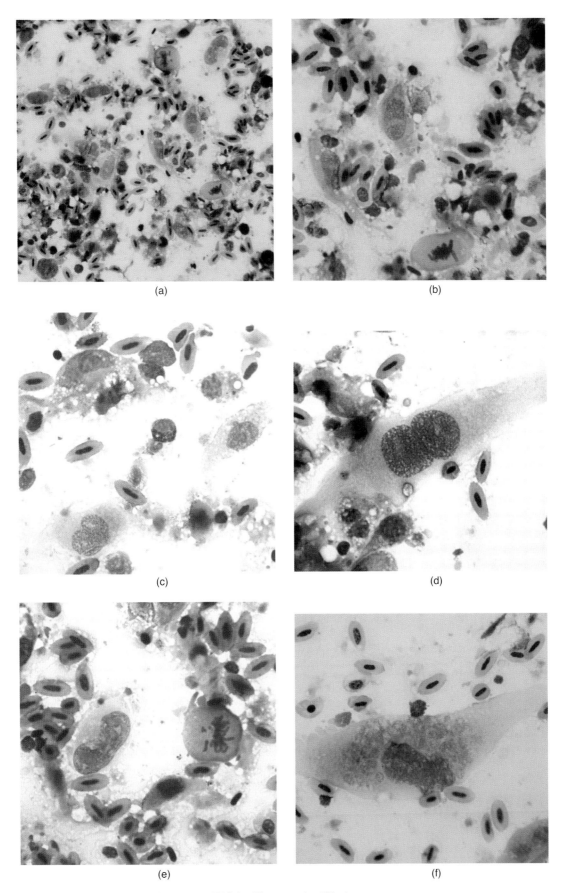

Fig. 53.4. (a–f) An aspirate of the left leg mass (Wright–Giemsa stain, 100×).

A 6-Year-Old Lovebird with Dystocia

54

Signalment

A 6-year-old intact female peach-faced lovebird (*Agapornis roseicollis*) was presented with possible dystocia.

History

The lovebird was presented as an emergency with a chief complaint of being egg bound according to the owner. It was noted on presentation that the bird's respiratory rate was slightly increased and the coelom was distended. The owner described the bird as being lethargic and stressed prior to bringing her to the hospital. The bird had a history of laying eggs but had not laid an egg in about a year.

Physical Examination Findings

On physical examination, the lovebird was alert and responsive. The coelom was moderately distended and the bird appeared uncomfortable. The coelom was distended and palpated firm but soft. No egg was identified (Fig. 54.1).

Recommendation for a diagnostic plan that included a complete blood count, plasma biochemistry profile, and a radiographic examination was declined by the client. Owing to a past history of egg laying and an enlarged coelomic cavity, egg-related coelomitis was suspected. Recommendation for coeliocentesis for cytodiagnosis was approved by the owner.

The coelomic aspiration was performed by inserting a 25-gauge needle on the ventral midline just caudal to the caudal margin of the keel. The needle was directed away from the ventriculus. The sample was collected but was not evaluated until the following day. The bird was released with a tentative diagnosis of egg-

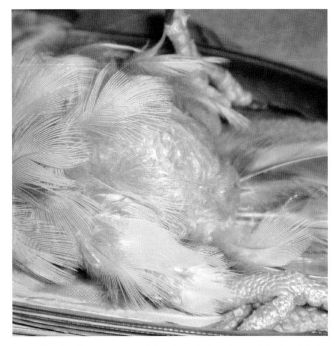

Fig. 54.1. An image of the distended coelom of the lovebird.

related coelomitis and treated at home with meloxicam (0.3 mg/kg, q 24 hours) (Figs. 54.2 and 54.3).

Interpretive Discussion

Figure 54.2 reveals a highly cellular sample that contains numerous erythrocytes, heterophils, and larger blue-staining cells that appear to be epithelial cells.

Figure 54.3a is a higher magnification that shows a cluster of large cells with abundant, lightly basophilic cytoplasm and round nuclei among numerous erythrocytes. The nuclei appear uniform in size and shape and have prominent large nucleoli and coarsely granular chromatin. The cells resemble hepatocytes.

225

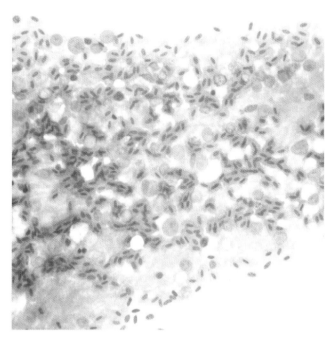

Fig. 54.2. The cytology from coeliocentesis (Wright– Giemsa stain, 40×).

Hepatocytes are easily damaged, especially in aspiration biopsy samples, and often appear as nuclei scattered in a background that resembles the cytoplasm of hepatocytes. A number of heterophils are also seen in this image.

Figure 54.3b shows heterophils intermingled with erythrocytes and cells that resemble hepatocytes.

The cytology sample that contained hepatocytes indicated that a fine-needle aspiration biopsy of the liver was accidentally obtained. Considering the location of the celiocentesis, it is likely the liver was enlarged. The presence of numerous heterophils suggests that either a heterophilic inflammation was associated with an enlarged liver or the peripheral blood had a marked heterophilia.

Summary

The owner was informed of the results but still declined further diagnostic testing. She was also informed that the meloxicam treatment may be contraindicated owing to possible hepatic disease. The client opted to continue the bird on the meloxicam because she felt it made the bird more comfortable. The bird was maintained comfortably on meloxicam for approximately 1 month at which time the owner felt it was time for euthanasia. The bird was submitted for necropsy.

Grossly, the liver was moderately enlarged and extended beyond the keel. The duodenum was reddened and severely distended with ingesta. All other organs appeared normal. Histologically, the small intestine lesions were consistent with enteritis with a bacterial etiology; however, no microbial culture or other testing was conducted.

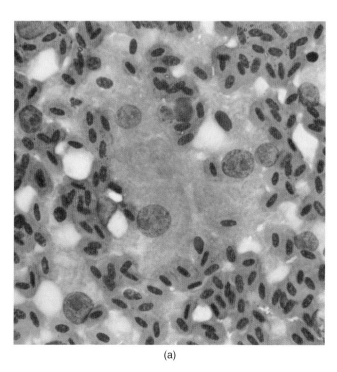

(a)

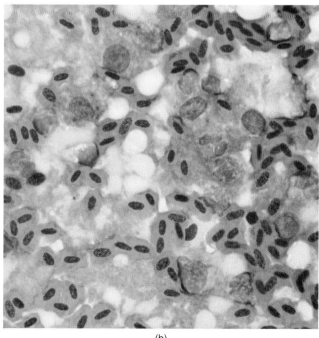

(b)

Fig. 54.3. (a and b) The cytology from coeliocentesis (Wright–Giemsa stain, 100×).

A 5-Year-Old Parrot with Dyspnea

55

Signalment

A 5-year-old intact male Eclectus parrot (*Eclectus roratus*) was presented as an emergency for dyspnea.

History

The owners reported that the parrot had started sneezing 5 days prior to presentation which had progressed to breathing difficulty. He was also more reclusive than normal but was eating and drinking well throughout the week. His diet consisted of nuts, fruits, and seeds. He was recently placed in a new cage $1^1/_2$ weeks prior to presentation. A bird from a different household lived in the cage previously.

The parrot was previously treated with tetracycline that was placed in the water. This was followed by treatment using tylosin in the water for the past 5 days. The client felt that the bird showed mild improvement with the second antibiotic. The bird suddenly developed dyspnea and wheezing at which point the client presented him to the emergency hospital where he was maintained in supplemental oxygen overnight.

Physical Examination Findings

On physical examination, the parrot exhibited open-mouth breathing and coughing. A 4 mm endotracheal tube was used for an air sac cannula that was immediately placed in the left abdominal air sac, which alleviated the bird's respiratory distress (Fig. 55.1).

Once the bird was stable the physical examination was completed. The bird weighed 376 g and was in good body condition. A small amount of clear discharge was observed in both nares.

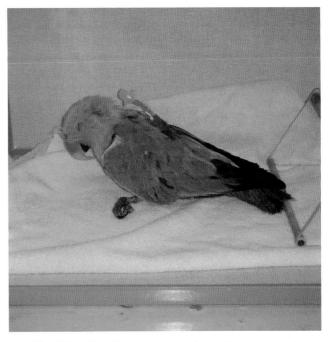

Fig. 55.1. The Eclectus parrot with an air sac cannula in the left abdominal air sac.

Other Diagnostic Information during Initial Visit

Radiographs revealed no significant findings and the lungs and air sacs appeared normal. Considering the bird's remarkable improvement after placing the air sac cannula, a lesion in the syrinx was suspected and an exploratory surgery of the syrinx was performed.

The bird was given atropine (0.015 mg) and butorphanol (0.112 mg) intramuscularly as preanesthetic agents. Anesthesia induction was made 5 minutes later using sevoflurane into the air sac tube.

The surgical approach to the syrinx was made with the patient in dorsal recumbency. A 4-cm incision was

227

made from the thoracic inlet in a cranial direction to expose the trachea and syrinx. The trachea was incised and a rigid arthroscope (1.9 mm) was used to better visualize the entire trachea and syrinx. A small, white, plaque was identified and removed from the ventral syrinx. An impression of the sample was taken for cytologic examination (Figs. 55.2 and 55.3) and the remainder of the sample was submitted for culture and sensitivity. The trachea and subcutaneous tissue were closed with a 5-0 glycomer 631 suture separately, and the skin was closed with 4-0 nylon suture in a cruciate pattern.

The parrot recovered well from surgery and remained hospitalized for 4 days. Blood was collected for evaluation of the hemogram and a plasma biochemistry profile (Figs. 55.4a and 55.4b; Tables 55.1 and 55.2).

Interpretive Discussion for the Initial Visit

A low-magnification image from the imprint of the material removed from the syrinx is shown in Fig. 55.2 revealing a marked number of inflammatory cells and erythrocytes. Higher magnification (Figs. 55.3a and 55.3b) reveals that the majority of the inflammatory cells are nondegenerate heterophils. A few of the heterophils exhibit cytoplasmic vacuolization. Extracellular bacteria can be seen in the background.

The blood film revealed toxic changes in the majority of the heterophils (Figs. 55.4a and 55.4b). These changes are noted by the dark basophilic cytoplasm and

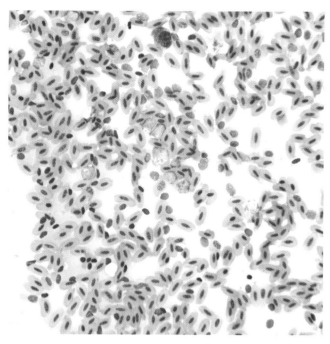

Fig. 55.2. A syrinx plaque imprint (Wright–Giemsa stain, 50×).

the decreased amount of granules present in the cytoplasm. Hypochromatic erythrocytes are also present (Fig. 55.4b).

The hemogram indicates a mild leukopenia; however, the presence on toxic heterophils in the peripheral

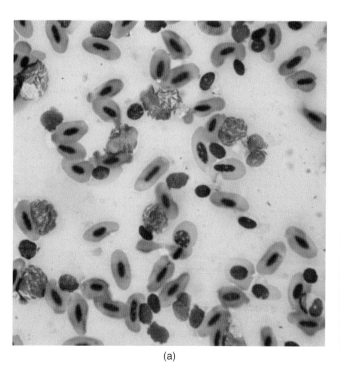

(a)

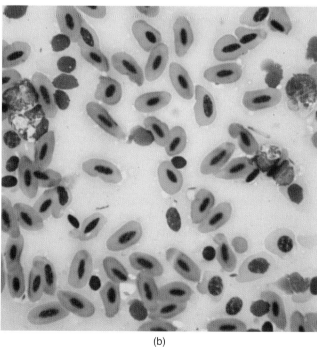

(b)

Fig. 55.3. (a and b) The syrinx plaque imprint (Wright–Giemsa stain, 100×).

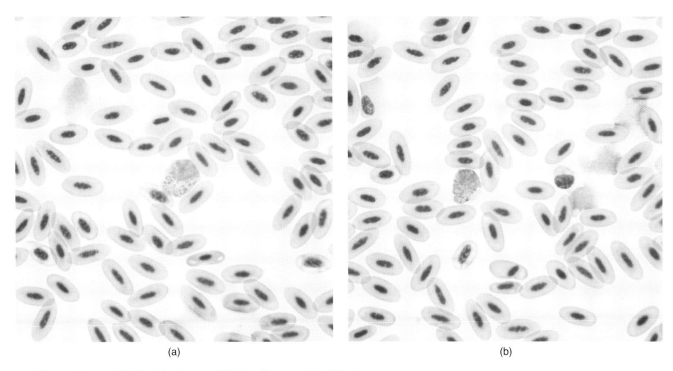

Fig. 55.4. (a and b) The blood smear (Wright–Giemsa stain, 100×).

blood film indicates a severe inflammatory response regardless of the actual cell count. This is likely a response to the inflammatory process in the syrinx. The plasma biochemistry panel revealed a marked increase in the aspartate aminotransferase (AST) and creatine kinase (CK) activities. The increased CK likely represents either skeletal muscle injury associated with the surgery or muscle exertion. The degree of increase in the AST likely indicates hepatocellular disease as it is too high to be associated with skeletal muscle involvement. A presumptive diagnosis of chlamydophilosis was made based on the evidence of a combination of hepatocellular disease and respiratory disease.

Summary for Initial Visit

The parrot was hospitalized for 4 days after surgery. During this time, a swab from the choanal slit, conjunctiva, and cloaca was submitted for *Chlamydophila* polymerase chain reaction (PCR) testing. The culture and the sensitivity obtained during surgery were pending at that

Table 55.1. Hematology results.

	Results	Normal range for Eclectus parrot[a]
WBC (10^3/μL)	3.5	5.5–25
Heterophils (10^3/μL)	1.4 (39%)	35–75%
Lymphocytes (10^3/μL)	1.5 (42%)	20–65%
Monocytes (10^3/μL)	0.5 (15%)	1–11%
Eosinophils (10^3/μL)	0.1 (2%)	0–1%
Basophils (10^3/μL)	0	0–3%
Plasma protein (g/dL)	3.5	—
PCV (%)	36	26–58
Thrombocytes	Clumped	—

[a]Carpenter (2005).

Table 55.2. Plasma biochemistry results.

	Initial visit	Recheck visit	Reference[a]
Glucose (mg/dL)	260	—	220–300
BUN (mg/dL)	3	—	0–6
Uric acid (mg/dL)	8.1	—	0.2–6.5
Total protein (biuret) (g/dL)	2.9	2.4	1.8–3.8
Albumin (g/dL)	<1.0	—	0.8–1.8
Globulin (g/dL)	1.9	—	0.8–2.2
Aspartate aminotransferase (IU/L)	2184	853	65–260
Creatine kinase (IU/L)	2186	2544	200–1600
Calcium (mg/dL)	8.7	—	8.5–10.2
Phosphorus (mg/dL)	5.3	—	4.5–9.0
Sodium (mEq/L)	152	—	138–158
Potassium (mEq/L)	3.6	—	2.0–4.6
Chloride (mEq/L)	106	—	100–120
Bicarbonate (mEq/L)	31.1	—	—
Anion gap (calculated)	19	—	—
Cholesterol (mg/dL)	177	—	125–450
Calculated osmolality	305	—	—

[a]Carpenter (2005).

time. As a precaution, the bird was treated with doxy-cycline (25 mg/kg PO BID), enrofloxacin (10 mg/kg PO BID), and meloxicam (0.5 mg/kg PO q 24 hours during hospitalization). He was also given enrofloxacin (8 mL of a 10 mg/mL enrofloxacin solution in 12 mL of saline) via 20-minute nebulization treatments twice daily.

The microbial culture from the lesion in the syrinx revealed a moderate growth of *Haemophilus* species. The organism was susceptible to all antibiotics except tetracycline on the antibiotic sensitivity profile. Although the bacterium was resistant to tetracycline, doxycycline was continued as it is considered to be the antibiotic of choice for chlamydophilosis.

The bird's condition quickly improved and the air sac cannula was removed after 24 hours. During the course of 3 days of treatment, the bird appeared to be recovering from its respiratory distress; however, on the fourth day of treatment, the bird began sneezing and exhibiting open-mouth breathing with audible respiratory sounds and had developed a moderate amount of subcutaneous emphysema on his head, back, and chest. He continued to eat and drink and the skin incision was healing.

Blood was collected to reevaluate the plasma AST activity (Table 55.2), and a tracheal aspirate was obtained for cytologic evaluation (Figs. 55.5 and 55.6). The *Chlamydophila* PCR results were obtained at this time and were shown to be negative.

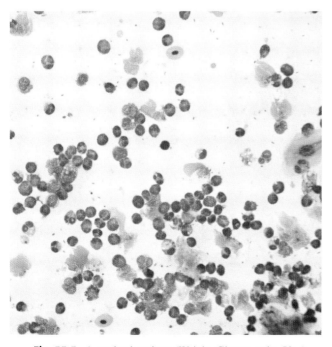

Fig. 55.5. A tracheal aspirate (Wright–Giemsa stain, 50×).

Interpretative Discussion

Figures 55.5 and 55.6a reveal a highly cellular sample consisting of primarily inflammatory cells. The inflammatory cells consist primarily of nondegenerate heterophils with a few macrophages and lymphocytes and support a cytodiagnosis of heterophilic inflammation. No etiologic agent can be seen in these images.

Figures 55.6b and 55.6c reveal fungal elements represented by septate branching hyphae, characteristics of *Aspergillus* sp.

The plasma AST activity had decreased significantly but remained elevated.

Itraconazole (10 mg/kg PO daily) and nebulization with clotrimazole were added to the daily treatments. A second tracheal aspirate was evaluated 24 hours following initiation of the antifungal treatments (Fig. 55.7).

Because of the continued presence of the fungal hyphae of the tracheal aspirate, clotrimazole was discontinued and replaced with amphotericin B owing to its fungicidal properties. The systemic itraconazole was continued. Amphotericin B (0.1 mL of 5 mg/mL) was combined with 0.9 mL of saline, of which 0.2 mL of the combination was directly applied into the trachea using a 5-French feeding tube. Another combination of amphotericin B (1 mL) and saline (4 mL) was used for nebulization twice daily. Nebulization with saline was also administered as needed.

The bird remained hospitalized for a total of 5 more days. Each day a tracheal aspirate was obtained for cytologic evaluation and treatment progress (Figs. 55.8–55.10).

Figure 55.7 reveals that robust, septate, branching hyphae are still present after 24 hours of antifungal treatment with itraconazole and clotrimazole.

Figure 55.8a shows degenerate fungal hyphae after 1 day of amphotericin B treatment. Figure 55.8b is an image from the same sample showing evidence of fewer degenerate heterophils with nondegenerate heterophils predominating the inflammatory response.

Figure 55.9 reveals a predominance of nondegenerate heterophils after 48 hours of amphotericin B treatments. Although not shown, the sample contained fewer degenerate hyphae than the sample obtained 24 hours prior.

Figure 55.10 reveals a predominance of nondegenerate heterophils after 72 hours of amphotericin B treatments. No fungal hyphae were observed at this time on the tracheal aspirate sample.

Along with the improvement seen cytologically, the bird's clinical signs of respiratory distress also improved. He continued to occasionally open-mouth breathe and exhibit respiratory noise, but these improved each day. Owing to financial concerns and the improvement of the parrot's overall condition, the client elected

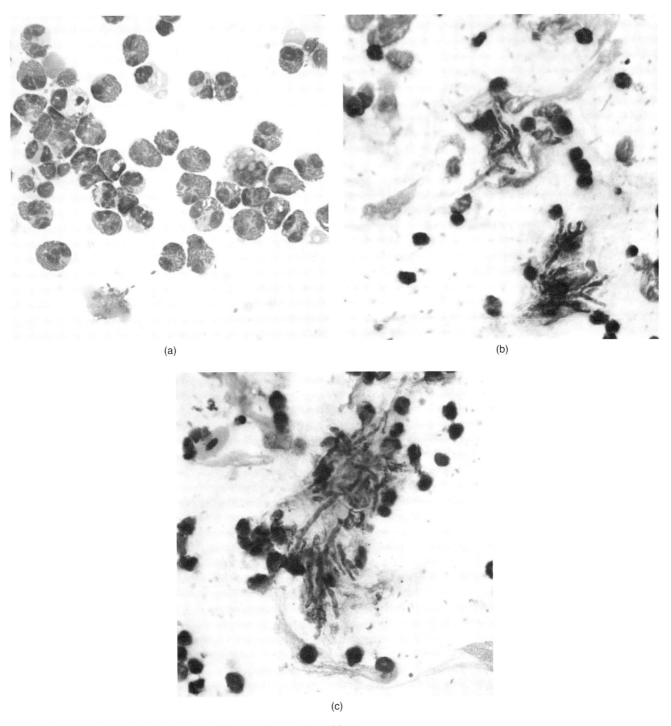

(a)

(b)

(c)

Fig. 55.6. (a–c) The tracheal aspirate (Wright–Giemsa stain, 100×).

to continue treatment at home and the bird was discharged 5 days after the initiation of the amphotericin B treatments. The client was unable to continue the nebulization treatments at home. The bird was treated at home with itraconazole (10 mg/kg PO q 24 hours) and trimethoprim-sulfa (20 mg/kg PO BID) and was to return in 2 weeks for reevaluation.

Summary

Ten days following his discharge from the hospital, the bird presented as an urgent care patient for respiratory distress. The owners reported that the bird ate a peanut the night before at which time he began sneezing uncontrollably. The parrot coughed up part of the peanut and had not been breathing well ever since. The

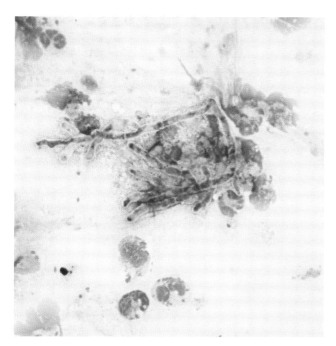

Fig. 55.7. Day 2 of antifungal treatment, tracheal aspirate after 1 day of itraconazole and clotrimazole treatment in an Eclectus parrot with a *Haemophilus* and fungal infection in the syrinx (Wright–Giemsa stain, 100×).

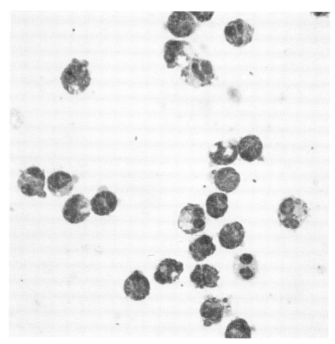

Fig. 55.9. Day 4 of antifungal treatment, tracheal aspirate after 2 days of amphotericin B treatment (Wright–Giemsa stain, 100×).

client was concerned that the bird had aspirated part of the peanut.

A physical examination revealed that the bird was open-mouth breathing and appeared to have an increased expiratory effort. Due to financial restrictions, the own-

ers opted against further diagnosis and the bird was euthanized.

Gross necropsy revealed opaque and thickened cranial thoracic air sacs filled with white plaques. The lesion was more prominent on the right side and

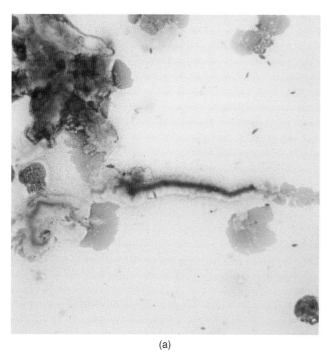

(a)

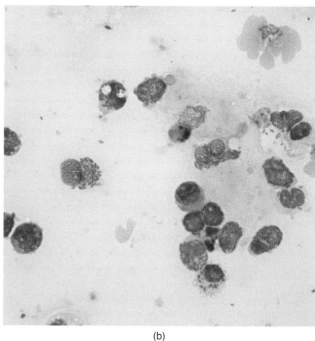

(b)

Fig. 55.8. (a and b) Day 3 of antifungal treatment, tracheal aspirate after 1 day of amphotericin B treatment (Wright–Giemsa stain, 100×).

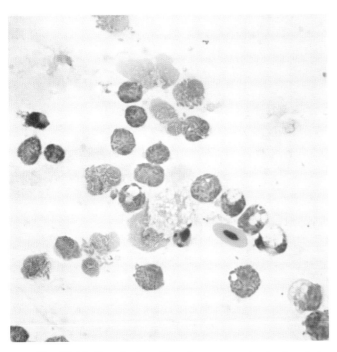

Fig. 55.10. Day 5 of antifungal treatment, tracheal aspirate after 3 days of amphotericin B treatment (Wright–Giemsa stain, 100×).

surrounded the heart base. The cranial thoracic cavity also displayed multifocal white plaques along the parietal pleura. There was a small food particle lodged within the syrinx but did not appear to obstruct the airway. Otherwise, the syrinx appeared normal. Histopathologic examination provided a diagnosis of fibrosing airsacculitis and ulcerative tracheitis, but no etiologic agent could be found.

The bird initially had a bacterial (*Haemophilus*) infection in the syrinx. The fungal lesion developed later. Aspergillosis is typically associated with immunosuppression in birds. It is likely that the cause of the compromised immune system in this bird was associated with the bacterial infection and handling for medication. In retrospect, addition of an antifungal therapy targeting aspergillosis may be an important addition to treatment of any bird with respiratory disease and potential immunosuppression.

A 2-Year-Old Macaw with Anorexia and Weight Loss

56

Signalment

A 2-year-old female Military macaw (*Ara militaris*) was presented with a 10-day history of anorexia and weight loss (Fig. 56.1).

History

The macaw began to exhibit partial anorexia approximately 2 weeks prior to presentation and was being tube fed a commercial nestling formula to support its nutritional intake. According to the owner, during the past 10 days, the bird appeared to be painful while being fed using a feeding tube. The macaw had been treated 2 weeks prior to presentation at another veteri-

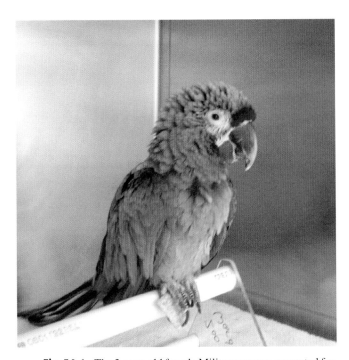

Fig. 56.1. The 2-year-old female Military macaw presented for chronic anorexia.

nary hospital where whole body radiographs, a blood profile, and a crop biopsy were obtained. The complete blood cell count and plasma chemistries were all within normal limits at that time. The veterinarian was concerned about an enlarged proventriculus on the whole body radiographs; therefore, a crop biopsy was obtained in an effort to confirm a suspected proventricular dilatation syndrome; however, the histopathologic examination revealed a normal ingluvies.

Physical Examination Findings

Physical examination findings revealed a 775 g Military macaw with moderate reduction of the pectoral muscle mass (body score of 2.5/5.0). A blood sample was obtained via jugular venipuncture and submitted for a complete blood cell count and plasma biochemical profile. Whole body radiographs were obtained with and without contrast material in the gastrointestinal tract. The macaw was tube fed 12 mL of a 36% barium sulfate suspension. A fecal sample was also obtained for cytologic examination (Tables 56.1 and 56.2 and Figs. 56.2–56.5).

Interpretive Discussion

Interpretation of the complete blood cell count depends on which published reference value is used. It is best to use reference values from the laboratory doing the testing, if available. Another alternative is to use previous blood profiles of the patient during times of normal health to compare during times of illness. Whenever these are not available, the clinician must rely on published reference values or use decision levels, threshold values of which the veterinarian responds. In this case, the macaw appears slightly anemic based on a packed cell volume (PCV) below 35% (a decision level used by the authors). The leukocyte count appears to be within normal limits for macaws; however, there is a relative

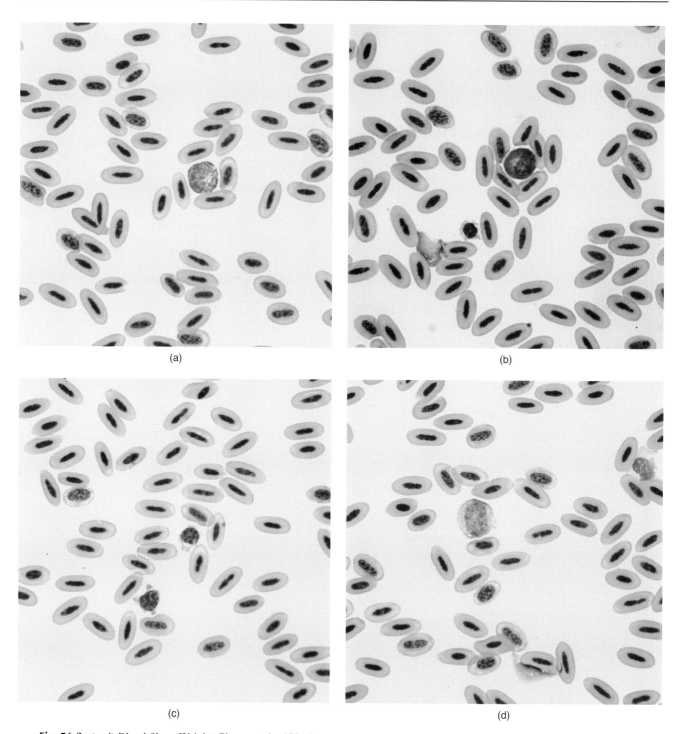

(a)

(b)

(c)

(d)

Fig. 56.2. (a–d) Blood films (Wright–Giemsa stain, 100×).

heterophilia and lymphocytosis. There also appears to be a slight hypoproteinemia and hypocalcemia, which likely result from inadequate dietary intake.

Figure 56.2a represents a typical heterophil on the blood film. The heterophil shows increased cytoplasmic basophilia, indicative of slight toxicity. Heterophil toxicity is indicative of an inflammatory response, re-

gardless of the cell count. The image also indicates a slight increase in polychromasia, indicating a regenerative response to the erythrocytes. A regenerative anemia can be seen with a hemolytic anemia or recovery from blood loss or depression anemia. Figure 56.2b shows a plasma cell and a thrombocyte. Figure 56.2c shows two small lymphocytes. Figure 56.2d shows a monocyte.

Table 56.1. Hematology results.

		Reference[a]	Reference[b]
PCV (%)	32	47–55	25–55
Leukocytes			
WBC ($10^3/\mu$L)	11.9	7.0–22.0	7.0–30.0
Heterophils ($10^3/\mu$L)	9.5	—	—
Heterophils (%)	80	40–60	37–75
Lymphocytes ($10^3/\mu$L)	1.6	—	—
Lymphocytes (%)	13	35–60	20–60
Monocytes ($10^3/\mu$L)	0.5	—	—
Monocytes (%)	4	0–2	1–10
Eosinophils ($10^3/\mu$L)	0.2	—	—
Eosinophils (%)	2	0–1	0–1
Basophils ($10^3/\mu$L)	0.1	—	—
Basophils (%)	1	0–1	0–3
Thrombocytes			
Estimated number	Adequate	1–5/1,000× field	
Morphology	Normal, clumped		
Plasma protein (refractometry) (g/dL)	1.9	3–5	

[a]Campbell and Ellis (2007).
[b]Carpenter (2005).

The coelomic, thoracic, soft tissue, and osseous structures are within normal limits on the whole body radiographs (Figs. 56.3 and 56.4). There is a focal accumulation of contrast seen within the pharyngeal region, crop, proventriculus, ventriculus, and intestinal structures. There is an irregularly marginated focal region of contrast material within the tissues adjacent to the left scapulohumeral joint. The focal accumulation of

Table 56.2. Plasma biochemical results.

		Reference[a]	Reference[b]
Glucose (mg/dL)	284	145–345	225–330
BUN (mg/dL)	2	3.0–5.6	0–6
Uric acid (mg/dL)	1.1	2.5–11	0.2–6.0
Total protein (biuret) (g/dL)	2.0	2.1–4.5	1.5–3.5
Albumin (g/dL)	0.7	1.2–3.1	0.6–1.7
Globulin (g/dL)	1.3	—	0.8–1.9
Aspartate aminotransferase (IU/L)	164	100–300	60–180
Creatine kinase (IU/L)	228	100–300	180–1,100
Calcium (mg/dL)	8.0	8.5–13	8.5–10.8
Phosphorus (mg/dL)	4.5	2.0–12.0	4.6–6.9
Sodium (mEq/L)	144	140–165	135–156
Potassium (mEq/L)	2.8	2.0–5.0	2.0–4.2
Chloride (mEq/L)	107	—	96–118
Bicarbonate (mEq/L)	21	14–25	—
Anion gap (calculated)	19	—	—
Cholesterol (mg/dL)	89	100–390	75–300
Calculated osmolality	290	—	—

[a]Johnston-Delaney and Harrison (1996).
[b]Carpenter (2005).

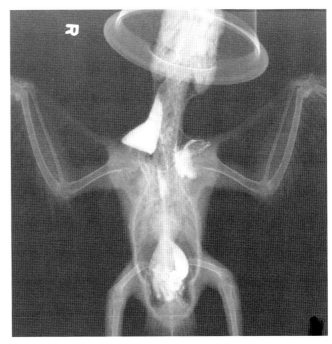

Fig. 56.3. The whole body ventral–dorsal radiograph taken 45 minutes following barium contrast delivered via tube into the ingluvies.

contrast within the pharyngeal region may represent reflux. The contrast adjacent to the left scapulohumeral joint is suggestive of subcutaneous accumulation. An esophageal or crop perforation leading to this accumulation is possible.

The fecal cytology reveals a marked number of *Candida*-like yeast (Figs. 56.5a and 56.5b). Figure 56.5b reveals budding forms of the yeast. The yeast has the morphology of *Candida albicans*, a common inhabitant of the gastrointestinal tract of psittacine birds and opportunistic pathogen.

Summary

Cytologic examination of the tube-feeding formula failed to reveal the food as being the source of the yeast. The cause of the yeast overgrowth as with most fungal diseases is often associated with immunosuppression. The cause of the immunosuppression in this case is not known. The yeast overgrowth can also be associated with a dysbiosis resulting from gastrointestinal disease. The apparent candidiasis can also cause a decrease in gastrointestinal motility and malabsorption and maldigestion. The macaw was treated with itraconazole (10 mg/kg, orally daily for 10 days). Thirty-six hours following the introduction of the itraconazole, a fecal sample was negative for yeast.

Because the radiographs revealed leakage of barium out of the crop, surgical exploration of the ingluvies was

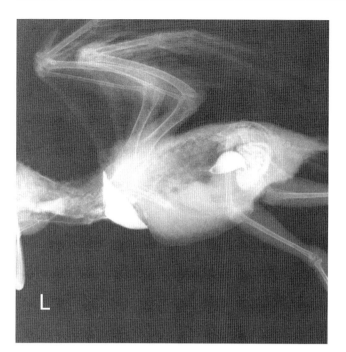

Fig. 56.4. The whole body lateral radiograph taken 45 minutes following barium contrast delivered via tube into the ingluvies.

performed. The macaw was given 0.23 mg midazolam, 0.015 mg atropine, and 0.76 mg butorphanol intramuscularly as a preanesthetic treatment 10 minutes prior to induction with sevoflurane. An opening in the crop

was discovered at the biopsy site, which was cleaned and closed. An attempt to remove the barium from the surrounding tissue failed owing to the adherence of the material. The opening in the crop was closed using a 4-0 absorbable suture in a simple continuous pattern. The skin was closed using a simple, interrupted 4-0 nylon suture. Recovery from the anesthesia was uneventful. The bird was placed on meloxicam (0.3 mg/kg, orally daily) for 5 days postoperatively.

The bird began eating a mix of nuts and fruits on her own the day following surgery. She continued to eat on her own during the next 2 days. She had an increase in fecal output and the appearance remained normal.

The bird continued to do well at home and made a complete recovery. Her skin sutures were removed by her local veterinarian 2 weeks after the surgery, and she was reported to have returned to normal at that time.

One month later, however, the macaw returned with the complaint of having edema around her eyes and yellow urates. She was still eating well and gaining weight (840 g) at that time, but had a mild leukocytosis (14,300/μL), elevated plasma aspartate aminotransferase (AST) activity (1,058 IU/L), and bile acid of 40 μmol/L. Although her titer for *Chlamydophila* was negative, she was treated with doxycycline for the possibility of a false-negative titer. After 2 weeks of doxycycline treatment, her AST decreased to 540 IU/L and her bile acid was 16 μmol/L; however, she was not

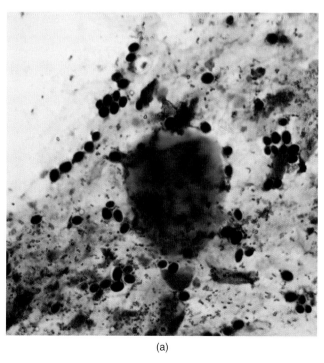

(a)

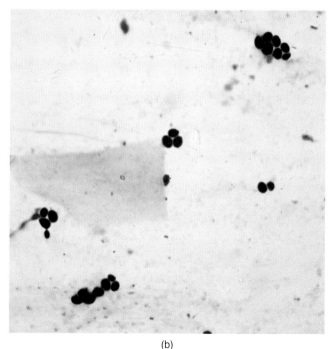

(b)

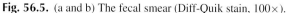

Fig. 56.5. (a and b) The fecal smear (Diff-Quik stain, 100×).

doing well and began showing weight loss (805 g) and lethargic behavior. She developed a significant leukocytosis (26,900/μL) and hypoproteinemia (1.7 g/dL) at that time. Repeat radiographs revealed an enlarged cardiohepatic silhouette, suggesting hepatomegaly, cardiomegaly, or both. A liver biopsy was performed for histopathologic examination that revealed bile duct hyperplasia, suggestive of aflatoxicosis and hepatocellular necrosis with intranuclear inclusions suggestive of herpesvirus infection. The bird was given a poor prognosis for survival and died 2 days later. Necropsy revealed cardiomegaly with hydropericardium and hepatomegaly. The likely etiology was psittacine herpesvirus infection.

57

An Adult Goose with a Mass on the Wing

Signalment

An adult female domestic goose (*Anser anser*) was presented for a mass on her left wing (Fig. 57.1).

History

The goose was presented 2 years earlier with complaint of dyspnea and loss of voice. At that time, an intratracheal pedunculated mass was found to be the cause of the dyspnea and vocal loss. The mass was removed surgically and determined to be a lipoma based on histopathologic examination.

The goose was fed a commercial diet prepared for domestic geese and a mixture of grains. The client did not know how long the mass had been on the wing.

Physical Examination Findings

The physical examination revealed an apparently healthy goose with a firm mass on the alula of the left wing. Blood was obtained from the medial metatarsal vein for a blood profile. A fine-needle aspiration biopsy

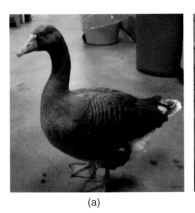
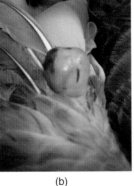

(a)   (b)

Fig. 57.1. (a and b) An image of the domestic goose with a mass on its left wing.

Table 57.1. Hematology results.

		Reference[a]
PCV (%)	35	42–54
Leukocytes		
WBC ($10^3/\mu$L)	25.1	20–22
Heterophils ($10^3/\mu$L)	19.8	—
Heterophils (%)	79	39
Lymphocytes ($10^3/\mu$L)	4.5	—
Lymphocytes (%)	18	46
Monocytes ($10^3/\mu$L)	0.8	—
Monocytes (%)	3	6
Eosinophils ($10^3/\mu$L)	0	—
Eosinophils (%)	0	2
Basophils ($10^3/\mu$L)	0	—
Basophils (%)	0	7
Thrombocytes		
Estimated number	Adequate	1–5/1,000× field
Morphology	Normal, clumped	
Plasma protein (refractometry) (g/dL)	Lipemia	3–5

[a]Campbell (2000) for the Canada goose.

was obtained from the mass for cytological evaluation (Tables 57.1 and 57.2 and Figs. 57.2a–57.2c).

Interpretive Discussion

The hemogram was evaluated based on reference values for Canada geese (*Branta canadensis*) because there is little information in the literature for normal blood profiles in domestic geese. The hemogram suggests that the bird is anemic; however, a packed cell volume (PCV) of 35% would be considered to be the low end of the normal range in many species of birds. The total leukocyte count would seem high for many species of birds; however, it is only slightly elevated when compared to normal Canada geese. The leukocyte differential, however, suggests a relative heterophilia

241

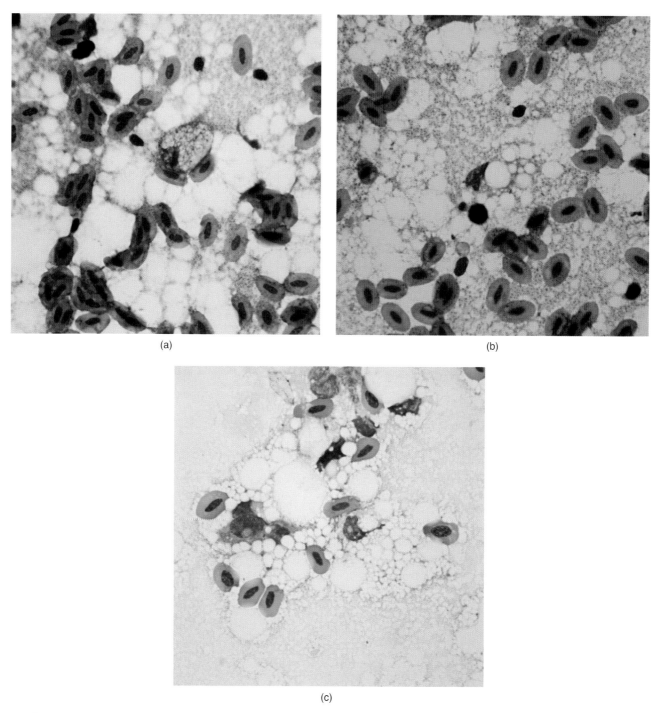

(a)

(b)

(c)

Fig. 57.2. (a–c) Images of imprint of the mass (Wright–Giemsa stain, 100×).

and lymphopenia. This suggests either a stress leuko-gram or perhaps a mild inflammatory response.

The only significant plasma biochemistry finding is a marked increase in cholesterol. The plasma sample was extremely lipemic, which required special separation of the plasma. The lipemia could affect the outcome of the biochemical profile, although the results of most analytes appear normal.

Figures 57.2a–57.2c reveal a cytology that contains a marked amount of fat vacuoles in the background of the sample. There are also numerous erythrocytes. There are a few foamy cells with eccentric nuclei that likely represent adipocytes. Normal avian adipocytes differ from those of mammals because they are typically highly vacuolated owing to fat that stains negatively with Wright–Giemsa stain. The nuclei of the cells in the

Table 57.2. Plasma biochemical results.

		Reference[a]
Glucose (mg/dL)	204	207–241
BUN (mg/dL)	—	—
Uric acid (mg/dL)	3.0	6.0–10.5
Total protein (biuret) (g/dL)	4.6	4.1–5.5
Albumin (g/dL)	1.6	1.9–2.3
Globulin (g/dL)	3.0	2.2–3.4
Aspartate aminotransferase (IU/L)	34	58–92
Creatine kinase (IU/L)	101	—
Calcium (mg/dL)	11.3	9.5–10.9
Phosphorus (mg/dL)	3.9	1.9–3.7
Sodium (mEq/L)	148	138–146
Potassium (mEq/L)	3.0	2.8–4.0
Chloride (mEq/L)	108	101–109
Bicarbonate (mEq/L)	18.4	—
Anion gap (calculated)	25	—
Cholesterol (mg/dL)	777	144–200
Calculated osmolality	—	—

[a]Johnston-Delaney and Harrison (1996) for the Canada goose.

sample are not as pyknotic as one would expect from normal adipocytes, suggesting the cells are young and likely represent hyperplasia or benign neoplasia. Gentle heat fixation of the slide prior to staining may have improved adherence of the adipocytes to the slide, thus increasing the number of cells to evaluate.

Summary

The mass was surgically removed from the bird under a general anesthetic using isoflurane. The histopathologic diagnosis of the mass was an angiolipoma.

A 14-Year-Old Budgerigar with Lethargy and Anorexia

58

Signalment

A 14-year-old intact female budgerigar (*Melopsittacus undulatus*) was presented with the complaint of lethargy and partial anorexia for the past 24 hours.

History

The budgerigar was presented because it had been sleeping more, eating less, and sitting puffed up during the past 24 hours. The budgerigar appeared off-balance and was unable or unwilling to lift her left leg off the perch. According to the owner, the bird was originally acquired from a breeder because she was unable to lay eggs. Although the client had owned the bird for 8 years, the actual age of the bird was 14 years according to the date on its leg band. The bird was fed a commercial brand pelleted diet supplemented with a variety of seeds,

vegetables, and powdered vitamin supplement. She lived alone in a commercial birdcage; however, there was a cockatiel (*Nymphicus hollandicus*) and lovebird (*Agapornis* sp.) housed in separate cages in the same room.

Physical Examination Findings

The physical examination revealed a 50 g female budgerigar with a moderate reduction of the pectoral muscle mass. Other than appearing weak, no other abnormalities could be found on physical examination. The droppings in the bottom of the cage appeared grossly normal; however, a sample was collected for cytologic evaluation (Fig. 58.4).

A small blood sample was obtained via jugular venipuncture for evaluation of a blood film (Fig. 58.3) and determination of the packed cell volume (PCV). The PCV was 38%. Whole body radiographs were also obtained (Figs. 58.1 and 58.2).

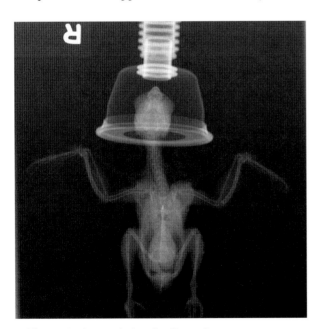

Fig. 58.1. A ventral–dorsal radiograph.

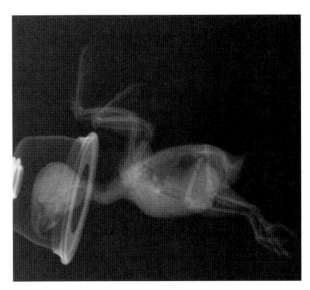

Fig. 58.2. A lateral radiograph.

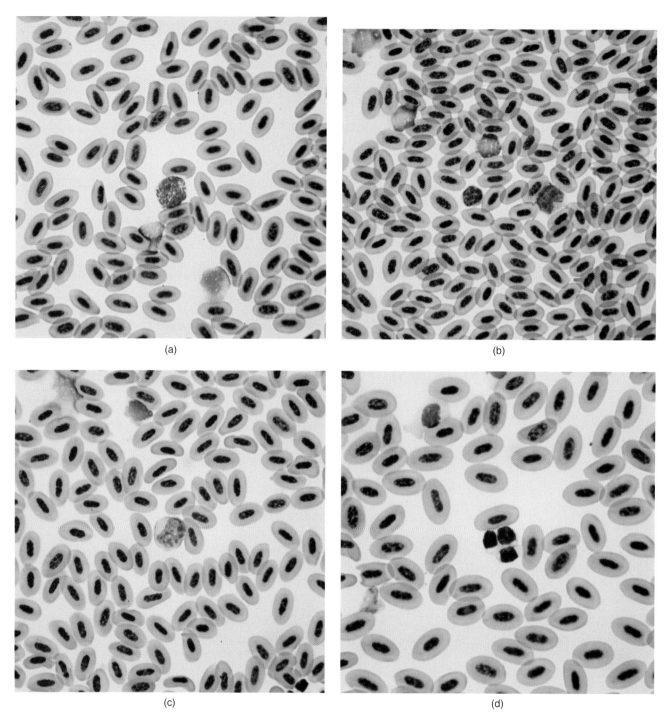

Fig. 58.3. (a–d) Blood films (Wright–Giemsa stain, 100×).

Interpretive Discussion

The body weight of this budgerigar is greater than one would expect for this species, especially one with reduction of the pectoral muscle mass.

The ventral–dorsal (VD) radiographs show loss of the normal appearance of the cardiohepatic silhouette as expected for a psittacine bird. The lateral view reveals a faint, curved opacity that projects over the ventral aspect of the thoracic air sacs. This could represent an enlarged proventriculus or other tissue in the space normally occupied only by the air sacs. On this same image, an ovoid soft-tissue opacity projects over the caudal air sacs at the level of the acetabulae. The dorsal and caudal margins

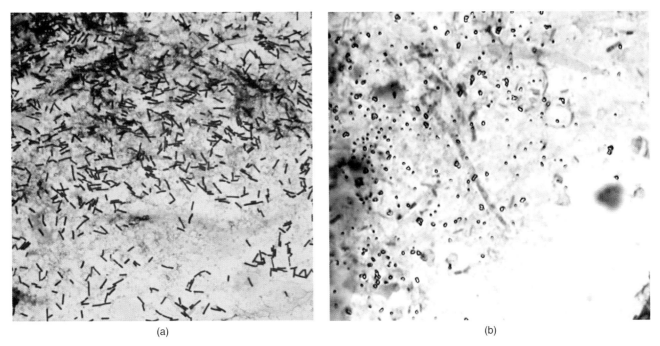

(a)   (b)

Fig. 58.4. (a and b) The fecal smear (Diff-Quik stain, 100×).

of this opacity are well delineated. This mass could be associated with the reproductive tract. On the VD image, the lateral margins of the soft tissues within the caudal aspect of the coelomic cavity extend a bit more laterally than expected. There is an increased opacity within the medullary cavities of both ulnas, both femurs, and both tibiotarsi. The increased opacity of the long bones suggests medullary hyperostosis, which could be a normal variant in an egg-laying hen. The radiographic findings could indicate an enlarged liver or proventriculus; however, the appearance of these structures could be influenced by the presence of a mass in the caudal aspect of the coelomic cavity. A gastrointestinal contrast study would be helpful in delineating the gastrointestinal tract in relationship to the mass.

Figure 58.3a shows a normal heterophil, and the erythrocytes exhibit a normal degree of polychromasia. Figure 58.3b shows a lymphocyte and a monocyte in the center of the image. Figure 58.3c shows a monocyte and Fig. 58.3d shows a clump of three thrombocytes. The blood film revealed no significant findings.

The fecal cytology revealed a uniform population of bacteria instead of a mixed population of morphological types (Fig. 58.4a). This is unusual and likely represents a dysbiosis of the bacterial population in the gastrointestinal tract. Figure 58.4b shows large rod-shaped to filamentous structures with mottling throughout. These organisms resemble the avian gastric yeast organism, the ascomycetous yeast of the genus *Macrorhabdus*.

Summary

An exploratory celiotomy was performed the next day to investigate the abnormal findings on the radiographic studies. The bird was given 0.05 mg butorphanol and 0.001 mg atropine intramuscularly as a preanesthetic treatment. Twenty minutes later, the bird was anesthetized using isoflurane via face mask. The bird was placed in right lateral recumbency, and a left flank approach was performed through a 1.5 cm incision through the skin and body wall. The proventriculus was enlarged and dilated. Although difficult to fully evaluate because of the enlarged proventriculus, other organs in the coelomic cavity appeared normal. An attempt to biopsy the proventriculus was not made because of the friable nature of the tissue. The body wall and subcutaneous tissues were closed independently using simple continuous 4-0 absorbable glycomer 631 suture, and the skin was closed using 4-0 nylon suture in a simple interrupted pattern.

The procedure lasted 20 minutes, and the bird made an uneventful recovery following delivery of naloxone HCl (10 mg/kg) via an intraosseous catheter placed in the bird's tibiotarsus.

Postoperatively, the bird was treated with meloxicam (0.5 mg/kg, orally, daily) for 3 days. She was also treated with trimethoprim-sulfa (20 mg/kg, orally, twice daily).

The dilated proventriculus likely resulted from gastric yeast disease (macrorhabdosis) as indicated by the presence of the organism in the feces. Neurogenic proventricular dilatation (proventricular dilatation syndrome) is another possible cause for the enlarged proventriculus; however, histopathologic examination of a gastric biopsy would have been needed to confirm that diagnosis. An obstruction distal to the proventriculus is an other possible cause for the enlarged proventriculus. The mass seen on the lateral radiograph was not identified during the surgery. The mass could have been an egg developing within the oviduct as there was radiographic evidence of hyperostosis of the long bones.

The client elected to euthanize the bird instead of pursuing additional diagnostic testing, such as contrast radiography, or trial treatment for macrorhabdosis. No necropsy was performed.

59

A 35-Year-Old Parrot with Weight Loss and Dyspnea

Signalment

A 35-year-old yellow-naped Amazon parrot (*Amazona auropalliata*) was presented with a complaint of weight loss and dyspnea.

History

The yellow-naped Amazon parrot of unknown gender was a wild-caught bird that was given as a gift from its previous owners to the client who had owned the bird for 18 years. The bird was fed a commercial pelleted diet along with fruits and vegetarian food. The bird was the only pet in the household and lived in a large commercial birdcage with corn cob bedding. The bird was currently being treated by another veterinarian with oral enrofloxacin for a sinus infection.

Physical Examination Findings

The 585 g bird was presented as a critical care patient because it was weak and exhibited a marked inspiratory and expiratory stridor with wheezing and pronounced expiratory push. The respiratory rate was 42 breaths/minute. The bird exhibited swelling in the sinus below each eye. The bird's right eye revealed phthisis bulbi from previous sinusitis. This, however, appeared benign. The bird was immediately placed inside a metabolism cage to provide warmth and supplemental oxygen. The examination was limited because of the bird's inability to withstand prolonged periods outside of supportive oxygen.

Once stable, a blood sample was obtained via jugular venipuncture for a blood profile. A tracheal wash sample was also obtained by quickly passing a sterile tube into the trachea to the level of the syrinx using 0.5 mL of sterile saline. The aspirated fluid was submitted for culture and cytologic examination (Tables 59.1 and 59.2 and Figs. 59.1 and 59.2).

Interpretive Discussion

Figure 59.1 reveals images of three heterophils and a thrombocyte on the blood film. The cytoplasm of the central heterophils shows a slight increase in cytoplasmic basophilia, suggestive of low-grade toxicity.

The increased packed cell volume (PCV) in the hemogram likely represents hemoconcentration because of dehydration, although polycythemia could be another possible explanation because of chronic oxygen depletion associated with chronic respiratory disease. The leukogram reveals a marked leukocytosis with a heterophilia and relative lymphopenia. This along with the presence of toxic heterophils indicates a severe inflammatory leukogram.

The plasma biochemical profile indicates an increased aspartate aminotransferase (AST) and marked increase in creatine kinase. This indicates skeletal muscle injury; however, one cannot rule out the possibility of coexisting hepatocellular disease. In general, plasma AST activity greater than 500 IU/L is suggestive of hepatocellular disease. Further testing with a plasma bile acid concentration or liver biopsy would help in the interpretation. The bird has a normal plasma total protein concentration. This is unexpected as both dehydration and inflammation would increase the plasma protein concentration. The albumin appears low; however, a protein electrophoresis would provide a better assessment of the plasma proteins. The bird also has an increase in the plasma bicarbonate concentration that reflects the metabolic component of the acid–base balance and suggests either a metabolic alkalosis or compensation for a respiratory acidosis.

The cytological specimen obtained from the tracheal wash as represented by Fig. 59.2 reveals a moderate number of nondegenerate heterophils, indicating a heterophilic tracheobronchitis. No etiological agent was identified.

249

Table 59.1. Hematology results.

		Reference[a]	Reference[b]
PCV (%)	62	45–55	37–50
Leukocytes			
WBC (10^3/µL)	31.3	6–11	6–11
Heterophils (10^3/µL)	26.6	—	—
Heterophils (%)	85	30–75	55–80
Lymphocytes (10^3/µL)	3.8	—	—
Lymphocytes (%)	12	20–65	20–45
Monocytes (10^3/µL)	0.9	—	—
Monocytes (%)	3	0–3	0–3
Eosinophils (10^3/µL)	0	—	—
Eosinophils (%)	0	0–1	0–1
Basophils (10^3/µL)	0	—	—
Basophils (%)	0	0–5	0–1
Thrombocytes			
Estimated number	Adequate	1–5/1,000× field	
Morphology	Normal, clumped		
Plasma protein (refractometry) (g/dL)	5.4	3–5	

[a]Campbell and Ellis (2007).
[b]Johnston-Delaney and Harrison (1996).

Summary

The bird was supported during the next 2 days with syringe feedings and oxygen supplementation. Nebulization treatments with enrofloxacin were also provided. The goal was to perform other diagnostic tests once the bird became more stable; however, after 2 days, the bird's respiratory efforts worsened. An air sac cannula using a 4.5 mm endotracheal tube inserted into the left caudal abdominal air sac was sutured in place with the bird under isoflurane anesthesia. The parrot began to breathe easier for about 1 hour post-tube placement; however, a serosanguineous fluid began to form within the air sac cannula. Within 30 minutes, the fluid completely occluded the tube. The bird died approximately 2 hours after air sac cannula placement because the bird was unable to ventilate effectively through its upper airway.

Table 59.2. Plasma biochemical results.

		Reference[a]	Reference[b]
Glucose (mg/dL)	240	190–345	220–350
BUN (mg/dL)	3	3.1–5.3	—
Uric acid (mg/dL)	5.6	2.3–10.0	2–10
Total protein (biuret) (g/dL)	3.9	3.0–5.0	3–5
Albumin (g/dL)	1.5	1.9–3.5	1.6–3.2
Globulin (g/dL)	2.4	—	—
Aspartate aminotransferase (IU/L)	676	130–350	100–350
Creatine kinase (IU/L)	7,102	55–345	45–265
Calcium (mg/dL)	8.8	8.5–14.0	8–13
Phosphorus (mg/dL)	4.3	3.1–5.5	3.1–5.5
Sodium (mEq/L)	151	125–155	136–152
Potassium (mEq/L)	3.3	3.0–4.5	3.0–5.0
Chloride (mEq/L)	111	—	—
Bicarbonate (mEq/L)	34.1	13–26	—
Anion gap (calculated)	9	—	—
Cholesterol (mg/dL)	318	180–305	—
Calculated osmolality	303	—	—

[a]Johnston-Delaney and Harrison (1996).
[b]Carpenter (2005).

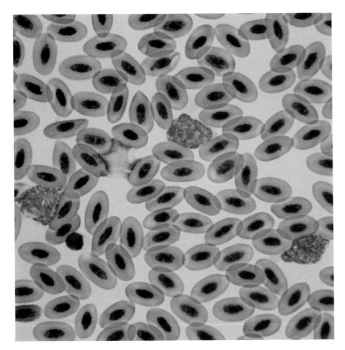

Fig. 59.1. A blood film (Wright–Giemsa stain, 100×).

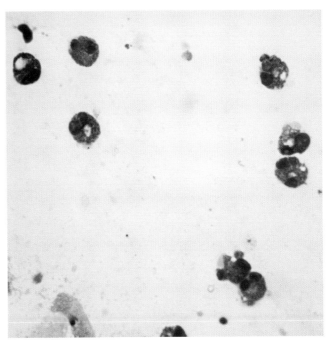

Fig. 59.2. A direct smear from the tracheal wash sample (Wright–Giemsa stain, 100×).

A necropsy revealed a parrot with minimally adequate fat stores and minimal autolysis. A granular to fibrinous, slightly firm 0.4 cm × 0.25 cm × 0.25 cm brown/gray mass was found at the tracheal–syringeal interface, occupying approximately 50–60% of the lumen. All other organs, including the air sacs, lungs, heart and central nervous system, were within normal limits grossly.

Histologic examination of the trachea revealed an ulcerated and pedunculated, round mass composed of a thick layer of degenerate polymorphonuclear and mononuclear cells, ghost cells, and karyorrhectic debris within a bright, eosinophilic granular to fibrillar substance flanked to each side by stratified squamous epithelium extending from the wall of the trachea to occupy approximately 50% of the tracheal lumen in two of the three sections. Within this region, most prominent in the periphery, there were large numbers of dimorphic parallel-walled hyphal structures that have frequent septae and regular branching (*Aspergillus*). Underlying the serocellular crusts of the mass, there is a short stalk composed of marked pyogranulomatous inflammation within a highly vascular fibrous stroma that extends transmurally between highly mineralized tracheal rings.

Abundant polymorphonuclear cells, macrophages, and amphophilic to basophilic mucinous debris were present within the tracheal lumen of the one section that did not contain a pedunculated mass. Other findings included a mild multifocal portal hepatitis and a moderate, chronic esophagitis with severe mucosal gland ectasia. The diagnosis based on histopathologic examination was a chronic multifocal pyogranulomatous and ulcerative tracheitis with intralesional fungal hyphae, presumed to be *Aspergillus*.

The tracheal wash sample cytology indicated a heterophilic inflammatory response that is usually interpreted as an acute inflammation. No mixed cell inflammation, macrophagic inflammation, or fungal elements were found that would support a diagnosis of fungal tracheitis in this case. In this case, the sample obtained from the tracheal wash was either not representative of the actual lesion or a secondary fungal infection developed after the sample was obtained. Occasionally, as with biopsy samples, the specimen may not reveal the actual pathology because of where the sample was actually obtained. In this case, the tube used to obtain the wash sample may not have reached the tracheal syrinx border.

A 29-Year-Old Parrot with Halitosis and Reduced Vocalization

60

Signalment

A 29-year-old orange-winged Amazon parrot (*Amazona amazonica*) was presented with a complaint of halitosis and reduced vocalization (Fig. 60.1).

History

The orange-winged Amazon parrot of unknown gender was presented with a 5-month history of halitosis, sinus congestion, and reduced vocalization. The bird was fed primarily a seed diet along with fruits and vegetarian food. It was the only bird in the household and lived in a large commercial birdcage. The bird was currently being treated by another veterinarian with an antibiotic (enrofloxacin), an antifungal agent (itra-

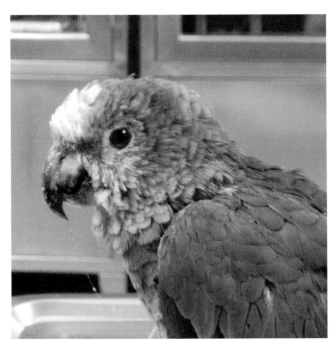

Fig. 60.1. The orange-winged Amazon parrot on presentation.

conazole), and intramuscular injections of vitamin A (0.25 mL of vitamin A 50,000 IU/mL given every 7 days) for an ulcerated mass with associated white plaques found on the roof of the bird's mouth. According to the owner, the symptoms improved for a period, before returning a short time later. The bird began to vocalize more following the treatments.

Physical Examination Findings

The bird weighed 400 g and appeared to be in relatively good condition and exhibited normal behavior. A mass was discovered in the roof of its mouth. The soft tissue mass covered the hard palate and extended to the back of his mouth, completely obliterating the choanal slit. This caused the bird to breathe entirely through an open mouth. The mass was encrusted with a white caseous exudate (Fig. 60.2a). The mass bled profusely when manipulated, and the tissue appeared to be proliferative (Fig. 60.2b).

Blood was collected via jugular venipuncture for a blood profile. A sample for cytodiagnosis was obtained by scraping the lesion after the majority of the covering exudate had been removed (Tables 60.1 and 60.2 and Figs. 60.3a and 60.3b).

Interpretive Discussion

The leukogram reveals a leukocytosis with a heterophilia, lymphopenia, and monocytosis. This is indicative of a significant inflammatory response. The plasma biochemistries reveal a slight decrease in potassium that is likely associated with decreased dietary intake of potassium and a slight increase in cholesterol, which is likely associated with increased fat intake from the predominate seed diet. The slight increase in creatine kinase is likely associated with skeletal muscle involvement following a long transport or struggle

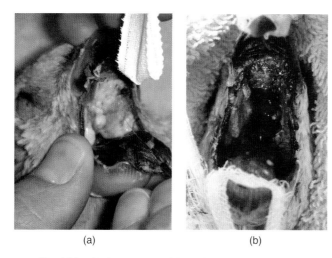

(a)   (b)

Fig. 60.2. (a) Appearance of the lesion in the roof of the mouth of the 29-year-old orange-winged Amazon parrot before swabbing mouth and (b) after removing the exudative coating.

during blood collection. The plasma chemistries are not significant findings.

Figure 60.3a reveals numerous erythrocytes, epithelial cells, and chains of bacterial cocci. Figure 60.3b reveals numerous erythrocytes, three large epithelial cells, nondegenerate heterophils, and lymphocytes. The epithelial cells in both figures exhibit squamous differentiation based on their polygonal shapes and baby blue cytoplasm indicating keratinization. The epithelial cells demonstrate anisokaryosis, pleomorphic nuclei,

Table 60.1. Hematology results.

		Reference[a]	Reference[b]
PCV (%)	53	45–55	37–50
Leukocytes			
WBC (10³/μL)	22	6–11	6–11
Heterophils (10³/μL)	16.7	—	—
Heterophils (%)	76	30–75	55–80
Lymphocytes (10³/μL)	0.2	—	—
Lymphocytes (%)	1	20–65	20–45
Monocytes (10³/μL)	5.0	—	—
Monocytes (%)	23	0–3	0–3
Eosinophils (10³/μL)	0	—	—
Eosinophils (%)	0	0–1	0–1
Basophils (10³/μL)	0	—	—
Basophils (%)	0	0–5	0–1
Thrombocytes			
Estimated number	Adequate	1–5/1,000× field	
Morphology	Normal, clumped		
Plasma protein (refractometry) (g/dL)	6.0	3–5	

[a]Campbell and Ellis (2007).
[b]Johnston-Delaney and Harrison (1996).

Table 60.2. Plasma biochemical results.

		Reference[a]	Reference[b]
Glucose (mg/dL)	295	190–345	220–350
BUN (mg/dL)	2	3.1–5.3	—
Uric acid (mg/dL)	1.6	2.3–10.0	2–10
Total protein (biuret) (g/dL)	4.8	3.0–5.0	3–5
Albumin (g/dL)	2.3	1.9–3.5	1.6–3.2
Globulin (g/dL)	2.5	—	—
Aspartate aminotransferase (IU/L)	218	130–350	100–350
Creatine kinase (IU/L)	416	55–345	45–265
Calcium (mg/dL)	10.1	8.5–14.0	8–13
Phosphorus (mg/dL)	3.4	3.1–5.5	3.1–5.5
Sodium (mEq/L)	151	125–155	136–152
Potassium (mEq/L)	2.3	3.0–4.5	3.0–5.0
Chloride (mEq/L)	112	—	—
Bicarbonate (mEq/L)	16.6	13–26	—
Anion gap (calculated)	25	—	—
Cholesterol (mg/dL)	334	180–305	—
Calculated osmolality	302	—	—

[a]Johnston-Delaney and Harrison (1996).
[b]Carpenter (2005).

nuclear chromatin clumping, high nucleus to cytoplasm ratio, and multinucleation. Some cells have a dark blue cytoplasm, suggestive of inappropriate keratinization (dyskeratosis). These findings are suggestive of a squamous cell carcinoma. The numerous erythrocytes and mixed cell inflammation are associated with the ulcerative nature of the lesion and the exudative nature of the surface of the lesion.

A vitamin A deficiency resulting in squamous metaplasia of the salivary glandular tissue that encircles the choanal slit as well as the lingual and sublingual salivary glands is common in Amazon parrots, especially those on primarily a seed diet. This disorder predisposes birds to secondary infections with bacterial and fungal organisms. Therefore, the use of vitamin A supplementation and antimicrobial agents was indicated. Cytologically, squamous metaplasia would reveal clusters or sheets of normal-appearing, cornified squamous epithelial cells.

Summary

Histologic examination of the affected oral mucosa obtained by punch biopsy revealed a proliferative mass of well-differentiated squamous epithelial cells that formed clusters and cords. The cells were large, polygonal with fairly distinct cell borders, and an abundant amount of darkly eosinophilic cytoplasm. The round to oval nuclei were moderately pleomorphic, had finely stippled chromatin, and contained a single prominent nucleolus. Mitoses were low, averaging one to two per ten 400× fields. There were multifocal areas

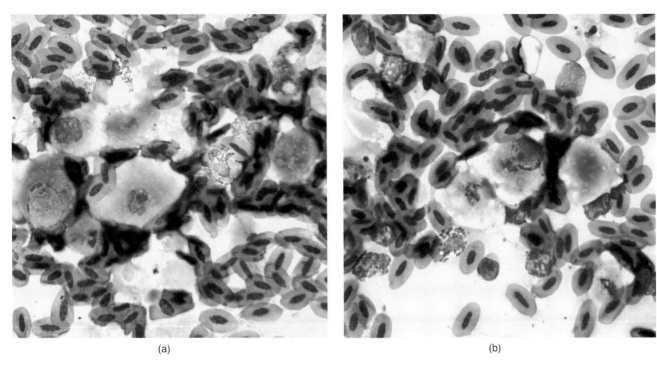

Fig. 60.3. (a and b) The imprint of the scraping from the mass (Wright–Giemsa stain, 100×).

of dysplasia and loss of orderly progression from basal cells to keratinized squamous epithelial cells.

There was mild anisokaryosis and anisocytosis, as well as mild dyskeratosis. Histologic examination of the exudative material covering the oral mass revealed a serocellular crust composed of abundant macrophages, heterophils, and sloughed squamous epithelial cells. Admixed throughout the section, there were numerous bacterial colonies.

Radiation therapy was considered to be the best treatment for the squamous cell carcinoma. The bird was anesthetized using intramuscular atropine (8 μg), butorphanol (0.4 mg), and midazolam (0.08 mg) as pre-anesthetic agents followed 30 minutes later with anesthetic induction with isoflurane. Computer tomography (CT scan) images were used as a staging tool for delivery of radiation therapy for the squamous cell carcinoma lesion in the bird's mouth. The 1 mm thick transverse images revealed that the rostral aspect of the mass was located at the base of the rhinotheca and extended 1.5 cm caudally in the right oral cavity. Owing to the location of the mass, curative radiation therapy was considered risky and likely to result in sloughing of the rhinotheca.

Cryosurgery was used as an alternative to radiation therapy. With the bird in dorsal recumbency, the mass was frozen using a conical shaped probe. Only one freeze-thaw cycle was performed owing to the significant swelling of the mass following the initial treatment.

Following anesthetic recovery, the bird was released to its owner and treated at home with trimethoprim-sulfa (30 mg/kg, orally, twice daily) for the secondary bacterial infection and meloxicam (0.3 mg/kg, orally, daily) for analgesia and partial treatment for squamous cell carcinoma.

The parrot was treated two more times using cryosurgery at 3-week intervals. Initially, the mass exhibited significant reduction in size and the once hidden choanal slit began to reappear; however, the mass persisted and use of radiation therapy was readdressed.

Palliative radiation was performed with 6 Gy times four fractions (treatments) delivered 1 week apart for a total of 24 Gy. The bird was anesthetized during each treatment as described for the CT scan procedure. The lesion nearly completely disappeared following the third radiation treatment.

Both cryosurgical and radiation therapies resulted in necrosis of the lesion. This led to significant epistaxis 1 or 2 days following treatment.

The parrot lived a relatively normal life for 1 year following initial presentation, but died unexpectedly during the night at home. The necropsy revealed moderate arteriosclerosis of the heart and associated great vessels, moderate pulmonary mineralization and edema, and mild lymphocytic centrilobular hepatitis. A 1 cm diameter mottled brown plaque was found in the choanal fissure. Histologic examination of this lesion revealed squamous cell carcinoma.

A 6-Month-Old Cockatiel with Labored Breathing

61

Signalment

A 6-month-old male cockatiel (*Nymphicus hollandicus*) was presented with labored breathing (Fig. 61.1).

History

The cockatiel was being housed at a local pet store with two other cockatiels of the same age. One of the cage mates was suspected to have psittacosis 2 weeks earlier; however, according to the pet store manager, the test results were negative. The cockatiels were fed a commercial pellet diet designed for their species and millet seeds. This bird was weaned from his hand-feeding formula 2 months prior to presentation. He

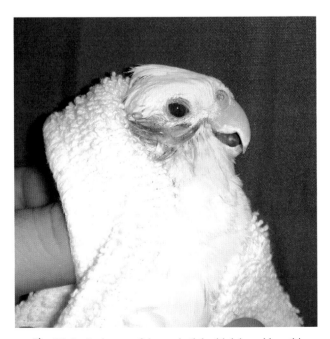

Fig. 61.1. An image of the cockatiel with labored breathing.

became acutely ill during the night. According to the pet store manager, the bird appeared normal until he suddenly appeared to be "gasping for air." The cockatiel had not been eating for 24 hours.

Physical Examination Findings

On arrival, the bird exhibited open-mouth breathing, kept his eyes partially closed, and although weak, managed to perch. A quick assessment of the bird's body condition was made by palpation of the keel bone, revealing a body condition score of 3/9. The cockatiel was weighed (68 g) and immediately placed inside a heated oxygen-enriched cage and remained there until it became more stable and while the history was being obtained. Approximately 2 hours later, the bird was active, showed less dyspnea, and began eating food that was provided by the pet store personnel. Droppings in the cage revealed a green color to the urinary component. The bird developed severe dyspnea immediately on removal from the oxygen-enriched environment. It was noted that the nares were occluded and the choanal slit in the mouth was reddened. The nares were opened by performing a sinus wash using physiological saline through a syringe held tightly against each nostril. A mucoid fluid was collected on a cotton-tipped applicator from the choanal slit for cytodiagnosis (Figs. 61.2a and 61.2b). An attempt to obtain a blood sample via jugular venipuncture for hematology and plasma AST, CK, and total protein values was abandoned because of the deteriorating condition of the bird during the brief handling to remove the material occluding the nares. A fecal sample was submitted for polymerase chain reaction (PCR) testing for *Chlamydophila psittaci*.

Interpretive Discussion

Figures 61.2a and 61.2b reveal nondegenerate heterophils with a thick background that is likely associated

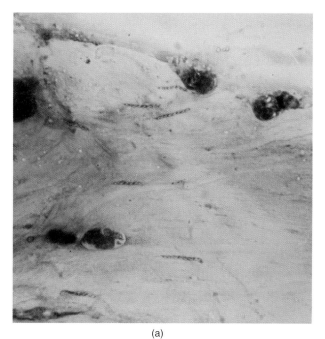
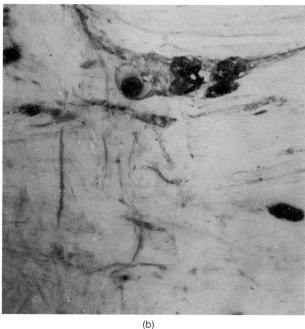

(a)   (b)

Fig. 61.2. (a and b) The image of the sinus wash sample (Wright–Giemsa stain, 100×).

with the mucoid nature of the material collected from the choanae. The sample was likely diluted with saline because it was collected from a wash procedure; therefore, the number of inflammatory cells may be higher than what appears on the sample. These images also reveal large spiral-shaped bacteria. The cytodiagnosis is a mild heterophilic inflammation likely associated with a spirochete infection.

Summary

The clinical signs of upper respiratory disease in this cockatiel exhibiting significant weight loss can be associated with a number of common infectious diseases of psittacine birds, which include chlamydophilosis (psittacosis) and aspergillosis. A blood profile would have been helpful in determining the extent of any systemic manifestation of the disease. A hemogram revealing a severe inflammatory leukogram with a marked leukocytosis, heterophilia, and monocytosis would be supportive of those two diseases. Severe inflammatory leukograms with a total leukocyte count approaching 50,000/µL or greater in psittacine birds are often associated with infections caused by *Mycobacterium, Aspergillus,* and *Chlamydophila.*

A plasma biochemical profile supportive of a diagnosis of chlamydophilosis would include a hyperproteinemia, hyperglobulinemia, an increased plasma aspartate aminotransferase (AST) with a normal creatine kinase (CK), and increased bile acids. The presence of biliverdinuria (green urine) as identified in this patient

would further support hepatobiliary disease and a presumptive diagnosis for chlamydophilosis.

The bird was treated for a spirochete infection with the choice of antibiotic treatment also targeting a presumptive diagnosis for an infection with *C. psittaci.* Spirochetes are difficult to culture; therefore, an antibiotic sensitivity is difficult to obtain. These organisms, however, respond to a variety of antibiotics. Therefore, an antibiotic protocol using doxycycline (2.1 mg PO BID) for 45 days and enrofloxacin (0.4 mg PO BID) for 14 days was initiated. The bird was maintained in an oxygen-enriched environment and also received 10 mg enrofloxacin per milliliter saline as a nebulization treatment for 30 minutes twice daily.

Spirochete infections in cockatiels are generally associated with young birds and result in an upper respiratory infection associated with excess mucus production in the choanae and trachea (Schmidt et al., 2003). Affected birds are often presented with oral lesions or an acute, mild rhinitis or sinusitis.

The fecal PCR testing for *C. psittaci* in this patient was positive, indicating that the bird was actively shedding the organism. It is possible that this bird had a mixed infection with *C. psittaci* and the spirochetes (presumed to be a *Helicobacter* sp.). Cockatiels can be asymptomatic carriers for both agents and break with the diseases associated with them during times of stress.

The bird died 24 hours after presentation. The body was returned to the pet store for a necropsy to be performed by the store's pathologist.

A 13-Year-Old Parrot with a Prolapsed Cloaca

62

Signalment

A 13-year-old intact female Ecteclus parrot (*Eclectus roratus*) was presented with a prolapsed cloaca.

History

This parrot was presented to the referring emergency clinic for acute hemorrhage from the vent and a cloacal prolapse. On presentation to the emergency clinic, the owner reported that the bird lost approximately one-eighth to one-fourth cup of blood. Two weeks prior, the bird suffered from a similar event, which resolved. On physical examination at the emergency clinic, the bird was stable although pale and had a prolapsed cloaca. The cloaca was irrigated with saline and lubricated with a water-based, water-soluble lubricant; however, manual reduction of the prolapse was unsuccessful. The bird was provided with supportive care, which included 4 days of hospitalization for subcutaneous fluid administration, enrofloxacin (25 mg/kg PO q 24 hours), cloacal flushing and lubrication, butorphanol as needed, and one injection of iron dextran (10 mg/kg). After the 4 days of hospitalization and supportive care, no additional hemorrhage was noted and the prolapsed cloaca reduced on its own. The bird was referred for further diagnostics and treatment.

On the initial presentation (day 1), the owner reported that the parrot normally laid three to four eggs per year; however, no clutch was produced this year during the time of her regular laying season. It was also noted that the bird's normal diet consisted of a variety of seed mixes, commercial pellets, fruits, vegetables, and occasionally eggs, meat, and potatoes. The bird was housed in a large cage in the living room of the house. Corn cob bedding was used as cage substrate. The client had owned the bird since it was a fledgling.

During the initial physical examination, the bird weighed 590 g and was in good body condition. The only

abnormality at that time was a distended coelom. The cloaca was not prolapsed. Initial diagnostics included a complete blood count (CBC) (day 1) and diagnostic profile (day 1) from a blood sample obtained via jugular venipuncture at the time the bird was under isoflurane anesthesia for obtaining whole body radiographs (Tables 62.1 and 62.2 and Figs. 62.1–62.3).

Interpretive Discussion 1

Figure 62.1a shows a heterophil, increased polychromasia, and numerous elliptical cells with a high nucleus–cytoplasm ratio and blue cytoplasm. Figure 62.1b shows two lymphocytes, increased polychromasia, and the elliptical cells shown in Fig. 62.1a. The non-erythrocytic elliptical cells are immature thrombocytes that have taken on the elliptical shape of the mature cell likely as a result of accelerated maturation in response to

Table 62.1. Hematology results.

	Day 1	Day 7	Normal range for Eclectus parrot[a]
WBC ($10^3/\mu L$)	9.5	9.3	5.5–25
Heterophils ($10^3/\mu L$)	7.7	4.5	—
Heterophils (%)	81	48	35–75%
Lymphocytes ($10^3/\mu L$)	1.5	3.1	—
Lymphocytes (%)	16	33	20–65%
Monocytes ($10^3/\mu L$)	—	1.2	—
Monocytes (%)	—	13	1–11%
Eosinophils ($10^3/\mu L$)	0.2	0.2	—
Eosinophils (%)	2	2	0–1%
Basophils ($10^3/\mu L$)	0.1	0.4	—
Basophils (%)	1	4	0–3%
Plasma protein (g/dL)	6.6	6.0	—
PCV (%)	19	31	26—58
Thrombocytes	—	Adequate	—

[a]Carpenter (2005).

259

Table 62.2. Plasma biochemical results.

	Day 1	Day 7	Reference[a]	Reference[b]
Glucose (mg/dL)	277	256	190–345	220–350
BUN (mg/dL)	3	3	3.1–5.3	—
Uric acid (mg/dL)	3.8	1.7	2.3–10.0	2–10
Total protein (biuret) (g/dL)	4.0	4.0	3.0–5.0	3–5
Albumin (g/dL)	1.7	1.8	1.9–3.5	1.6–3.2
Globulin (g/dL)	2.3	2.2	—	—
A/G ratio	0.7	0.8	—	—
Aspartate aminotransferase (IU/L)	178	305	130–350	100–350
Creatine kinase (IU/L)	513	2461	55–345	45–265
Calcium (mg/dL)	11.1	9.2	8.5–14.0	8–13
Phosphorus (mg/dL)	5.3	4.6	3.1–5.5	3.1–5.5
Sodium (mEq/L)	150	148	125–155	136–152
Potassium (mEq/L)	3.4	2.8	3.0–4.5	3.0–5.0
Chloride (mEq/L)	118	114	—	—
Bicarbonate (mEq/L)	21.7	27.7	13–26	—
Anion gap (calculated)	14	10	—	—
Cholesterol (mg/dL)	668	632	180–305	—
Calculated osmolality	301	296	—	—

[a]Johnston-Delaney and Harrison (1996).
[b]Carpenter (2005).

a thrombocytopenia from consumption of mature thrombocytes because of the bleeding episodes.

The plasma biochemistry profile on day 1 reveals a hypercholesterolemia that suggests an increase in cholesterol synthesis or decreased excretion or catabolism of cholesterol by the liver.

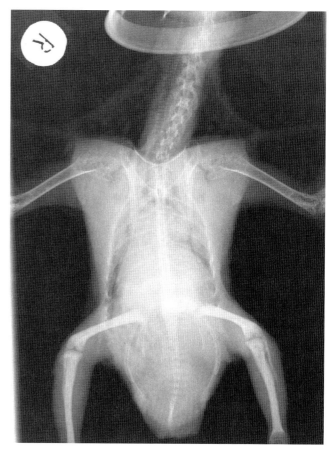

Fig. 62.2. The radiograph of ventral–dorsal position.

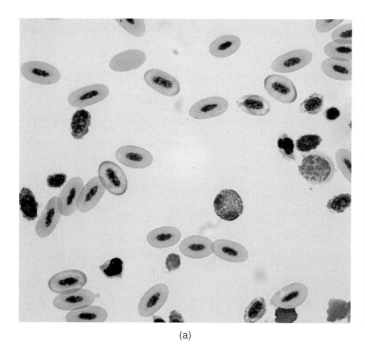
(a)

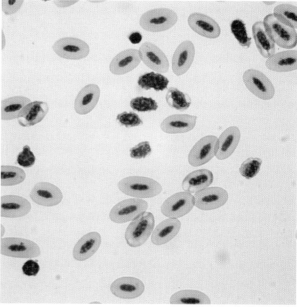
(b)

Fig. 62.1. (a and b) The blood film (Wright–Giemsa stain, 100×).

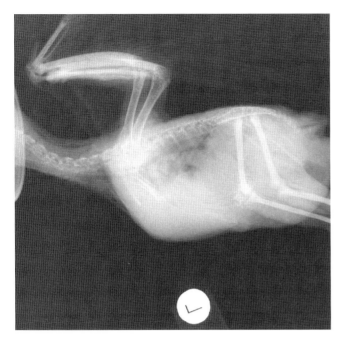

Fig. 62.3. The radiograph of lateral position.

The radiographs show increased soft-tissue opacity within the mid to caudal aspects of the coelomic cavity. This opacity likely caused the mass effect with resultant caudal and ventral bowing of the caudoventral body wall, prominence of the vent, and slight craniad displacement of the ventriculus. On the ventral–dorsal radiograph, there is loss of the normal hour-glass appearance of the cardiohepatic silhouette. On that same view, there is a lobular soft-tissue opacity that overlies the hepatic silhouette. There is also increased opacity of the femurs and tibiotarsi (also in the radius and ulna of each wing, but not shown), which indicated medullary hyperostosis seen with female birds undergoing active folliculogenesis.

Summary 1

An exploratory surgery was performed 2 days following presentation. When the coelomic cavity was entered, a mass was detected in the region of the infundibulum of the oviduct. This structure was covered with a thin membrane containing yolk material. This was considered to be an ectopic egg and the cause of the soft-tissue opacity observed on the radiographs. A salpingohysterectomy was performed and the oviduct was submitted for histological evaluation and culture. Histologically, the tissue was normal oviduct and uterus, and there was no growth reported on the culture. The bird was discharged with instructions to continue the enrofloxacin treatments, and meloxicam (0.5 mg/kg PO BID for 5 days) was provided.

The bird returned 5 days postoperative because of another episode of hemorrhaging from the vent. The client reported that the bird had intermittent episodes of cloacal prolapse since her surgery. She also continued to bleed although not to the degree that she experienced previously. The bird's cloaca remained reduced for less than 12 hours following surgery, according to the client. Despite her condition, the bird continued to eat well but was not able to pass feces normally.

Physical Examination Findings on Day 7

Upon physical examination, the bird was bright, alert, and responsive. She appeared to be in good body condition and weighed 509 g. The sutures were still in place from surgery and the incision was healing. The cloaca was prolapsed and a small amount of blood dripped from the prolapse. Along the right ventral aspect of the mucosal surface of the cloaca, there was a mass, approximately 1.5 cm in diameter, with a necrotic center (Fig. 62.4). It was noted that the bird was able to pass normal droppings when the mass was prolapsed.

The bird was placed under general anesthesia using isoflurane by face mask in order to better evaluate the cloaca. The cloacal mass was irrigated with saline (Fig. 62.5). An impression of the mass was obtained for cytodiagnosis (Fig. 62.6).

Silver sulfadiazine was applied topically to the mass, and the cloaca was reduced. Two stay sutures using 4-0 nylon suture were placed adjacent to each lateral commissure of the vent. Blood was collected via jugular venipuncture to reevaluate the CBC (Table 62.1, day 7) and diagnostic profile (Table 62.2, day 7). The bird was hospitalized for treatment.

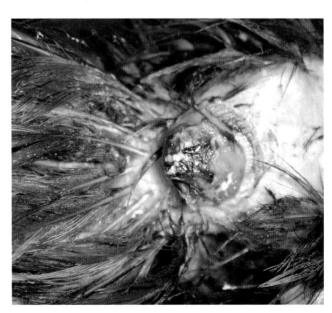

Fig. 62.4. The cloacal prolapse at presentation.

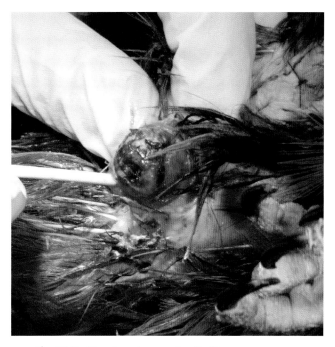

Fig. 62.5. The cloacal mass after flushing.

Three days after the second presentation, the bird was placed under general anesthesia to obtain a biopsy of the cloacal mass and samples were submitted for histological evaluation. An impression of the biopsy of the mass was made for cytological evaluation (Figs. 62.7 and 62.8).

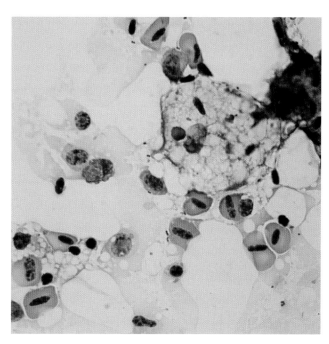

Fig. 62.7. The impression of the biopsy taken of the cloacal mass (Wright–Giemsa stain, 100×).

Interpretive Discussion 2

The cytologic examination of the surface of the cloacal mass (Fig. 62.6) shows an inflammatory response that consists primarily of nondegenerate heterophils with macrophages, erythrocytes, and a lymphocyte. This is indicative of an inflammatory response and no indication for neoplasia.

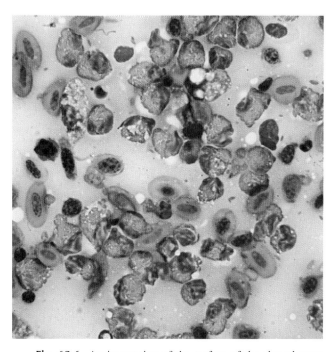

Fig. 62.6. An impression of the surface of the cloacal mass (Wright–Giemsa stain, 100×).

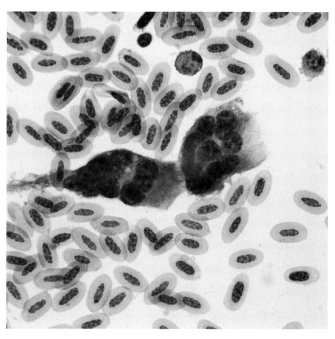

Fig. 62.8. The cloacal mass 3 days after the biopsy.

The cytology of the deeper aspects of the cloacal mass obtained from an imprint of the biopsy reveals large foamy macrophages (Fig. 62.7) and multinucleated giant cells (Fig. 62.8). These findings support a different type of inflammatory response (macrophagic) than what was observed on the surface of the lesion.

The hemogram shows improvement in the packed cell volume (PCV), indicating the bird is responding to her anemia. A slight monocytosis indicates a mild inflammatory response. On both day 1 and day 7 of the hemogram, the refractometric protein concentration is elevated; however, this is not supported by the normal plasma protein concentration found on the biochemical profile. The apparent decreased albumin and increased globulin concentrations shown on the biochemical profile would be best evaluated using protein electrophoresis. The plasma creatine kinase activity has increased on day 7, which is likely associated with the surgery, skeletal muscle trauma, or muscle exertion. The increased aspartate aminotransferase activity, although considered normal, is likely associated with the muscle involvement.

Summary 2

The bird was hospitalized for 7 days. Treatment included meloxicam (0.5 mg/kg PO BID), enrofloxacin (20 mg/kg PO q 24 hours), metronidazole (50 mg/kg PO BID), silver sulfadiazine applied topically to cloaca, and assisted defecation. Because the bird was unable to pass droppings on her own and she required assistance, this was performed by placing a lubricated cotton-tipped applicator into her cloaca and pressing the mass to one side, allowing the waste to pass through the vent. This was performed two to three times daily.

During the biopsy procedure, the mass was shown to be continuous with the cloacal mucosa; therefore, an aggressive debulking of the mass was not done. Histopathologic examination revealed tissue sections of infiltrated sheets of histiocytes with foamy to vacuolated cytoplasm. There were numerous multinucleate giant cells as well as multifocal areas of necrosis present throughout the sample. No organisms were identified.

The mass reduced in size over the course of 1 week and by the seventh day was approximately half the size that it was on presentation (Fig. 62.8). The bird also began defecating small amounts on its own.

The bird was discharged on the eighth day, and by the following day, the owner reported that the bird was defecating on her own without problems.

The cause of the abscess was unknown, although self-inflicted trauma during a previous cloacal prolapse episode was possible. The bird was likely experiencing reproductive problems with the ectopic egg during this laying season and, in straining to pass it, prolapsed her cloaca. The hemorrhagic episodes likely were associated with trauma to the cloaca when prolapse occurred. The abscess likely developed in association with the trauma.

A 17-Year-Old Cockatoo with Broken Blood Feathers

63

Signalment

A 17-year-old female Umbrella cockatoo (*Cacatua alba*) was presented with a recent history of broken blood feathers.

History

The cockatoo had broken four pin feathers associated with the primary flight feathers on both wings the night prior to presentation. The bleeding had stopped; however, several broken flight feathers on both wings resulted in dried blood, covering the feathers on the wings and body coverts.

The client reported that the bird had been picking her feathers for the past 2 years, and this behavior had gotten worse during the past year. She also reported that the bird was presented to a veterinarian who specializes in birds a year earlier for a mass just cranial to the cloaca on the ventral side of the bird. At that time, the mass was considered to be benign and of no concern, according to the veterinarian. The "mass" had increased dramatically in size since that time. The bird laid a normal clutch of two eggs 4 months prior to presentation.

The bird was housed in a commercial birdcage and fed a diet of commercial pellets and nuts. Other pets in the household included three dogs, a cat, and a Rosella parrot (*Platycercus* sp.).

Physical Examination Findings

The 1.1-kg cockatoo was extremely nervous and exhibited frightened behavior and signs of stress in the examination room. Although it did not vocalize, it tried to escape capture. The bird exhibited severe alopecia owing to feather picking, resulting in a large area of missing feathers on the enlarged abdominal area. A large herniated area just cranial to cloaca was observed. Palpation of this area indicated soft-tissue structures and no

hard mass. The droppings appeared normal, suggesting normal gastrointestinal and urinary function.

Blood was collected via jugular venipuncture for a blood profile while the bird was placed under isoflurane anesthesia via face mask for whole body radiograph evaluations. A fine-needle aspiration biopsy of an intracoelomic mass was obtained for cytodiagnosis. The sample appeared clear and greasy when placed on the microscope slides (Figs. 63.1–63.5 and Tables 63.1 and 63.2).

Interpretive Discussion

The initial whole body radiographs (Figs. 63.2a and 63.3a) reveal a large soft-tissue opaque mass in the caudal dorsal aspect of the coelomic cavity, causing cranial and ventral displacement of the coelomic

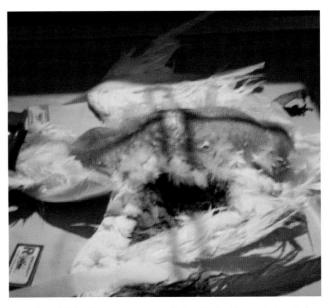

Fig. 63.1. The appearance of the Umbrella cockatoo being positioned for whole body radiographs.

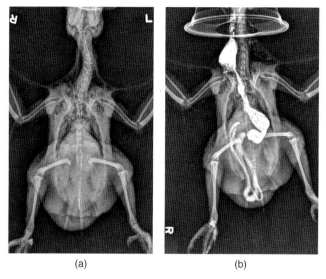

Fig. 63.2. The whole body ventral–dorsal radiographs of the Umbrella cockatoo: (a) the initial radiograph and (b) the 85-minute contrast radiograph.

structures. This likely represents a neoplastic mass arising from the reproductive tract. There appears to be a marked enlargement of the hepatic silhouette, extending beyond the margins of the coxofemoral joint on the ventrodorsal view. The enlarged hepatic silhouette can be

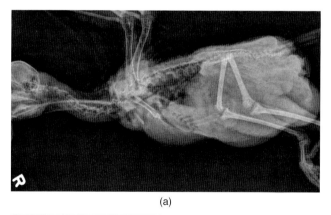

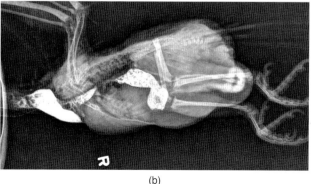

Fig. 63.3. The whole body lateral radiographs of the Umbrella cockatoo: (a) the initial radiograph and (b) the 85-minute contrast radiograph.

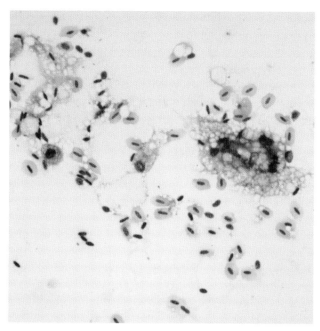

Fig. 63.4. A fine-needle aspiration biopsy of the intracoelomic mass (Wright–Giemsa stain, 50×).

associated with hepatomegaly, proventricular dilation, or an intracoelomic mass. There is a rounded soft-tissue opacity, extending beyond the caudal ventral aspect of the vent correlating with this patient's described history of having a hernia. The hernia is likely due to the space occupying mass in the caudal dorsal coelomic cavity. A rounded, oblong soft-tissue opacity ventral to the synsacrum can be seen on the lateral view. This likely represents either renomegaly or gonadomegaly. There is increased opacity within the long bones, representing medullary hyperostosis associated with follicular genesis.

A continued radiographic study (Figs. 63.2b and 63.3b) of the bird is compared with the initial study made the same day 85 minutes following the administration of 25 mL of a 92% liquid barium suspension diluted 1:2 with water via gavage. The proventriculus is normal in size. Owing to the limited progress of the barium's travel through the gastrointestinal tract after 85 minutes, the bird likely has decreased gastrointestinal motility. There is contrast within the small intestines, which is being ventrally displaced by the previously described soft-tissue mass in the caudodorsal coelomic cavity. There is a loop of small intestine (likely duodenum based on its shape) incorporated into the previously described hernia. The radiographic studies in this bird indicate herniation of small intestines owing to displacement by a soft-tissue mass in the coelomic cavity. Differentials include neoplasia arising from the urinary system or reproductive tract.

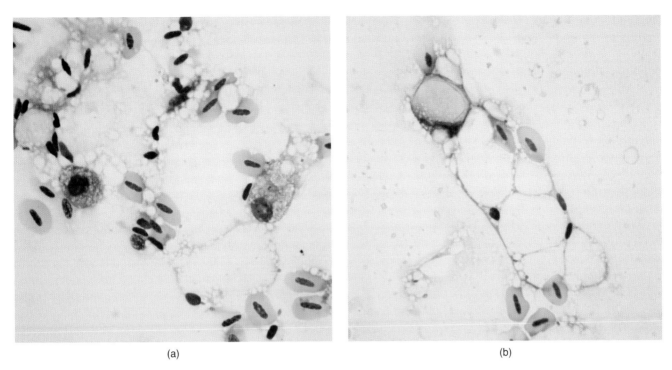

(a)

(b)

Fig. 63.5. (a and b) The fine-needle aspiration biopsy of the intracoelomic mass (Wright–Giemsa stain, 100×).

The blood profile reveals a nonregenerative anemia. This is likely associated with an anemia of chronic disorders. There is no evidence of inflammation. The glucose is elevated, which is likely associated with a stress response. The plasma creatine kinase activity is increased owing to muscle exertion during handling or possible recent trauma to the skeletal muscles (the bird fell from the examination table onto the floor landing on her keel when being examined). The marked increase in the plasma calcium concentration is likely associated

Table 63.1. Hematology findings.

		Reference[a]	Reference[b]
PCV (%)	29	42–54	38–48
Leukocytes			
WBC ($10^3/\mu$L)	6.3	5–10	5–11
Heterophils ($10^3/\mu$L)	4.8	—	—
Heterophils (%)	76	55–80	55–80
Lymphocytes ($10^3/\mu$L)	1.4	—	—
Lymphocytes (%)	23	20–45	20–45
Monocytes ($10^3/\mu$L)	0	—	—
Monocytes (%)	0	0–2	0–1
Eosinophils ($10^3/\mu$L)	0.1	—	—
Eosinophils (%)	1	0–1	0–2
Basophils ($10^3/\mu$L)	0	—	—
Basophils (%)	0	0–3	0–1
Thrombocytes			
Estimated number	Adequate	1–5/1,000× field	
Morphology	Normal, clumped		
Plasma protein (refractometry) (g/dL)	8.5	3–5	

[a]Campbell and Ellis (2007).
[b]Johnston-Delaney and Harrison (1996).

Table 63.2. Plasma biochemical results.

		Reference[a]	Reference[b]
Glucose (mg/dL)	453	185–355	200–300
BUN (mg/dL)	4	3.0–5.1	0–6
Uric acid (mg/dL)	6.2	3.5–10.5	0.2–8.5
Total protein (biuret) (g/dL)	3.7	3.0–5.0	1.5–4.0
Albumin (g/dL)	1.5	1.8–3.1	0.3–1.6
Globulin (g/dL)	2.4	—	0.8–2.5
Aspartate aminotransferase (IU/L)	370	145–355	50–400
Creatine kinase (IU/L)	1,798	95–305	140–1,000
Calcium (mg/dL)	25.6	8.0–13.0	8–11
Phosphorus (mg/dL)	6.2	2.5–5.5	3.5–8.0
Sodium (mEq/L)	142	130–155	135–155
Potassium (mEq/L)	2.5	2.5–4.5	2.5–5.5
Chloride (mEq/L)	114	—	97–120
Bicarbonate (mEq/L)	15	14–25	—
Anion gap (calculated)	15	—	—
Cholesterol (mg/dL)	406	145–355	100–500
Calculated osmolality	295	—	—

[a]Johnston-Delaney and Harrison (1996).
[b]Carpenter (2005) for cockatoos.

with current folliculogenesis activity as indicated by the hyperostosis of the long bones in the radiographic examinations.

Figures 63.4 and 63.5 show a moderately cellular sample that contains a slight number of erythrocytes. There are large cells that occur in aggregates or singly. These cells have an abundant vacuolated cytoplasm and an eccentrically located oval nucleus. The background contains numerous round, clear spaces. These spaces and the clear vacuoles in the cells likely represent fat that does not stain with the Wright–Giemsa stain. The large cells are adipocytes and the cytology is representative of a lipoma or liposarcoma. The clear, oily appearance of the specimen on the slide indicates that the sample is from fatty tissue.

The blood profile and radiographic evidence of hyperostosis indicating active folliculogenesis and the history of the bird laying a clutch of normal eggs 5 months prior to presentation suggest a normal female reproductive tract. The intracoelomic mass seen on radiographs likely does not involve the gastrointestinal tract, urinary tract, or reproductive tract. The cytologic examination of the sample aspirated from the coelomic mass indicates fatty tissue and supports a diagnosis of an intracoelomic lipoma, infiltrative lipoma, or liposarcoma.

Summary

The cockatoo was admitted for an intracoelomic exploratory surgery to investigate the nature of the intracoelomic mass and repair the hernia.

The cockatoo was given 1.1 mg butorphanol, 0.33 mg midazolam, and 0.033 mg atropine intramuscularly as a preanesthetic treatment. Twenty minutes later, the bird was induced and maintained with isoflurane anesthesia following endotracheal intubation using a 4.0 mm tube. During the 1 hour and 24 minutes surgery, the bird was given 48.8 mL lactated Ringer's solution intravenously via a catheter placed in the basilic vein. The bird also received 5 mL of an esterified amylopectin-containing starch (hetastarch) intravenously during the procedure. Prior to recovery, the bird received 0.5 mg meloxicam intramuscularly and 1.0 mg butorphanol intramuscularly.

The bird was placed in dorsal recumbency, and radiocautery was used to create a skin incision extending 2 cm from the caudal point of the keel to just cranial to the herniated area cranial to the cloaca. A body wall incision was made using radiocautery to expose the contents of the coelomic cavity. A large amount of yellow fat was found, occupying the majority of the coelomic cavity and encircling the ventriculus (Fig. 63.6). A large amount of fat along with the duodenum was found herniated through the body wall. As much as possible, the fat was carefully removed using blunt dissection. A cloacopexy using 5-0 polytrimethylene carbonate suture was used to close the body wall in a simple continuous pattern in the area of the hernia. The rest of the body wall was closed using the same material and pattern. The skin was closed using a 4-0 glycomer 631 suture in a

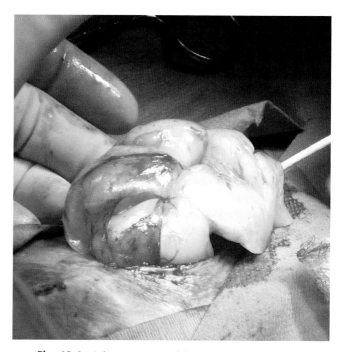

Fig. 63.6. A large amount of intracoelomic fat found during surgery.

simple interrupted pattern. A portion of the fatty tissue removed from the bird's coelomic cavity was submitted for histopathologic evaluation.

The bird made an uneventful recovery from anesthesia and surgery and was placed in the critical care facility for close observation for 12 hours. She was treated with meloxicam (0.5 mg PO daily) postoperatively. Although she made no attempt to remove her sutures, she was sent home with an Elizabethan collar designed for birds in the event she pull at the sutures. At home the bird was less active than normal; however, she was eating and playing with her toys according to the client. The bird died 29 hours following her surgery possibly as a result of reperfusion problems or lipid embolism. No necropsy was performed.

Histopathologic evaluation revealed sheets of normal adipocytes with moderate infiltration by lymphocytes, macrophages, multinucleated giant cells, and fewer heterophils. Frequently at the junction of the adipose lobules, there were areas of moderate degeneration and necrosis. A histologic diagnosis of necrotic lipoma was made.

64

An Adult Duck with a Mass on the Rhinotheca

Signalment

An adult male white-winged wood duck (*Cairina scutulata*) was presented with a mass on the rhinotheca (Fig. 64.1).

History

The duck was a member of a large group of waterfowl housed in a public zoological park. This species of duck is highly endangered, and this drake was part of the breeding program. The duck was housed in a large wetlands exhibit with other waterfowl and was fed a commercial duck food supplemented with small fish and insects. The keeper was unsure of the duck's age.

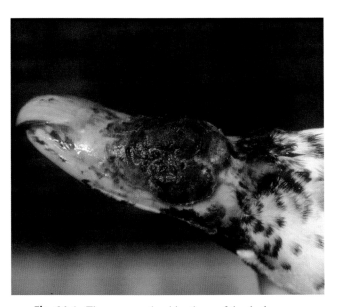

Fig. 64.1. The mass on the rhinotheca of the duck.

The mass was noted a month prior to presentation and had grown considerably in size since then, according to the keeper.

Physical Examination Findings

The duck appeared to be in good condition. The only abnormality found was a large, firm, painless mass on the rhinotheca, growing throughout the entire thickness of that structure. A fine-needle aspiration biopsy was performed for cytodiagnosis. A blood sample was collected from the medial metatarsal vein for a blood profile (Tables 64.1 and 64.2 and Figs. 64.2 and 64.3).

Interpretive Discussion

The hemogram appears to be within normal limits based on references for other species of Anseriformes. Figure 64.2a shows a heterophil (granulocyte on top of the image) and an eosinophil (granulocyte on bottom of the image). Figure 64.2b shows a lymphocyte, a thrombocyte (cell in the center of the image), and a monocyte. Figure 64.2c shows a heterophil and a lymphocyte. The images show a normal degree of polychromasia for a nonanemic bird, and the heterophil morphology is normal.

The plasma biochemistry profile appears to be within normal limits for Anseriformes, according to the limited references.

Figures 64.3a and 64.3b show few to moderate numbers of erythrocytes and a population of large pleomorphic nucleated cells that appear to be related (having a common source). These cells are round to spindle-shaped and exhibit anisocytosis and anisokaryosis. Many of the cells have one or more nuclei. The nuclear

Table 64.1. Hematology results.

		Reference[a]	Reference[b]	Reference[c]
PCV (%)	44	42–54	32–48	40–51
Leukocytes				
WBC ($10^3/\mu$L)	13.8	20–22	6–34	14–38
Heterophils ($10^3/\mu$L)	4.6	—	3–7	2–14
Heterophils (%)	33	39	—	—
Lymphocytes ($10^3/\mu$L)	8.1	—	9–17	7–19
Lymphocytes (%)	59	46	—	—
Monocytes ($10^3/\mu$L)	0.6	—	0–3	0–2
Monocytes (%)	4	6	—	—
Eosinophils ($10^3/\mu$L)	0.4	—	0–1	0–1
Eosinophils (%)	3	2	—	—
Basophils ($10^3/\mu$L)	0.1	—	0–1	0–1
Basophils (%)	1	7	—	—
Thrombocytes				
Estimated number	Adequate	—	—	—
Morphology	Normal, clumped			
Plasma protein (refractometry) (g/dL)				

[a]Campbell (2000) for the Canada goose.
[b]Mulley (1979).
[c]Mulley (1980).

chromatin is coarsely clumped at times, and the cells often reveal prominent large nucleoli. The cytoplasm is often abundant, gray, and contains vacuoles. One small cell in Fig. 64.3b contains numerous golden brown cytoplasmic granules. Figure 64.3c shows two of these cells containing numerous golden brown cytoplasmic granules, indicative of melanin pigment. The cytology indicates a poorly differentiated melanoma.

Table 64.2. Plasma biochemical results.

		Reference[a]	Reference[b]
Glucose (mg/dL)	224	207–241	122–230
BUN (mg/dL)	0.5	—	0.7–2.3
Uric acid (mg/dL)	1.5	6.0–10.5	—
Total protein (biuret) (g/dL)	4.7	4.1–5.5	3.5–5.2
Albumin (g/dL)	2.4	1.9–2.3	2.4–3.6
Globulin (g/dL)	2.3	2.2–3.4	—
Aspartate aminotransferase (IU/L)	54	58–92	0–116
Creatine kinase (IU/L)	211	—	—
Calcium (mg/dL)	10.3	9.5–10.9	—
Phosphorus (mg/dL)	3.9	1.9–3.7	0.8–5.6
Sodium (mEq/L)	148	138–146	—
Potassium (mEq/L)	3.0	2.8–4.0	—
Chloride (mEq/L)	108	101–109	—
Bicarbonate (mEq/L)	18.4	—	—

[a]Johnston-Delaney and Harrison (1996) for the Canada goose.
[b]Mulley (1979).

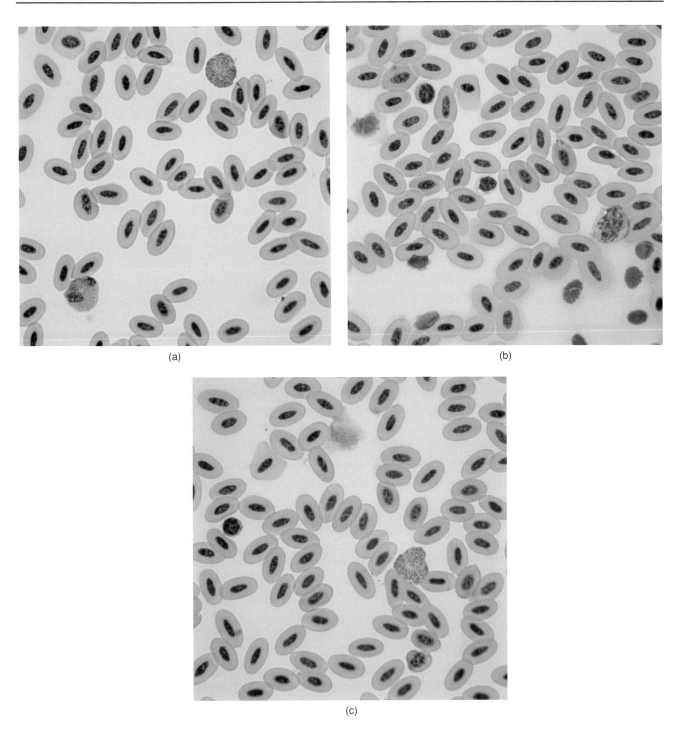

(a)

(b)

(c)

Fig. 64.2. (a–c) Blood films (Wright–Giemsa stain, 100×).

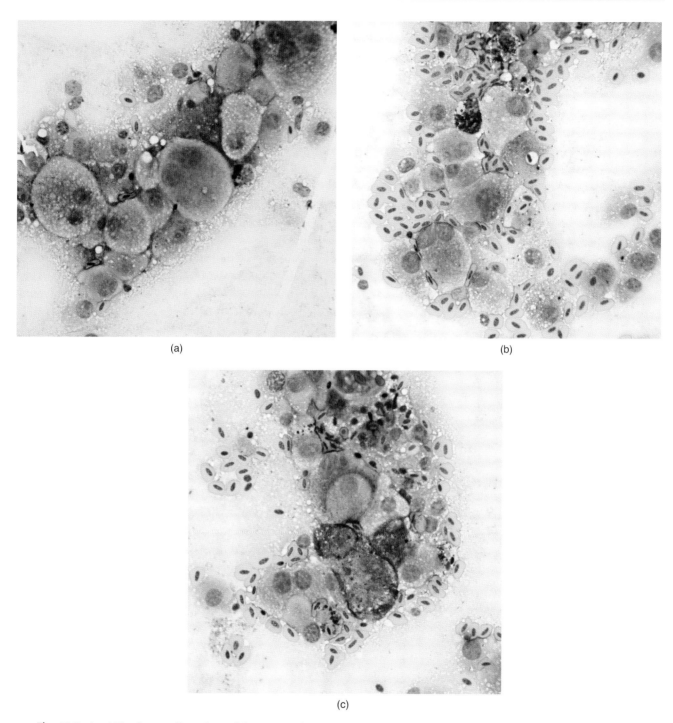

(a)

(b)

(c)

Fig. 64.3. (a–c) The fine-needle aspirate of the mass (Wright–Giemsa stain, 50×).

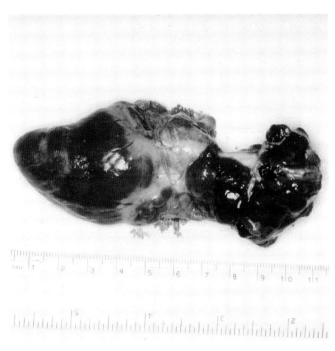

Fig. 64.4. A large mass (melanoma) involving the great vessels at the base of the duck's heart.

Summary

The bird was given a poor prognosis for response to therapy and survival based on a highly invasive and poorly differentiated melanoma on the rhinotheca. The duck died 1 month later. The necropsy and histopathologic examination confirmed the diagnosis of a malignant melanoma. The melanoma had metastasized to the base of the heart, incorporating the great blood vessels in that area, which likely contributed to the duck's death (Fig. 64.4).

A 3-Month-Old Flamingo with a Mass on the Rhinotheca

65

Signalment

A 3-month-old Chilean flamingo (*Phoenicopterus chilensis*) was presented with a mass on the rhinotheca (Fig. 65.1).

History

The flamingo chick was one of a number of chicks hatched in a colony of Chilean flamingos kept at a zoological park. The keepers noticed this flamingo chick as well as a few others had developed "sores" on their beaks or feet. The flamingos were housed in an outdoor exhibit that contained a large shallow pond, sandy beach area, and numerous trees and shrubs. They were fed a commercially made pelleted diet for flamingos supplemented with krill.

Physical Examination Findings

The flamingo chick appeared to be in good condition. The only abnormality found was a large, firm, painless, multilobulated mass on the dorsal aspect of the rhinotheca. The surface of the mass was covered with scabs. A fine-needle aspiration biopsy was performed for cytodiagnosis (Figs. 65.2 and 65.3).

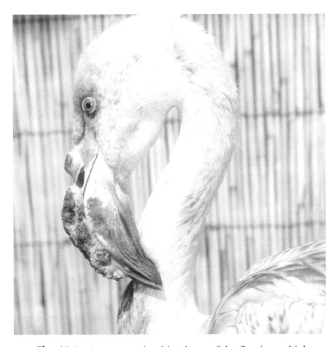

Fig. 65.1. A mass on the rhinotheca of the flamingo chick.

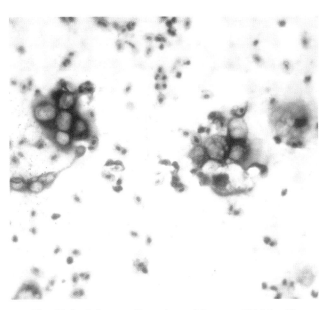

Fig. 65.2. A fine-needle aspirate of the mass (Wright–Giemsa stain, 50×).

277

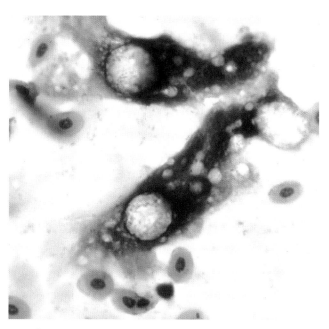

Fig. 65.3. A fine-needle aspirate of the mass (Wright–Giemsa stain, 100×).

Interpretive Discussion

Figure 65.2 shows a highly cellular sample that contains many erythrocytes. There are also squamous epithelial cells that contain large, round inclusions. Closer inspection of these epithelial cells (Fig. 65.3) reveals the larger round inclusions contain smaller inclusions. These findings are consistent with pox inclusions where the large cytoplasmic inclusion bodies within the squamous epithelial cells are known as Bollinger bodies that contain the smaller Borrel bodies.

Summary

The flamingo chick survived the pox infection. The lesions eventually healed resulting in minimal scarring. There was no specific treatment provided.

Section 7
Herptile Cytology Case Studies

A 2-Year-Old Lizard with Difficulty Breathing

66

Signalment

A 2-year-old male intact Green iguana (*Iguana iguana*) presented as an emergency for difficulty breathing.

History

This iguana presented to the emergency service for having respiratory difficulty. The emergency staff found and removed a large amount of mucous and hair lodged in the back of his mouth that partially occluded his glottis after which his respiratory status stabilized and he began to breathe normally.

The iguana had free roam in a single room in a house. The temperature was maintained at 76–77°F and he had access to two heating pads and heat lamp. His diet was primarily romaine lettuce but was also fed dog food on occasion when the lettuce is unavailable.

Physical Exam Findings

The 730-g male Green iguana presented the following morning for a more complete evaluation. The lizard was in fair to poor body condition and was undersized for his age. He was gray in color and exhibited generalized weakness. A mucoid nasal discharge was noted. Examination of his mouth and oral cavity revealed areas that were inflamed and ulcerated. There was still a small amount of hair, string, and mucus coating the affected regions. A swab of mucus from the oral cavity was prepared for cytological evaluation (Figs. 66.1–66.4).

Other Diagnostic Information

A blood sample was obtained from the caudal vein using the lateral approach on the tail. The sample was submitted for a blood profile (Tables 66.1 and 66.2).

Interpretive Discussion

The cytologic sample from the oral swab is highly cellular and consists primarily of heterophils indicating a severe heterophilic inflammation. Figure 66.2 reveals a heterophil exhibiting bacterial phagocytosis and supports the cytodiagnosis of septic heterophilic inflammation and stomatitis.

Additional information provided by the blood film is helpful in further assessment of the condition of the lizard. Figure 66.3 reveals a monocyte (large cell on the left), two lymphocytes, and two intact heterophils. A broken heterophil is located in the lower right. The heterophils have a slightly basophilic cytoplasm. It should be noted that the relative high number of leukocytes found in this image supports a leukocytosis. Figure 66.4 reveals two heterophils and a basophil. The heterophils have a basophilic and vacuolated cytoplasm indicating

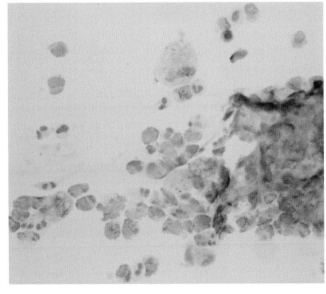

Fig. 66.1. A smear from swab of the oral cavity (Wright–Giemsa stain, 50×).

281

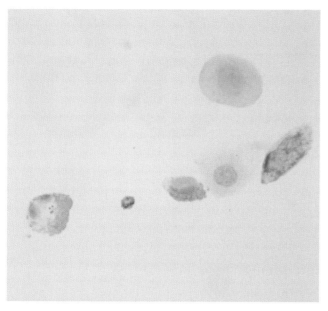

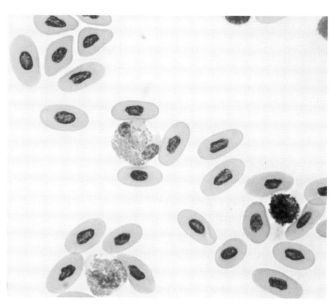

Fig. 66.2. A smear from swab of the oral cavity (Wright–Giemsa stain, 100×).

Fig. 66.4. A blood film (Wright–Giemsa stain, 100×).

toxicity. Heterophil toxicity is often found in association with inflammatory responses resulting in accelerated heterophilic production.

The hematology results revealed a moderate leukocytosis, heterophilia, lymphocytosis, and monocytosis (Table 66.1). This inflammatory leukogram likely coincides with the stomatitis.

The plasma biochemical profile indicates a mild hyperphosphatemia and hypocalcemia that are likely associated with the poor husbandry conditions that include a lack of unfiltered UVB lighting and calcium-poor diet resulting in nutritional hyperparathyroidism. The increased protein from the dog food is of a concern as it often leads to renal failure in the herbivorous iguanas whose kidneys do not tolerate excessive animal protein, which could be another explanation of the hyperphosphatemia. The elevated AST activity may be from muscle exertion or injury or hepatocellular disease. Because the plasma CK activity was high, it is likely that the AST activity is elevated owing to muscle exertion or injury as a result from restraint; however, one cannot rule-out coexisting hepatocellular disease. The hyperkalemia suggests a disturbance in potassium metabolism as might be found with increased intake, decreased urinary excretion, or acidosis (metabolic or respiratory).

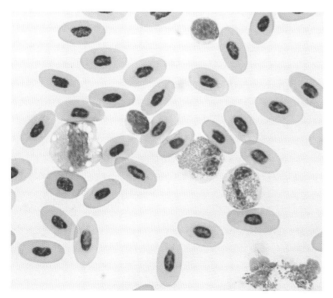

Fig. 66.3. A blood film (Wright–Giemsa stain, 100×).

Table 66.1. Hematology results.

	Results	Normal range for Green iguanas[a]
WBC ($10^3/\mu$L)	22.8	3–10
Heterophils ($10^3/\mu$L)	10.0	0.35–5.2
Lymphocytes ($10^3/\mu$L)	9.1	0.5–5.5
Monocytes ($10^3/\mu$L)	2.7	0–0.1
Eosinophils ($10^3/\mu$L)	0.5	0–0.3
Basophils ($10^3/\mu$L)	0.5	0–0.5
Plasma protein (g/dL)	6.1	—
PCV (%)	30	25–38
Adequate thrombocytes	Exist	—

[a]Diethelm (2005).

Table 66.2. Plasma biochemistry results.

	Results	Normal range for Green iguanas[a]
Glucose (g/dL)	246	169–288
BUN (mg/dL)	2	0–4
Uric acid (mg/dL)	5.5	<6.7
Phosphorus (mg/dL)	7.3	4–6
Calcium (mg/dL)	8.1	8.8–14.0
Total protein (g/dL)	6.3	5.0–7.8
Albumin (g/dL)	3.0	2.1–2.8
Globulin (g/dL)	3.3	2.5–4.3
A/G ratio	0.9	—
Cholesterol (mg/dL)	293	104–333
CK (IU/L)	2038	1947 ± 2058
AST (IU/L)	113	5–52
Sodium (mg/dL)	160	158–183
Potassium (mg/dL)	5.1	1.3–3.0
Chloride (mg/dL)	115	117–122
Bicarbonate (mg/dL)	21.8	—
Anion gap	28	—
Calculated osmolality	322	—

[a]Diethelm (2005).

Repeating the blood profile after a few days of treatment would be helpful in the assessment of this iguana. Likewise, radiographic evaluation would be helpful in the assessment of the patient in regards to bone density, such as osteopenia or pathologic fractures associated with a metabolic calcium deficiency, and presence of renal disease.

Summary

This iguana was sent home with systemic antibiotics (ceftazidime, 20 mg/kg IM every 72 hours) and topical treatment (silver sulfadiazine) for the stomatitis. A diet change that included the addition of dark green leafy vegetables, a calcium supplement, and removal of the dog food in the diet was recommended. Environmental changes, such as periodic exposure to unfiltered sunlight and better temperature control, were also recommended. According to the owner, the iguana was doing well 2 weeks later, but declined returning for a repeat blood profile.

A 3-Year-Old Lizard with Vomiting and Weight Loss

67

Signalment

A 3-year-old female leopard gecko (*Eublepharis macularius*) was presented for vomiting and weight loss.

History

The gecko was presented with 1-week duration of lethargy, anorexia, weight loss, and regurgitation. It was also noted that she had not defecated for 2 days. She laid one egg 1 month ago and, according to the owner, had not been the same since then. Because the gecko was acquired only 6 months prior to presentation, any previous history was unknown. She was acquired along with a male leopard gecko that appeared healthy.

Physical Examination Findings

The lizard was quiet, yet responsive, and weighed 50 g. She was very thin as denoted by the severe decrease in tail mass (Fig. 67.1). Her coelomic cavity palpated normal. There was a small white mass noticed on the cornea of her eyes. A scraping of this mass was collected (Fig. 67.2) for cytodiagnosis.

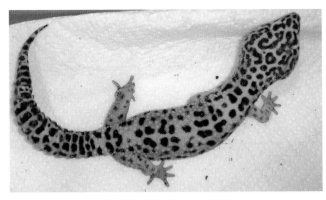

Fig. 67.1. The leopard gecko with decreased tail mass.

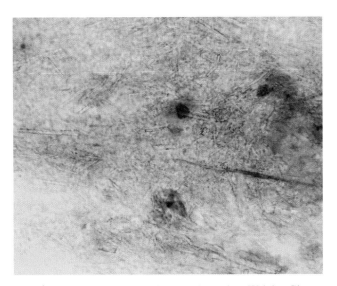

Fig. 67.2. The cytology of a corneal scraping (Wright–Giemsa stain, 100×).

Other Diagnostic Information

A gastric wash was performed and evaluated cytologically. There appeared to be an overpopulation of bacteria as well as inflammatory cells. On the basis of the cytology of the gastric wash, gastritis was suspected. There was no evidence of *Cryptosporidia*; however, that disease, a common cause of weight loss in this species, could not be ruled out based on this finding alone.

Interpretive Discussion

Figure 67.2 reveals a poorly cellular sample that contains numerous long, golden colored, needle-shaped crystals. These crystals were refractile under polarized light (not shown) and indicative of uric acid crystals. This unusual finding was suggestive of a possible systemic hyperuricemia as would be found with gout.

285

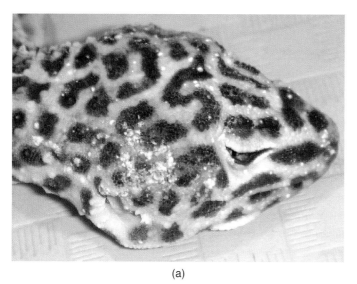

(a)

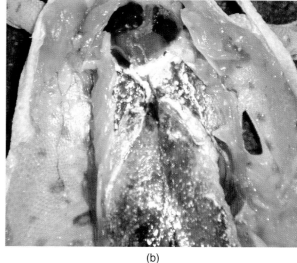

(b)

Fig. 67.3. The image of gross necropsy findings.

Summary

Further diagnostics, such as plasma uric acid and phosphorus concentrations, and whole body radiographs may have aided in the diagnosis of gout likely associated with renal failure. Because of the lizard's poor condition and prognosis for survival, the client elected to support the animal at home instead of euthanasia. The gecko was sent home with tube feeding instructions and an antibi-otic for the gastritis. The gecko died 2 weeks later and the body was returned for necropsy. The body was speckled with pinpoint white to cream-colored masses on the skin (Fig. 67.3a). During the necropsy, the visceral organs were also covered with gout tophi (Fig. 67.3b), confirming visceral gout. Causes of visceral gout in this lizard include renal failure associated with a diet too high in protein, chronic dehydration, or renal infection.

A 9-Year-Old Lizard with a Mass near the Vent

68

Signalment

A 9-year-old male leopard gecko (*Eublepharis macularius*) was presented for a mass near the vent.

History

The owner noticed the mass 2 days earlier. The gecko was anorexic for 2 weeks and had not defecated for several days. According to the owner, the gecko shed the week prior to presentation. A heat lamp was added the day prior to presentation, and the gecko had been basking ever since. The owners also added an additional water container for the lizard to soak in an effort to help the vent.

The gecko was housed in a 20-gallon glass terrarium with walnut substrate. Decorations included rocks and a bark hut. Water was available at all times and was changed every other day. The cage was cleaned as needed. The gecko's diet consisted of crickets and mealworms with a powdered vitamin and mineral supplement.

Physical Examination Findings

The slightly thin, 72-g leopard gecko had a large ulcerated mass surrounding, and possibly involving, the vent (Fig. 68.1). An aspirate of the mass was taken for cytologic examination (Fig. 68.2).

Interpretive Discussion

Figure 68.2 reveals a highly cellular sample. The majority of the cells are inflammatory cells with a predominance of macrophages. Intracellular bacteria can be found within phagosomes of the macrophages, indicating septic inflammation. The macrophagic inflammation is likely associated with a chronic bacterial infection (abscess) and response to necrotic tissue.

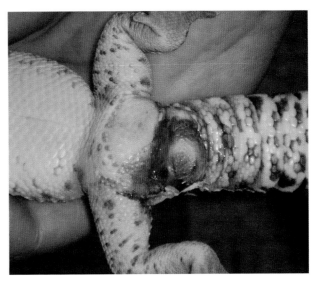

Fig. 68.1. An image of the lesion adjacent to the vent.

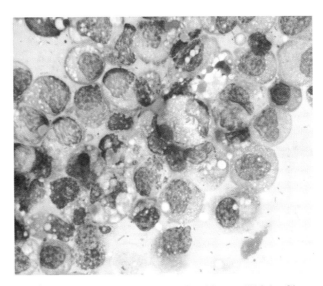

Fig. 68.2. A fine-needle aspiration biopsy (Wright–Giemsa stain, 100×).

287

Summary

The abscess was surgically removed, and the area was flushed and irrigated with saline. The wound was left open and the gecko was placed on a broad-spectrum systemic antibiotic. The client had declined antimicrobial culture owing to the expense. The owner was also instructed to remove the walnut substrate and replace it with paper. Twice daily flushing of the wound was also part of the lizard's care. The wound had completely healed when examined 6 weeks later.

A 19-Year-Old Lizard with a Large Mass on Its Leg

69

Signalment

A 19-year-old intact male green iguana (*Iguana iguana*) was presented with a large mass on its left hind leg.

History

The iguana was initially seen by another veterinary clinic 18 months prior to presentation. There, the mass was diagnosed and treated as an abscess using surgical debridement, saline irrigation, and antibiotics. When the mass recurred, a biopsy was obtained and submitted for histopathologic examination. The iguana was referred for treatment options.

Despite the large mass on his leg, the iguana exhibited normal behavior and activity at home. He had been eating, drinking, and defecating normally. Review of his care revealed excellent husbandry conditions at home. The diet consisted of a variety of fresh vegetables such as yellow squash, zucchini, apples, sweet potatoes, carrots, spinach, spring mix lettuce, peas, green beans, bok choy, and cabbage and dandelions. The lizard was housed in a habitat that provided the recommended captive environmental requirements for the species.

Physical Examination Findings

The iguana was bright, alert, and responsive. He weighed 4.2 kg and was in good body condition. There were no other abnormalities noted aside from the mass on his left rear limb. The mass was located on the ventral aspect of his thigh and appeared to be associated with one or more of the femoral pores. It was approximately 4 cm in diameter and ulcerated (Fig. 69.1).

Other Diagnostic Information

Blood was drawn from the caudal vein using the lateral approach and submitted for a complete blood count (CBC) and diagnostic profile (Tables 69.1 and 69.2).

Radiographs that were taken 3 months prior to presentation accompanied the patient (Fig. 69.2).

The mass was surgically removed on the day of admission into the veterinary hospital. Anesthetic induction was provided by intravenous propofol (10 mg/kg) and maintained using isoflurane following intubation (2.0 mm tube).

During surgery, a sterile marking pen was used to determine the appropriate surgical margins that would allow tissue apposition once the mass was excised. A number 15 blade was used to incise the skin around the mass in order to make a fusiform-shaped defect. The mass was superficial to the underlying musculature and was well encapsulated. Metzenbaum scissors and electrocautery were used to excise the mass within the capsule. The one large vessel entering the proximal aspect of the mass was occluded with hemoclips and

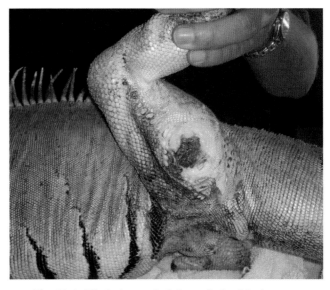

Fig. 69.1. The lesion on the left rear limb of the iguana.

289

Table 69.1. Hematology results.

	Results	Normal range for green iguanas[a]
WBC ($10^3/\mu L$)	4.2	3–10
Heterophils ($10^3/\mu L$)	3.2	0.35–5.2
Lymphocytes ($10^3/\mu L$)	0.7	0.5–5.5
Monocytes ($10^3/\mu L$)	0.1	0–0.1
Eosinophils ($10^3/\mu L$)	0	0–0.3
Basophils ($10^3/\mu L$)	0.2	0–0.5
Plasma protein (g/dL)	4.4	—
PCV (%)	26	25–38

[a]Diethelm (2005).

transected. Careful dissection around the mass was completed, and the mass was successfully removed within its capsule (Fig. 69.3a). Prior to placing the mass in 10% neutral buffered formalin for histology, an imprint was made from the freshly cut surface for cytodiagnosis (Fig. 69.3b). The skin was closed in two layers. The subcutaneous layer was closed using 3-0 glycomer 631 suture, with a few simple interrupted tension sutures followed by a more superficial simple continuous pattern. The skin layer was closed using 3-0 nylon suture using a horizontal mattress pattern. The lizard recovered from anesthesia and surgery without complications (Figs. 69.3 and 69.4).

Interpretive Discussion

Results of the CBC were within normal limits. The plasma biochemistry profile revealed hypoglycemia, hypoproteinemia, hypoalbuminemia, hypophos-

Table 69.2. Plasma biochemistry results.

	Results	Normal range for green iguanas[a]
Glucose (g/dL)	126	169–288
BUN (mg/dL)	2	2 ± 2
Phosphorus (mg/dL)	2.6	4–6
Calcium (mg/dL)	11.8	8.8–14.0
Total protein (g/dL)	4.2	5.0–7.8
Albumin (g/dL)	1.7	2.1–2.8
Globulin (g/dL)	2.5	2.5–4.3
A/G ratio	0.7	—
Cholesterol (mg/dL)	67	104–333
CK (IU/L)	220	1,947 ± 2,058
AST (IU/L)	16	5–52
Sodium (mg/dL)	131	158–183
Potassium (mg/dL)	4.1	1.3–3.0
Chloride (mg/dL)	94	117–122
Bicarbonate (mg/dL)	29.1	—
Anion gap	12	—
Calculated osmolality	259	—

[a]Diethelm (2005).

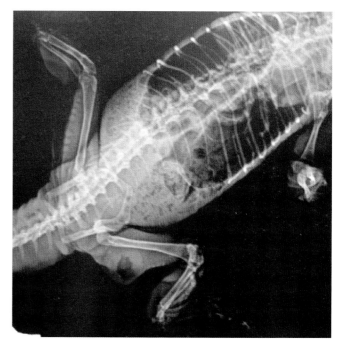

Fig. 69.2. The whole body dorsoventral radiograph of the iguana.

phatemia, hypocholesterolemia, hyponatremia, and hypochloremia. Explanation for these findings in an otherwise healthy-appearing iguana was challenging. It is possible that the published reference values used do not represent reference values that might have been obtained from the laboratory used to analyze the plasma sample. These findings may have resulted from anorexia owing to long transport associated with recent travel to the veterinary hospital. Lymphatic fluid dilution of the plasma sample would be another possible explanation; however, this was not supported by the CBC findings performed on the same blood sample. The hyperkalemia does not fit with the last two explanations, and if true, suggests either excessive intake of potassium, acidosis, or decreased urinary excretion of potassium. Repeat examination of these plasma analytes would be in order.

The radiograph in Fig. 69.2 revealed a soft-tissue mass on the left rear limb with no evidence of bone involvement.

The cytology of the imprint of the mass (Figs. 69.4a–69.4c) revealed a highly cellular sample. There are numerous erythrocytes and nondegenerate heterophils. The background contains a marked number of bacteria. These findings are likely associated with the ulcerative nature of the lesion. The images also reveal a highly pleomorphic population of squamous epithelial cells. The cells vary from clearly squamous cell in appearance to spindle shaped. The cells exhibit anisokaryosis, nuclear pleomorphism, multinucleation, and nuclear chromatin clumping. Some of the cells have

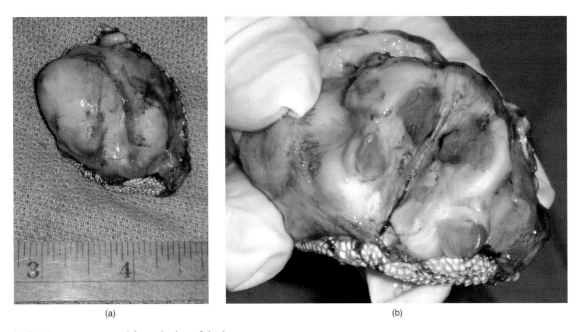

Fig. 69.3. The mass removed from the leg of the iguana.

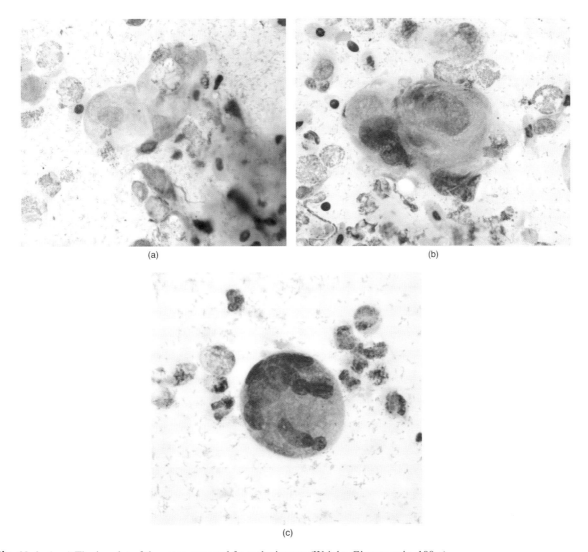

Fig. 69.4. (a–c) The imprint of the mass removed from the iguana (Wright–Giemsa stain, 100×).

cytoplasmic basophilia and perinuclear vacuolation. These cells are considered to be neoplastic squamous epithelial cells.

Summary

The iguana was discharged on the day of surgery and placed on meloxicam (0.5 mg/kg given orally daily for 30 days) for pain and chemotherapy in the event that the entire mass was not removed. The histology confirmed a squamous cell carcinoma. Neoplastic cells extended to within 2 mm of the inked margin of the mass, indicating that the mass was completely removed. The cytology in this case was somewhat academic because the histology of the biopsy obtained by the referring veterinarian had already identified the neoplasia. An aspirate of the mass may have revealed the same cytological findings under a different circumstance.

An 11-Year-Old Lizard with an Oral Mass

70

Signalment

An 11-year-old intact male Green iguana (*Iguana iguana*) was presented with an oral mass.

History

The iguana was recently surrendered to the local reptile humane society. On presentation to the shelter, the iguana had gingivitis and an oral mass.

Physical Examination Findings

The 3.7-kg Green iguana was in good body condition. A malocclusion of the maxilla and mandible that was especially prominent at the rostral end of the mouth was noted. A 1 cm ulcerated mass was found on the right rostral maxilla. There also appeared to be inflamed tissue extending to the left maxilla as well as the rostral mandible (Fig. 70.1).

A fine-needle aspirate of the mass was taken for cytologic examination (Figs. 70.2–70.4).

Other Diagnostic Information

Because of financial concerns, a recommendation for a blood profile was declined by the client; however, radiographs of the skull were obtained to evaluate the invasiveness of the mass (Fig. 70.5).

Interpretive Discussion

The cytologic results revealed a marked number of erythrocytes and one thrombocyte present in Fig. 70.2,

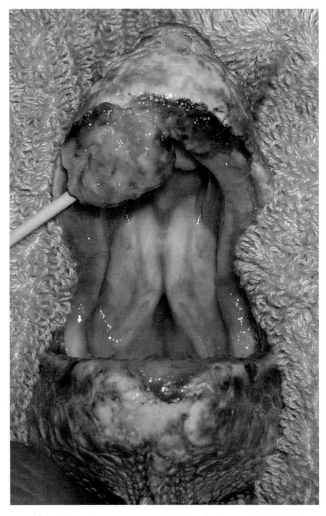

Fig. 70.1. The appearance of lesions in the mouth of the Green iguana.

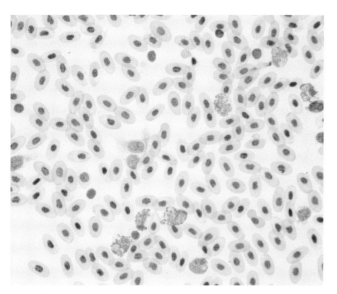

Fig. 70.2. A fine-needle aspiration biopsy of the oral mass (Wright–Giemsa stain, 50×).

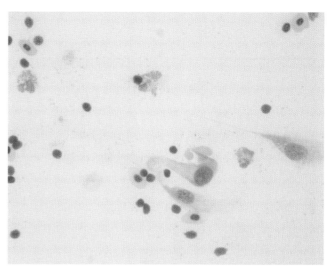

Fig. 70.4. A fine-needle aspiration biopsy of the oral mass (Wright–Giemsa stain, 50×).

indicating peripheral blood contamination of the sample. Seven heterophils are present in Fig. 70.2 along with two small lymphocytes and two spindle-shaped cells. Higher magnification of the cytology sample in Fig. 70.3 reveals three heterophils and a monocyte. A second aspirate (Fig. 70.4) was less contaminated by blood and revealed a moderately cellular sample with heterophils and spindle-shaped cells. The heterophils suggest an inflammatory lesion. The fusiform cells have an oval nucleus, moderately granular chromatin, small nucleoli, pale blue cytoplasm, and indistinct cell margins. These cells are fibroblasts, which often occur in chronic inflammatory lesions. Fibroblasts proliferate in

mature lesions to lay down collagen (Campbell and Ellis, 2007).

The radiograph findings included an increase in focal soft tissue along the rostral aspect of the maxilla. It was also noted that there is a focal region of lysis along the nasal bone, and on the rostral caudal projection there is a focal region of increased mineralization. The osseous changes may represent previous trauma or dystrophic mineralization. An infectious process or neoplasia is possible.

Summary

The iguana was placed under general anesthesia. Intravenous propofol (10 mg/kg) was used for induction. The iguana was intubated and maintained with 2.5% isoflurane. The mass was surgically removed using a CO_2 laser. Histopathologic examination revealed that the mass was composed of loose proliferating fibrous and granular connective tissues, containing numerous blood vessels, heterophils, and areas of hemorrhage. On the surface of the mass, and sometimes deep into the mass, there were lakes of fibrin and degenerate heterophils, containing numerous coccobacilli. Some of the blood vessels within the mass contained thrombi. The diagnosis was an inflammatory polyp with intralesional coccobacilli. The lesion was nonneoplastic but did extend to the margins.

An aerobic and anaerobic culture and sensitivity revealed a mixed bacterial infection with a light growth of *Escherichia coli*, *Pasteurella multocida*, and *Beta streptococcus*.

The iguana was treated with a broad-spectrum antibiotic (ceftazidime, 20 mg/kg IM 72 hours) for 21 days. According to the shelter manager, the iguana remained

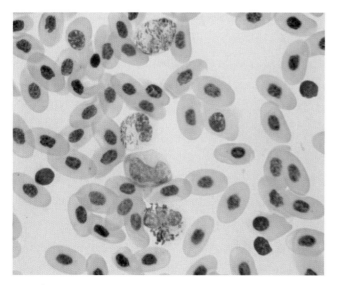

Fig. 70.3. A fine-needle aspiration biopsy of the oral mass (Wright–Giemsa stain, 100×).

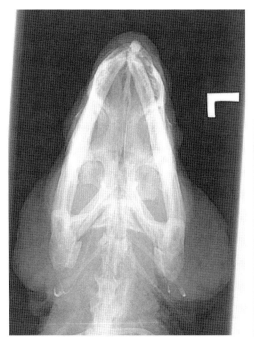 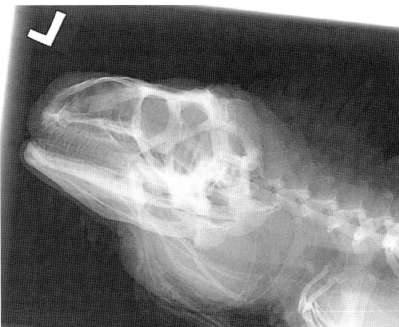

Fig. 70.5. The radiographs of the iguana's skull.

healthy until he returned approximately 1 year later for a recurrence of the mass. The mass was removed again and the iguana was placed on ceftazidime (20 mg/kg IM q 72 hours, seven treatments). The malocclusion of the mouth caused the gingiva to be constantly exposed, predisposing this iguana to chronic exposure gingivitis. Chronic low-grade osteomyelitis in the area is another possibility.

71

A 10-Year-Old Snake with a Coelomic Mass and Concern of Intestinal Impaction

Signalment

A 10-year-old intact male corn snake (*Elaphe guttata guttata*) was presented for a coelomic mass and concern of intestinal impaction.

History

The corn snake was presented with a coelomic mass considered to be an intestinal impaction. The mass was first noticed by the owner over 1 month prior to presentation and had been slowly increasing in size. The snake had been anorexic and had not defecated since the occurrence of the mass.

Physical Examination Findings

The corn snake was lethargic and dull. Tags of retained skin indicated dysecdysis. A 5-cm coelomic mass just cranial to the vent could be seen and palpated (Fig. 71.1).

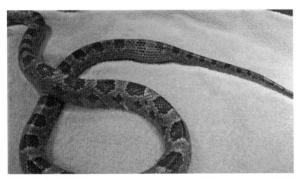

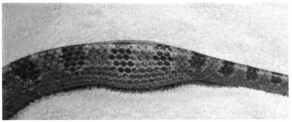

Fig. 71.1. The appearance of lesions in the body of the snake.

A fine-needle aspiration biopsy was obtained for cytological evaluation (Figs. 71.2 and 71.3).

Interpretive Discussion

Figure 71.2 reveals numerous erythrocytes, a heterophil, and macrophages. One macrophage has phagocytized material in the cytoplasm. The others are highly vacuolated. A higher magnification (Fig. 71.3a) reveals numerous erythrocytes and thrombocytes, indicating that the sample is primarily peripheral blood. It also reveals four heterophils and four monocytes (azurophilic). Figure 71.3b shows sodium and potassium urate crystals that were found in another area on the slide. These

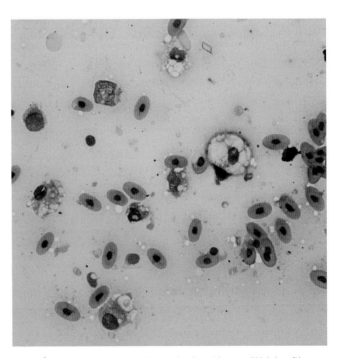

Fig. 71.2. A fine-needle aspiration biopsy (Wright–Giemsa stain, 50×).

297

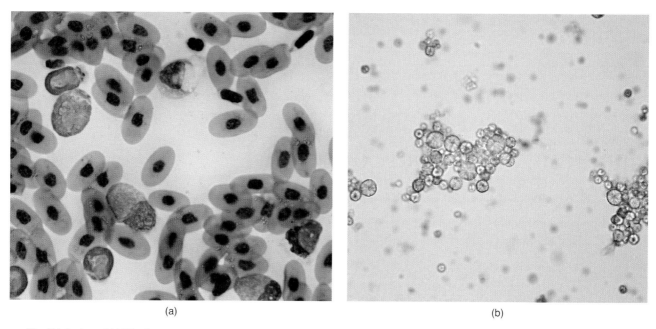

(a)　　　　　　　　　　　　　　　　　(b)

Fig. 71.3. (a and b) The fine-needle aspiration biopsy (Wright–Giemsa stain, 100×).

findings indicate an inflammatory response (macrophagic) associated with urate crystals.

Summary

The snake was anesthetized using ketamine and medetomidine intramuscularly as an induction and maintained on isoflurane following intubation. Exploratory surgery was performed in an effort to remove the mass. The mass was inherently associated with the left ureter and could not be removed alone without compromising urate flow out of the body; therefore, the left kidney was removed along with the associated ureter and mass. Both kidneys appeared normal grossly. Large firm fecal material was found in the intestinal tract just proximal to the mass. This fecal material had become too large owing to the obstructive nature of the mass, and an attempt to massage it into the cloaca failed. The fecal material was removed following an enterotomy. The en-

terotomy site was closed, and the coelomic cavity was thoroughly irrigated with saline. The body wall and skin were closed using standard procedures for reptiles.

The corn snake was tube fed a gruel made from dog food before he left the hospital the following day. The sutures were removed 6 weeks following the surgery. At that time, the snake had completely healed and was eating small mice on his own.

A blood profile would have been helpful in this case to provide a better prognosis; however, the client refused diagnostic testing owing to the cost. A blood film alone may have provided useful information. On the basis of the number of inflammatory cells present in the cytology sample that appeared to be primarily peripheral blood, the leukocyte count appeared high and the snake likely had an inflammatory leukogram. Histologic examination of the mass indicated a urate granuloma likely associated with leakage of urine from the ureter into the coelomic cavity.

A 9-Month-Old Lizard with Anorexia and Weight Loss

72

Signalment

A 9-month-old male leopard gecko (*Eublepharis macularius*) was presented for anorexia and weight loss (Fig. 72.1).

History

The gecko was purchased from a pet store 3 weeks prior to presentation and had not eaten for the past 2 weeks.

Physical Examination Findings

The 4 g lizard exhibited evidence of marked weight loss as depicted by the thin appearance of the tail. Although the gecko resisted restraint, it appeared weak. Because the gecko had not defecated for a number of days, a fresh fecal sample was not available for examination. Instead, a gastric wash was performed for gastric cytology (Figs. 72.2 and 72.3).

Interpretive Discussion

The gastric cytology stained with Wright–Giemsa stain (Fig. 72.2) revealed numerous round, clear to pale blue extracellular organisms that measured approximately 4–6 μm in diameter. These organisms stained positive with acid-fast stain (Fig. 72.3). These findings are supportive of a *Cryptosporidium* infection.

Summary

The client was informed of the potentially zoonotic nature of this disease. Because an effective treatment

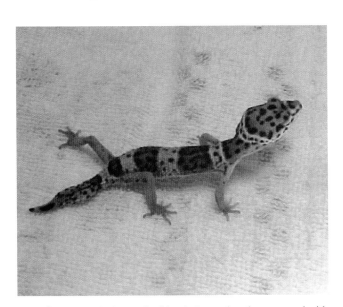

Fig. 72.1. The 9-month-old male leopard gecko presented with weight loss.

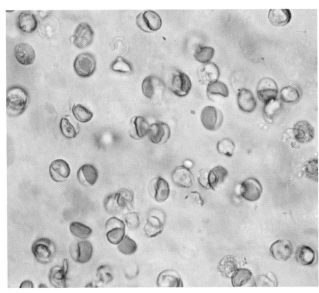

Fig. 72.2. A gastric wash sample (Wright–Giemsa stain, 100×).

299

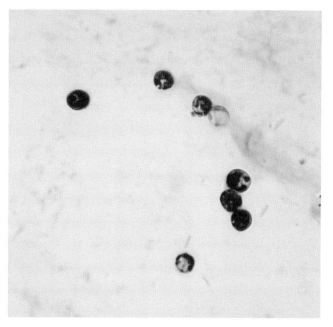

Fig. 72.3. A gastric wash sample (acid-fast stain, 100×).

for a *Cryptosporidium* infection in reptiles could not be offered and the gecko was extremely debilitated with a poor prognosis for survival, the client elected to euthanize her pet. A necropsy revealed the following: The lizard was thin with minimal fat and little to no autolysis. There was 0.75 mL of serosanguineous fluid within the abdomen. The colon was markedly distended with an intralumenal mucinous clot. There were no formed feces present in the intestine and/or rectum. All other organ systems appeared normal. Within the lumen of the intestines, there was a coagulum of fibrin, mucus, heterophils, sloughed epithelium, and necrotic debris. Multifocally, intestinal crypts were disorganized and contained an occasional vacuolated epithelium and intralumenal necrotic debris. Attached to the villous surface epithelium and occasionally intracellular, there were numerous, small, 1–5 μm in diameter, circular basophilic foci that were consistent with *Cryptosporidium*. Therefore, a diagnosis of intestinal cryptosporidiosis was made.

A 6-Year-Old Lizard with a Tail Mass

73

Signalment

A 6-year-old spayed female Green iguana (*Iguana iguana*) was presented with a mass at the base of the tail.

History

The iguana was presented for evaluation of a swelling or mass at the base of the tail. The iguana had been examined at another veterinary hospital 3 weeks prior for reevaluation of a possible intracoelomic mass that was diagnosed 5 months earlier. According to the owner, the blood profile performed at the other facility was considered to be normal; however, a radiograph taken at that time revealed an intracoelomic mass. No further workup had been performed and the iguana had been doing well since then. According to the owner, an ovariohysterectomy had been performed on the iguana 4 years earlier when the lizard developed dystocia.

The owner noticed a small swelling on the right side of the dorsal aspect of the tail base. The swelling had increased in size during the past few days and now involved the other side of the tail along the dorsal midline.

Physical Examination Findings

The iguana was bright, alert, and responsive and appeared to be in good body condition. No abnormalities were noted other than a small swelling at the base of the tail. An aspirate of the swelling was obtained for cytologic examination. A blood sample was collected via caudal venipuncture for a complete blood count and plasma biochemistry profile. Whole body radiographs were also obtained (Tables 73.1 and 73.2 and Figs. 73.1–73.3).

Interpretive Discussion

The current hemogram (Table 73.1) revealed significant changes compared with 3 weeks prior that

Table 73.1. Hematology results.

	Initial visit	Recheck 3 weeks later	Normal range for Green iguanas[a]
WBC ($10^3/\mu L$)	5.3	1.9	3–10
Heterophils ($10^3/\mu L$)	4.8	1.3	0.35–5.2
Lymphocytes ($10^3/\mu L$)	0.1	0.3	0.5–5.5
Monocytes ($10^3/\mu L$)	0.3	0.3	0–0.1
Eosinophils ($10^3/\mu L$)	0	0	0–0.3
Basophils ($10^3/\mu L$)	0.1	0	0–0.5
Plasma protein (g/dL)	6.5	4.0	—
PCV (%)	24	10	25–38
Thrombocytes	Clumped	Clumped	—

[a]Diethelm (2005).

Table 73.2. Plasma biochemistry results.

	Initial visit	Recheck 3 weeks later	Normal range for green iguanas[a]
Glucose (g/dL)	188	141	169–288
BUN (mg/dL)	2.0	2.0	0–4
Uric acid (mg/dL)	4.8	6.7	<6.7
Phosphorus (mg/dL)	3.0	3.2	4–6
Calcium (mg/dL)	13.6	11.9	8.8–14.0
Total protein (g/dL)	5.8	3.8	5.0–7.8
Albumin (g/dL)	2.7	1.9	2.1–2.8
Globulin (g/dL)	3.1	1.9	2.5–4.3
A/G ratio	0.9	1.0	—
Cholesterol (mg/dL)	—	—	104–333
CK (IU/L)	3,343	8,278	1,947 ± 2,058
AST (IU/L)	34	37	5–52
Sodium (mg/dL)	155	157	158–183
Potassium (mg/dL)	3.8	4.6	1.3–3.0
Chloride (mg/dL)	98	102	117–122
Bicarbonate (mg/dL)	28.7	28.1	—
Anion gap	33	31	—
Calculated osmolality	307	309	—

[a]Diethelm (2005).

301

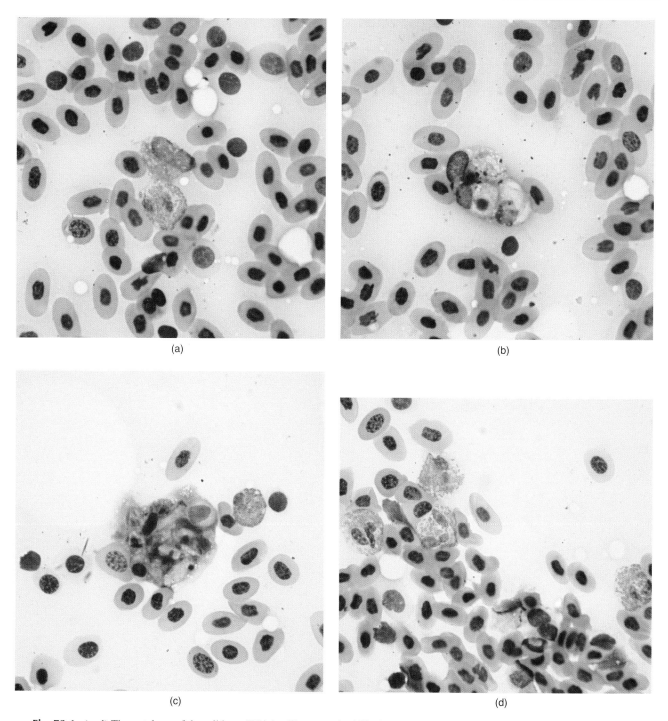

Fig. 73.1. (a–d) The cytology of the tail base (Wright–Giemsa stain, 100×).

included leukopenia, lymphopenia, a slight monocyto-sis, anemia, and drop in the plasma protein. It is possible that the blood sample was diluted with lymphatic fluid, a common occurrence when sampling blood from rep-tiles. The hemogram could also signal blood loss anemia along with an overwhelming inflammatory response that has resulted in consumption of heterophils. The signif-

icant plasma biochemistry profile changes indicated a loss to plasma protein supporting the drop in plasma protein (refractometric) found on the hemogram.

The fluid aspirated from the swelling on the left side of the tail base resembled blood. Figure 73.1a shows a heterophil and a monocyte with numerous erythro-cytes. There appears to be an increase in the degree

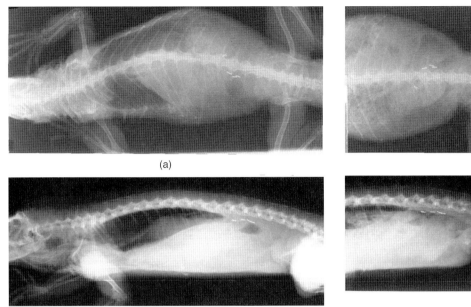
(a)

(b)

Fig. 73.2. The whole body radiographs: dorsoventral view (a) and lateral view (b).

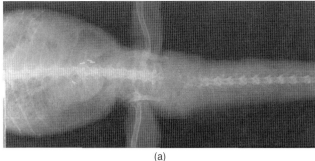
(a)

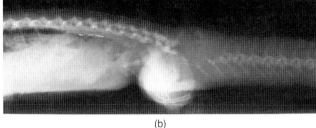
(b)

Fig. 73.3. The radiographs for the evaluation of the tail base lesion: dorsoventral view (a) and lateral view (b).

of polychromasia, suggesting a regenerative response. Figure 73.1b shows a multinucleated giant cell that has phagocytized cells that appear to be remnants of erythrocytes. Figure 73.1c shows a multinucleated giant cell that is clearly demonstrating erythrophagocytosis and a heterophil. Figure 73.1d shows four nondegenerate heterophils and numerous erythrocytes. The cytologic examination indicates peripheral blood contamination of the sample; however, it also demonstrates erythrophagocytosis and perhaps an increased number of inflammatory cells indicating previous hemorrhage into the lesion.

The packed cell volume (PCV) from the blood obtained from the tail vein was 10%. The PCV of the aspirated fluid was 30%. This finding is supportive of hemorrhage into the lesion and the hemogram findings, suggesting a blood loss anemia. The lesion, therefore, could represent a hematoma, hemangioma, or hemangiosarcoma.

The radiographic changes (Figs. 73.2 and 73.3) between the current radiographs and the ones obtained 3 weeks prior include a large, poorly circumscribed soft tissue mass surrounding the sacrococcygeal junction. There is gas seen within the soft tissues in this area. There are multiple areas of bone lysis of the vertebrae, laminae, and the dorsal spinous processes in this area. There is also some dystrophic mineralization seen within the mass. These findings are consistent with an aggressive neoplasia. The hemoclips seen in the

sublumbar area are consistent with this iguana's previous surgery.

Summary

The iguana was treated with a fluorinated chloramphenicol (30 mg/kg PO q 24 hours for 10 days), and an exploratory surgery of the coelomic cavity and tail mass was performed. The mass seen on the radiographs was a retained egg that may have been left in the coelomic cavity 4 years prior when an ovariosalpingohysterectomy was performed for dystocia. Surgical debridement of the tail mass revealed a large amount of clotted blood and a broken tail. A biopsy was obtained for histopathologic examination. The tail was bandaged and the iguana was hospitalized for 1 day. One week later, the iguana returned for examination of the fracture site. It was noted at that time that the iguana was exhibiting paresis of the tail and hind limbs and she was not able to defecate. There was no improvement in the appearance of the tail lesion. The owner elected euthanasia of the iguana and a necropsy was performed.

Histopathologic examination of the tail lesion revealed a severe chronic caseous, granulomatous, and heterophilic myositis and osteomyelitis with myelomalacia. The inflammatory process was likely associated with an infectious agent according to the report; however, no organism was visualized with special stains or culture.

74

A 27-Year-Old Snake with a Snout Lesion

Signalment

A 27-year-old male common boa constrictor (*Boa constrictor*) was presented with an infection on its snout.

History

The snake was presented to the hospital for swelling on the right side of the face. The swelling was first noticed approximately 2 months prior to presentation. The snake was treated with enrofloxacin by another veterinary hospital for 2 weeks with no improvement. The snake last shed and ate 3 days prior to presentation.

The owner feeds the snake live rats every 1–2 weeks. The snake lived in a wood and plexiglass enclosure where he was exposed to natural sunlight. Newspaper was used as cage substrate and the temperature was kept between 80 and 85°F. Water changes and overall enclosure cleanings using a commercial disinfectant were performed once weekly.

Physical Examination Findings

The 6.05-kg snake was bright, alert, and responsive on physical examination. The right side of the face was swollen just caudal to the right eye. The cloudy appearance of the spectacles over the eyes suggested that the snake was preparing to shed. There was also swelling near the region of the hemipenes.

An aspirate of the facial swelling was performed for cytological evaluation as well as a microbial culture and sensitivity. A swab of the right eye was also taken for culture and sensitivity. Other diagnostics included skull radiographs and a plasma biochemistry profile (Table 74.1 and Figs. 74.1–74.3).

Table 74.1. Plasma biochemistry results.

	Results	Normal range for boa constrictors[a]
Glucose (g/dL)	105	7–47
BUN (mg/dL)	27	1–3
Phosphorus (mg/dL)	4.6	3.9–6.5
Calcium (mg/dL)	9.0	11.8–15.6
Total protein (g/dL)	6.1	5.1–7.9
Albumin (g/dL)	2.8	2.1–3.7
Globulin (g/dL)	3.3	3.1–4.7
A/G ratio	0.8	—
Cholesterol (mg/dL)	—	146–304
CK (IU/L)	195	0–343
AST (IU/L)	49	0–85
Sodium (mg/dL)	151	149–165
Potassium (mg/dL)	4.1	2.2–5.0
Chloride (mg/dL)	121	105–133
Bicarbonate (mg/dL)	21.3	—
Anion gap	13	—
Calculated osmolality	304	—

[a]Diethelm (2005).

Other Diagnostic Information

The culture and sensitivity results showed a 1+ and 3+ growth of *Clostridium sporogenes* in the eye and swelling, respectively.

Interpretive Discussion

Low magnification of the cytology sample (Fig. 74.1) revealed a highly cellular sample that consisted of numerous heterophils and macrophages with a few erythrocytes indicating a mixed cell inflammation. Higher magnification of the sample revealed erythrophagocytosis (Fig. 74.2a) and leukophagocytosis (Fig. 74.2b). No etiologic agent could be found.

Radiographic findings (Fig. 74.3) included a moderate amount of soft-tissue swelling along the right aspect

305

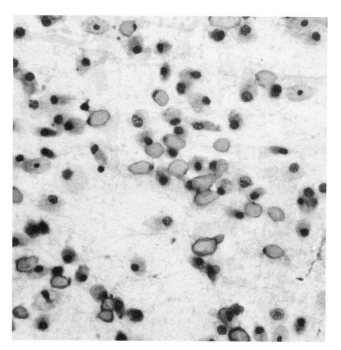

Fig. 74.1. An aspirate of the swelling (Wright–Giemsa stain, 40×).

of the head. There was no evidence of bony abnormalities. The findings were attributed to an inflammatory or infectious process along the right aspect of the head.

The significant findings on the plasma biochemistry panel included a hyperglycemia and increased urea ni-

trogen concentration. These findings could be associated with recent feeding.

Overall, the results are consistent with infectious stomatitis, a condition normally associated with a mixed bacterial infection.

Summary

The snake was treated with triple antibiotic ophthalmic drops (one drop in right eye, TID) realizing that this medication would not contact the cornea if the spectacle is intact. Intramuscular ceftazidime (20 mg/kg, q 72 hours) for seven treatments was also part of the treatment plan for the infectious stomatitis. During the following 5 months, the infection in the mouth worsened despite the ceftazidime treatments. Radiographs were repeated during this time to evaluate the presence of bony involvement (Fig. 74.4).

The radiographs revealed that the soft-tissue swelling on the right side of the face was still evident, but there was no significant evidence of osteolysis; however, a bone scan was performed to better evaluate the skull for osteomyelitis (Figs. 74.5).

Three mCi of Tc-99m HDP (technetium-99 high-density plasma) were injected via intracardiac injection. Delayed-phase imaging of the head was performed after 2 hours (Fig. 74.5). Both ventral and dorsal images of the head were taken. Increased uptake was recognized in the rostral half of the right maxilla; this region corresponds with the area of increased soft-tissue

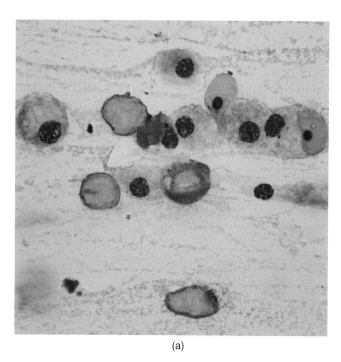

(a)

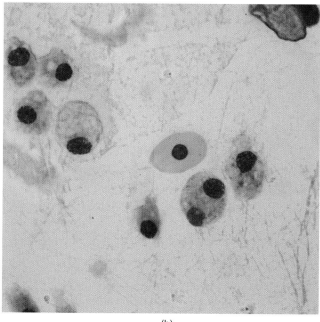

(b)

Fig. 74.2. (a and b) The aspirate of the swelling (Wright–Giemsa stain, 100×).

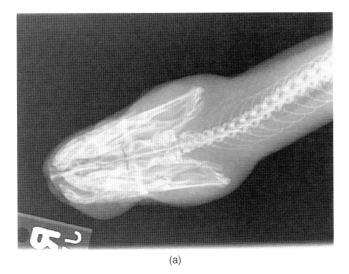

(a)

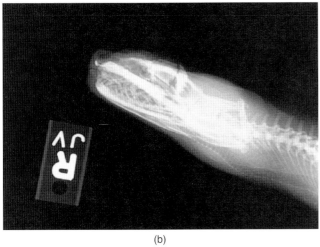

(b)

Fig. 74.3. The skull radiographs: dorsoventral (a) and lateral (b) views.

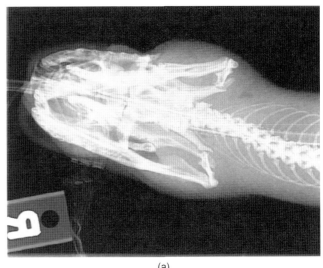

(a)

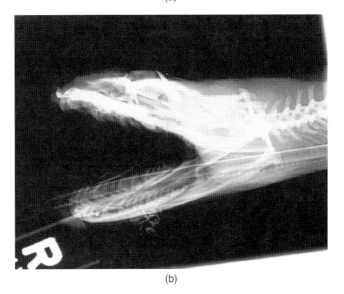

(b)

Fig. 74.4. The skull radiographs of snake: dorsoventral (a) and lateral (b) views.

proliferation noted previously by radiograph. The findings on this study are consistent with increased osteoblastic activity in the rostral right maxilla and likely associated with an infectious process or neoplasia. Another less likely differential, due to chronicity, would be a traumatic lesion.

The snake was placed under general anesthesia for surgical debridement. The abscess along the right side of the face was debrided, and antibiotic (ceftazidime) impregnated polymethyl methacrylate beads were implanted into the area of the lesion. A sample of the bone and soft tissue was submitted for histologic examination.

Histologically, the lesion was diagnosed as a moderate, regionally extensive, heterophilic stomatitis with osteonecrosis.

Two months later, the snake returned for suture removal. It was noted at that time that the lesion was healing and the snake appeared to be healthy.

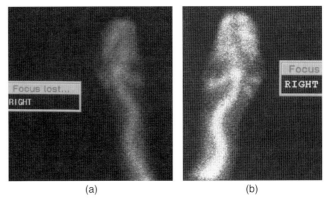

(a)   (b)

Fig. 74.5. The bone scan of the skull: ventral (a) and dorsal (b) views.

A 1-Year-Old Lizard with Multiple Infections

75

Signalment

A 1-year-old intact male leopard gecko (*Euble-pharis macularius*) was presented with a chief complaint of multiple infections (Fig. 75.1).

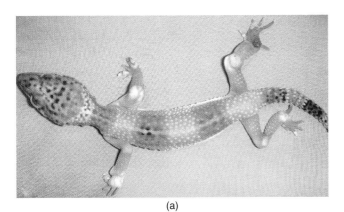

(a)

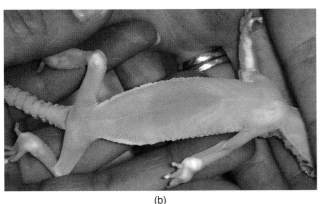

(b)

Fig. 75.1. The leopard gecko on presentation.

History

The gecko was relinquished to a nearby reptile shelter 3 days prior to presentation due to sudden anorexia and lethargy. The shelter staff noticed the swollen joints and presented him to the hospital. They reported that the previous owner claimed this was a sudden onset and that the lizard had not been eating well. The animal had not eaten at all while at the shelter.

Physical Examination Findings

On physical examination, the leopard gecko was thin, weighing only 20 g with a body condition score of 1/5. Several joints in all four limbs were swollen and surrounded by a white material that had congregated subcutaneously. The animal was ambulatory but appeared slow and hesitant when walking as though he was uncomfortable.

A fine-needle aspirate of the ventral left shoulder was obtained for cytodiagnosis. The material was gritty and difficult to aspirate (Fig. 75.2).

Interpretative Discussion

Figure 75.2 shows an acellular sample that contains only needle-shaped crystals. The crystals were birefringent under polarized light (not shown). These are uric acid crystals and support a diagnosis of articular gout.

309

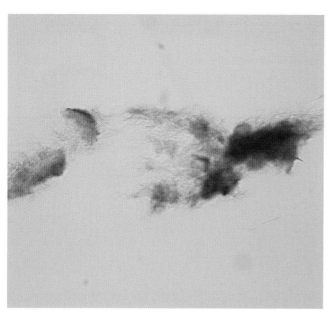

Fig. 75.2. An aspirate of the shoulder joint (Wright–Giemsa stain, 100×).

Summary

Articular gout or other forms of gout in lizards are the result of precipitation of uric acid from increased levels of uric acid due to dehydration, renal disease, or other chronic disease processes (Nevarez, 2009). Due to the advanced lesions in this case, euthanasia was elected. A full necropsy was not pursued; however, closer examination of the shoulder lesion revealed that the white material surrounding the left shoulder joint was chalky and extended deep within the joint.

76

An Adult Snake with Severe Dyspnea

Signalment

An adult Ball python (*Python regius*) was presented with severe dyspnea (Fig. 76.1).

History

The Ball python had a 3-month history of dyspnea that included open-mouthed breathing. The client had scheduled an appointment to have the snake examined 1 month prior to presentation; however, that appointment was cancelled. The client acquired the snake as an adult and owned the snake for 4 years. She did not know its exact age or its gender. The snake routinely ate an adult mouse once a week. The snake began exhibiting noisy breathing approximately 6 months earlier, but its respiratory effort became more noticeable during the past 3 months.

Physical Examination

The snake was presented in a state of severe respiratory distress. It positioned itself with the head and neck held in a vertical position as it breathed through an opened mouth. An obvious respiratory noise was made with each rapid breath as if made through a constricted airway. The ventral scutes were creased along the midline in the area of the lungs, indicating chronic labored breathing. The snake's overall body condition appeared normal.

A 2.0 mm endotracheal tube was inserted through the body wall and placed into the air sac (saccular lung) to provide immediate respiratory relief. A 3.0 mm rigid laparoscope was inserted through the glottis and into the trachea. A white glistening tracheal mass occluding nearly 95% of the tracheal lumen was found approximately 2.5 cm distal to the rima glottis. A flexible biopsy instrument was inserted into the trachea in an attempt to remove the mass; however, only a small portion of the mass was sampled. A small blood sample was obtained via caudal venipuncture and submitted for hematologic examination (Table 76.1 and Figs. 76.2a–76.2c).

Interpretive Discussion

The hemogram reveals a monocytosis and an elevated plasma protein (normal plasma protein values using the biuret method for most snakes is less than 8 g/dL). This suggests an inflammatory response; however, a monocytosis without a coexisting leukocytosis and heterophilia is unusual. The monocytosis is likely

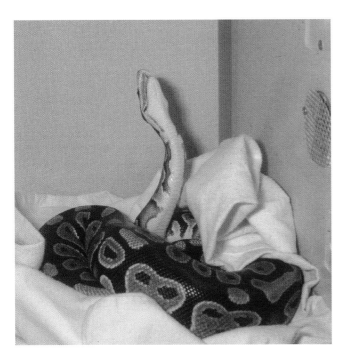

Fig. 76.1. An image of the Ball python with severe dyspnea.

311

Table 76.1. Hematology results.

	Results	Normal range for Ball pythons[a]
WBC (10^3/μL)	14.7	7.9–16.4
Heterophils (10^3/μL)	7.8	—
Heterophils (%)	53	56–67
Lymphocytes (10^3/μL)	1.2	—
Lymphocytes (%)	8	7–21
Monocytes (10^3/μL)	5.8	—
Monocytes (%)	39	0–1
Eosinophils (10^3/μL)	0	—
Eosinophils (%)	0	0
Basophils (10^3/μL)	0	—
Basophils (%)	0	0–2
Protein (g/dL)	9.0	—
PCV (%)	23	16–21
Thrombocytes	Adequate, clumped	

[a]Diethelm (2005).

associated with mobilization of monocytes because of peripheral demand for macrophages. Perhaps other cells were misidentified as monocytes because of their unusual morphology, such as toxic heterophils, if present. A blood film in this case, however, was not available for review.

Figures 76.2a–76.2c show mesenchymal cells, with basophilic cytoplasm often containing fine eosinophilic granules. These cells are embedded in an eosinophilic background material. The nuclei are frequently positioned at one edge of the cell and have coarsely granular chromatin with occasional prominent nucleoli. The cells exhibit moderate anisocytosis and variable nucleus–cytoplasm ratios. The cytologic examination indicates a mesenchymal cell neoplasm that is producing either chondroid or osteoid, therefore, likely has its origins in cartilage or bone. A chondroma or

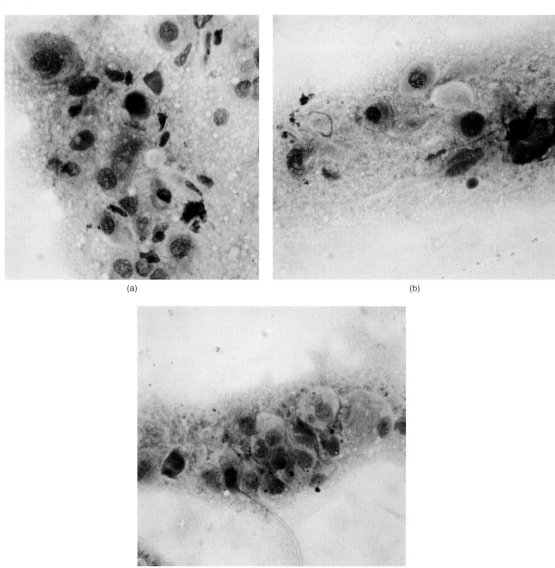

(a)

(b)

(c)

Fig. 76.2. (a–c) The imprint of the tracheal mass sample (Wright–Giemsa stain, 100×).

chondrosarcoma is more likely than an osteogenic sarcoma, owing to the lack of cells having the typical appearance of osteoblasts.

Summary

The snake died before it could be prepared for surgical removal of the tracheal mass. The plan was to remove the mass by transection of the involved section of the trachea followed by anastomosis of the healthy tracheal ends.

The gross necropsy revealed a 1 cm white glistening intratracheal mass occluding the lumen. Histopathologic findings revealed an increased number of normal-appearing chondrocytes within lacunae in a disorganized chondroid matrix. Mitotic figures were rare. The mass was focally continuous with the mineralized cartilaginous ring indicating that it arose from the tracheal ring. The diagnosis was a benign chondroma of the trachea.

An Adult Newt with a White Skin Lesion

77

Signalment

An adult rough-skinned newt (*Taricha* sp.) was presented with a white patchy area on the skin (Fig. 77.1).

History

The rough-skinned newt was housed in a 30-gallon terrarium. The bottom of the terrarium contains small, smooth natural rocks that were constantly covered in water. The terrarium contains artificial plants, larger rocks, and wooden structures for the newt's climbing and hiding behavior. According to the client, the water was changed once a month. The terrarium was kept at room temperature that varied from 70 to 80°F. The newt was subjected to a 12-hour photoperiod provided by a standard fluorescent lamp and a timer. The newt was fed a commercial pelleted food for newts, small feeder fish (i.e., guppies), and brine shrimp. The lesion appeared within the past 24 hours.

Physical Examination Findings

On physical examination, the newt appeared healthy and exhibited normal escape behavior. A small area of white discoloration of the skin was found on the dorsum. Gentle scraping of the lesion provided a sample for a wet mount preparation that was later stained with Wright–Giemsa stain (Figs. 77.2 and 77.3).

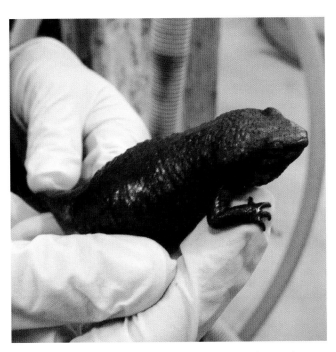

Fig. 77.1. The rough-skinned newt with a white patchy area on the dorsal skin.

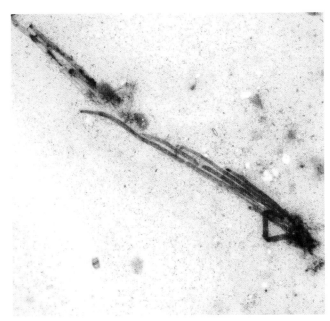

Fig. 77.2. A skin scraping (Wright–Giemsa stain, 20×).

315

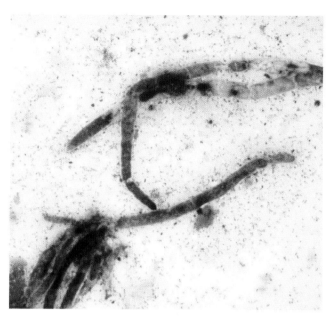

Fig. 77.3. A skin scraping (Wright–Giemsa stain, 50×).

Interpretive Discussion

Figure 77.2 shows septate, nonbranching fungal hyphae. Higher magnification (Fig. 77.3) of the fungi shows no apparent cellular response to the large fungal hyphae. The morphology of the fungal hyphae is compatible with that of a *Saprolegnia* sp.

Summary

Saprolegnia is a ubiquitous saprophytic water mold that lives off decaying organic material in aquariums and ponds (Fernandez-Beneitez et al., 2008). The organism is an opportunistic pathogen and will live on the skin of stress or injured fish, or in this case, a newt (Mylniczenko, 2009).

Maintaining healthy water quality is just as important to aquatic or semiaquatic animals as it is to fish. In this case, the newt lived in a terrarium without proper filtration to the water in the habitat. If water filtration was not being provided, then more frequent water changes was recommended. It is likely the water mold built up in the terrarium because of high levels of organic material in the water. The newt likely became infected through either a skin abrasion or a stressed immune system.

The newt was treated with malachite green (0.1 mg/L of water) as prolonged immersion treatment every 3 days for three treatments. The lesion disappeared following the first treatment.

78

An Adult Frog in a Moribund Condition

Signalment

An adult poison dart frog (*Dendrobates* sp.) was presented in a moribund condition (Fig. 78.1).

History

The client, a hobbyist, successfully raised a variety of poison dart frogs (*Dendrobates* sp.) and red-eyed tree frogs (*Agalychnis callidryas*). The *Dendrobates* spp. were kept in 12 different 30-gallon terrariums, each containing eight to ten frogs. The terrariums contained soil, moss, live plants, and a shallow pool of water with small pebbles. They were arranged in three rows of four, with each group of four sharing a common ventilation system (cross-draft ventilation). Each terrarium had its own misting system. The temperature of the habitats varied from 82°F during the day to 69°F at night. The

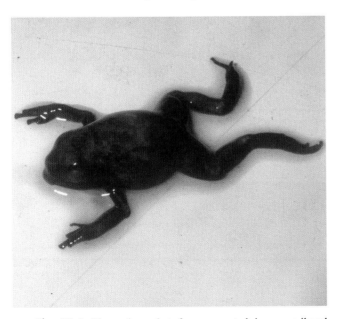

Fig. 78.1. The poison dart frog presented in a moribund condition.

frogs were maintained on a daily full spectrum light cycle between 7 AM and 5 PM. The frog habitats were cleaned every 3 weeks at which time more compost was added to the substrate. The frogs were fed a variety of insects, such as fruit flies (*Drosophila melanogaster*), meal worms (*Tenebrio molitor*), wax worms (Pyralidae), beetle larvae (Coleoptera), and Springtails (Collembola).

Recently, the client had been experiencing approximately 5% mortality in his frog population. The normal mortality was death of a frog once a month. Five frogs were found dead the week prior to presentation of this frog, and he had lost three frogs the previous week. It was noted that the frogs became thin before they died or thin dead frogs were found in the habitats.

Physical Examination Findings

On physical examination, the frog was poorly responsive. Its skin appeared dry and had a granular texture. Gentle scraping of the skin provided a sample for a wet mount preparation that was later stained with Wright–Giemsa stain. The wet mount preparation revealed several tiny motile organisms when viewed under a 100× objective (Figs. 78.2a and 78.2b).

Interpretive Discussion

Figure 78.2a shows a highly cellular sample with numerous erythrocytes. The background contains a variety of extracellular bacteria. A heterophil can be found in the upper right-hand corner of the image. The oval structures in the center have a distinct cell wall and multiple nuclei. These structures resemble the thalli or zoosporangia of the chytrid fungus, *Batrachochytrium dendrobatidis*, when they contain multiple discrete zoospores (Pessier et al., 1999). Figure 78.2b is a highly cellular sample that also contains what appears to be the zoosporangia of the chytrid fungus.

317

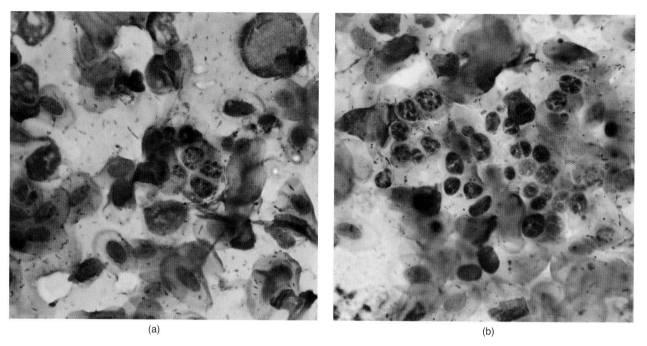

(a)   (b)

Fig. 78.2. (a and b) The skin scraping (Wright–Giemsa stain, 100×).

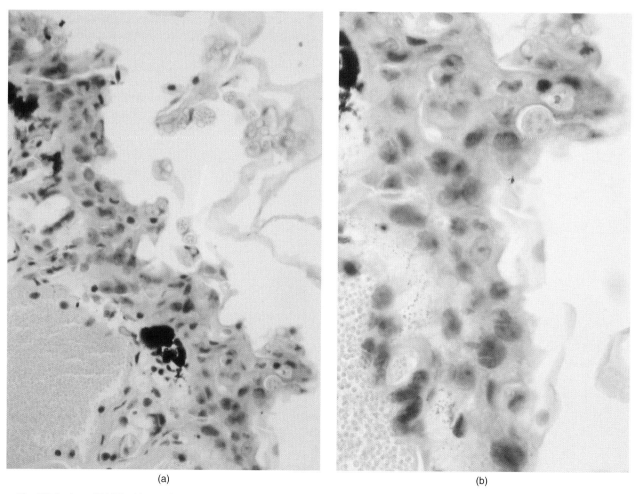

(a)   (b)

Fig. 78.3. (a and b) The histopathology of the skin lesion from the poison dart frog (a—HE stain, 20×; b—HE stain, 40×).

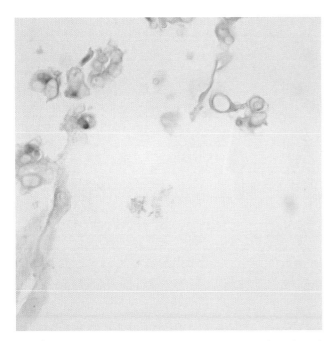

Fig. 78.4. The histopathology of the skin lesion from the poison dart frog (HE stain, 40×).

Summary

The frog died shortly after presentation and was submitted for necropsy that revealed no gross necropsy lesions other than thickening of the skin.

Histopathologic examination revealed focal aggregates of round 4–5 μm tear-drop-shaped, encapsulated, single-celled organisms embedded within the epithelium but only to the basal membrane. Often, a narrow tubular structure like a spout was located on one end of the capsule. Some contained multiple 1–2 μm basophilic spores. Areas infested with the organisms were thickened and revealed hyperkeratosis with sloughing of the outer layers of the skin. There was no underlying dermal inflammation. These histologic findings were indicative of the chytrid fungus, *B. dendrobatidis*. The chytrid zoosporangia that appeared as circular spaces with a homogenous appearance in the thickened epidermis likely represented immature stages of the sporangium, whereas those containing multiple discrete spores contained the mature zoospores ready to be released. The empty spaces represented the sporangia that have discharged their zoospores (Figs. 78.3 and 78.4).

Figures 78.3a and 78.3b reveal chytrid zoosporangia in the sloughed stratum corneum of the skin of the poison dart frog. Figure 78.4 shows an empty chytrid zoosporangium with a discharge tube or papillum.

Skin scrapings from frogs contain epithelial cells, soil debris, algae, and nonchytrid fungi. Congo red stain has been shown to delineate the chytrid zoosporangia from these structures and can be used as a rapid screening test for chytridiomycosis (Briggs and Burgin, 2003).

The client likely introduced the chytrid fungus into his collection when he recently obtained a shipment of new frogs from another breeding facility. The fungus uses keratin as substrate and its growth is restricted to highly keratinized structures. This results in hyperkeratosis of the skin, and death of the frog is related to disruption of the skin's osmotic regulation and supplementary respiration function. The adult frogs in the collection were treated topically using an antifungal agent (1% itraconazole suspension diluted to 0.01% with 0.6% saline as daily 5-minute immersions for 10 days). Also, the frogs were maintained at 37°F for 24 hours in an effort to kill the temperature-sensitive zoospores in the environment and to boost the immune system of the frogs. Larval stages (tadpoles) were treated using 0.1 ppm malachite green 24-hour baths. It was recommended that the habitats be thoroughly cleaned by removing all the plants and substrate and treated with a 0.4% bleach solution followed by leaving them to remain dry for 1 month. The client did not follow the habitat cleaning advice, but continued to treat tadpoles using the malachite green baths. His frog collection experienced no further deaths from the chytrid fungus.

A 10-Year-Old Lizard with Anorexia

79

Signalment

A 10-year-old female Green iguana (*Iguana iguana*) was presented with anorexia.

History

The iguana was presented with a 1-week history of anorexia. According to the owner, the iguana had been constipated and at times appeared to be straining during the past week. The iguana had been passing only urine and no feces. The client reported that the iguana had been "plugged up before" and she usually responded to soaking in the bathtub; however, this had not helped this time. The iguana was fed a diet that consisted of a variety of green leafy vegetables, apples, beans, and squash. The iguana was housed in a large homemade cage that was equipped with four heat lamps and a long ultraviolet light bulb suspended across the top. The iguana had not been ill at any time in the past.

Physical Examination Findings

The 2.6-kg female iguana had an enlarged coelomic cavity for a lizard that had not eaten for 1 week. She was active and responsive with a respiratory rate of 30 breaths/minute. The joint on the fourth digit of the right front foot was fused at the metacarpus, likely from a previous injury. The coelomic cavity appeared to be fluid-filled on palpation.

The client declined a recommendation for whole body radiographs and a blood profile, but did approve of aspiration of the coelomic cavity for fluid evaluation. A 20-gauge needle was used to aspirate a thick yellow fluid from the coelomic cavity (Figs. 79.1 and 79.2).

Interpretive Discussion

Figures 79.1 and 79.2 show a highly cellular sample containing numerous inflammatory cells on a thick basophilic background. The inflammatory cells are a mix of heterophils and large foamy macrophages, indicative of a mixed cell inflammation. The background contains round fat droplets, and Fig. 79.1 shows a large blue "protein" body. These findings are consistent with an egg-related coelomitis.

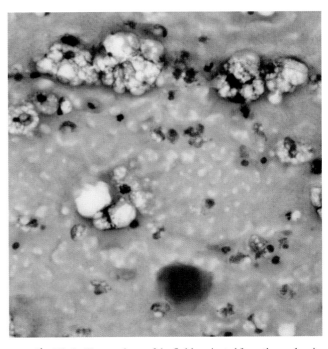

Fig. 79.1. The cytology of the fluid aspirated from the coelomic cavity (Wright–Giemsa stain, 50×).

321

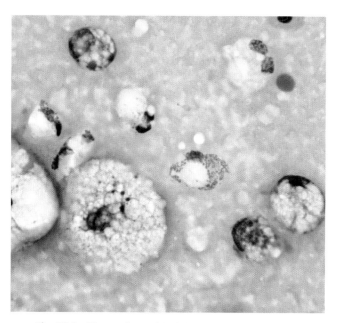

Fig. 79.2. The cytology of the fluid aspirated from the coelomic cavity (Wright–Giemsa stain, 100×).

Summary

Owing to a diagnosis of egg-related coelomitis and the poor prognosis for survival, the iguana was euthanized using a euthanasia solution delivered in the caudal vein. The gross necropsy revealed a thick yellow fluid (yolk material) filling the coelomic cavity. All internal organs were coated with a yellow fibrinous material. Both ovaries contained numerous large follicles. Three of these had ruptured and were likely the source of the yellow fluid in the coelom.

Section 8
Fish Cytology Case Studies

80

An Adult Eel with Anorexia and Skin Lesions

Signalment

An adult female Wolf eel (*Anarrhichthys ocellatus*) was presented with an 8-month history of anorexia and skin lesions (Figs. 80.1 and 80.2).

History

This Wolf eel was originally housed in an exhibit in a public aquarium. She was moved to a quarantine aquarium when cutaneous lesions were first noted. She exhibited an 8-month duration of multiple cutaneous ulcers that often progressed to granulomatous lesions. While in quarantine, she underwent a series of multiple prolonged treatments with antibiotics that included enrofloxacin and a fluorinated chloramphenicol. Three weeks after the initiation of the chloramphenicol treatment, the skin lesions showed improvement and the smaller ones on her side resolved into small white cutaneous scars. The larger lesion around the vent, however, progressed in size and for the most part was unresponsive to antibiotics.

Physical Examination Findings

The female Wolf eel exhibited a large ulcerated skin lesion that surrounded her vent (Fig. 80.2) and smaller skin ulcerations on other areas. Several small circular white scars on the body appeared to be remnants of previous ulceration sites. The fish was weak and provided little struggling when netted. A blood sample was obtained via caudal venipuncture for hematology and chemistry; however, the sample clotted in the EDTA (ethylenediaminetetraacetic acid) tube and only a chemistry profile was obtained. A 4 mm punch biopsy sample was obtained from the lesion surrounding the vent for histology. An imprint of the punch biopsy was obtained

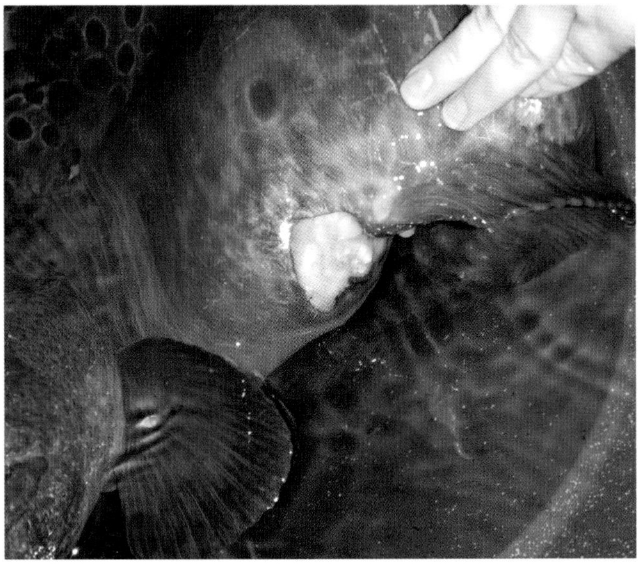

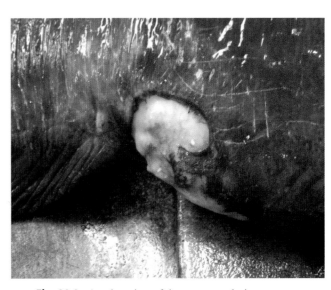

Fig. 80.1. The female Wolf eel with cutaneous ulcerations.

Fig. 80.2. Another view of the cutaneous lesion.

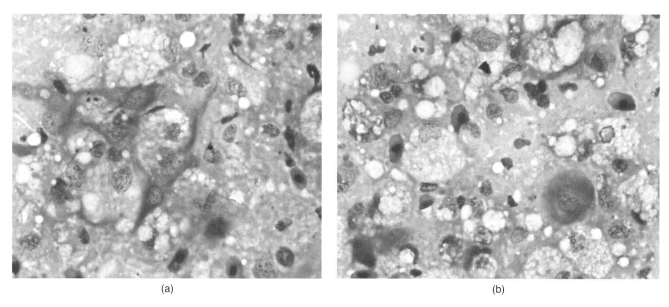

(a)   (b)

Fig. 80.3. (a and b) The imprint of skin lesion biopsy (Wright–Giemsa stain, 100×).

for cytological examination (Figs. 80.3a and 80.3b and Table 80.1).

Interpretive Discussion

The cytologic sample was highly cellular and contained primarily macrophages. Figures 80.3a and 80.3b reveal numerous foamy macrophages with fat droplets in the noncellular background. No etiologic agent could be found. A macrophagic inflammation with fat droplets is suggestive of a lipid disorder of the skin, such as xanthomatosis (although no cholesterol crystals were seen); however, a macrophagic inflammation could also be associated with an unidentified etiology such as *Mycobacterium*, fungal organism, or a foreign body.

Because no reference values were available for Wolf eels, interpretation of the plasma chemistry was based on experience with the plasma biochemistries of other animals. The blood glucose concentration was not compatible with life and indicated a poor prognosis for survival if not corrected or represented an erroneous number that needed to be repeated. The calcium value appeared to be reasonable for a normal value, but could also represent a female undergoing folliculogenesis. The hyperphosphatemia was a concern and may represent excessive phosphorus intake (either dietary or through the gills). Excessive dietary intake was unlikely because of the fish had been chronically anorectic. Renal failure was another possible explanation for the hyperphosphatemia; however, there was a possibility that this was a normal value for this species. The calcium–phosphorus ratio was inverted for most healthy animals and because the calcium appeared normal suggested either excessive

Table 80.1. Plasma biochemical results.

Glucose (mg/dL)	3.0
BUN (mg/dL)	5.0
Creatinine (mg/dL)	0.5
Phosphorus (mg/dL)	12.3
Calcium (mg/dL)	10.2
Total protein (g/dL)	3.6
Albumin (g/dL)	1.2
Globulin (g/dL)	2.4
A/G ratio	0.5
Cholesterol (mg/dL)	961
Total bilirubin (mg/dL)	0
CK (IU/L)	45
ALP (IU/L)	35
ALT (IU/L)	17
AST (IU/L)	25
GGT (IU/L)	0
Sodium (mg/dL)	150
Potassium (mg/dL)	5
Chloride (mg/dL)	136.2
Bicarbonate (mg/dL)	5
Anion gap	14
Calculated osmolality	290
Amylase	2.9
Iron	101
TIBC	596
Saturation percent	17
UIBC	495
Lipemia (mg/dL)	10
Hemolysis (mg/dL)	15
Icterus (mg/dL)	0

phosphorus intake or decreased phosphorus excretion. The total protein concentration appeared low, but could be normal for this species. The cholesterol concentration seemed high and was suggestive of a lipid disorder that supported the cytological and histological findings on the skin biopsy.

Summary

Histology of the biopsy indicated a chronic granulomatous dermatitis and offered a primary dyslipidosis as the cause. Microbial culture of the biopsy site revealed a mixture of bacteria that grew in low numbers and included *Citrobacter* sp., *Aeromonas hydrophila*, *Escherichia coli*, and *Flavobacterium* sp. These organisms were likely contaminants and not significant. *Mycobacterium* culture was negative.

Because the fish was chronically ill and had not eaten for a long while, the possibility that the lesions may indeed represent mycobacteriosis, a potentially zoonotic disease, and the severity of the animal's condition and poor prognosis, the aquarists elected to euthanize the patient and submit the body for a necropsy. The fish was euthanized with an overdose of tricaine methanesulfonate.

There was minimal autolysis observed during the necropsy examination. Significant gross necropsy findings included multiple, round, ulcerative lesions on the skin. The largest skin lesion measured 2.5 cm in diameter and was circumferentially around the vent. Some lesions had hemorrhagic areas, while others were white and firm (fibrosis). Within the coelomic cavity, there was approximately 100 mL of yellow-tinged, opaque fluid. The liver was diffusely pale and small pieces floated in formalin.

Fluid analysis revealed a yellow cloudy fluid with a clear supernatant. The nucleated cell count was 12,800 cells/μL with an erythrocyte count of 20,000 RBCs/μL. The refractometric protein concentration was 4.8 g/dL. The cytology revealed a moderate cellularity represented by 27% heterophils, 13% lymphocytes, and 60% monocytes. No microorganisms or evidence of neoplasia was found; therefore, the fluid cytology represented a mixed cell inflammation of unknown etiology.

Histologic examination of the skin revealed innumerable numbers of macrophages with multifocal areas of concentrated macrophages forming discrete granulomas, extending from the superficial dermis into the deep dermis. Multiple sections of skin contained this granulomatous inflammation. Multifocal areas containing moderate numbers of heterophils mixed within the large population of macrophages were also found. The inflammation extended into the subcutaneous tissues, but not the muscular layers of the body wall. One section of the largest skin mass revealed an abundance of cholesterol clefts, moderate numbers of vascular profiles, and numerous macrophages. Special stains (GMS, acid-fast, and gram stain) did not reveal any organisms within the granulomatous lesions; therefore, the etiology of this disease remained uncertain. Although mycobacteriosis was not identified with special stains, a diagnosis of that disease cannot be definitively ruled out. Culture attempts for mycobacterium later failed to demonstrate the presence of a *Mycobacterium* species.

Other significant histologic findings included a severe chronic diffuse hepatic lipidosis, mild chronic focal branchitis (inflammation of the gills), and moderate multifocal to coalescing chronic oophoritis.

A 1^1/$_2$-Year-Old Goldfish
with Dropsy

81

Signalment

A 1^1/$_2$-year-old goldfish (*Carassius auratus*) of unknown gender was presented with the primary complaint of dropsy (a layman's term for a distended coelomic cavity) (Fig. 81.1).

History

This fish was kept in a 55-gallon aquarium along with a number of freshwater tropical fish. The aquarium water was kept at approximately 72°F. Water quality appeared adequate, with ammonia and nitrite levels reported to be zero. The water was on the alkaline side of neutral with a pH of 8.4. Other fish in the aquarium were normal. Previous ineffective treatments performed at home included a 3% saltwater bath and a praziquantel bath.

Physical Examination Findings

A 50 ppm solution of tricaine methanesulfonate was used to sedate the patient for a physical examination. The coelomic cavity was moderately distended, and ulcerative lesions were found near the right pectoral fin (Fig. 81.2). Blood was collected for a complete blood count using the lateral approach to the caudal vein. Approximately 8 mL of clear yellow fluid was aspirated from the coelomic cavity and submitted for fluid analysis (Table 81.1 and Figs. 81.3 and 81.4).

Interpretive Discussion

Although the reference does not provide a normal range for the total leukocyte count, there is an increased heterophil–lymphocyte ratio and increase in monocyte numbers. This is supportive of an inflammatory leukogram and the packed cell volume (PCV) indicates anemia. Figure 81.3a shows three toxic heterophils and a

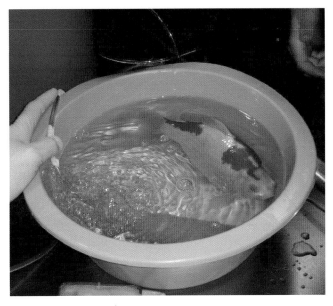

Fig. 81.1. The 1^1/$_2$-year-old goldfish presented with dropsy.

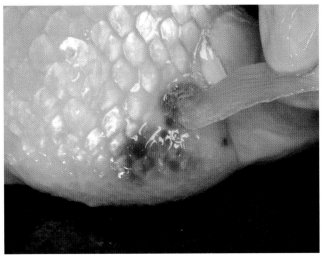

Fig. 81.2. The lesion near the right pectoral fin found on physical examination.

329

Table 81.1. Hematology results.

		Reference[a]
WBC ($10^3/\mu$L)	20	—
Heterophils ($10^3/\mu$L)	14.6	—
Heterophils (%)	73	26–32
Lymphocytes ($10^3/\mu$L)	0.6	—
Lymphocytes (%)	3	65–75
Monocytes ($10^3/\mu$L)	4.8	—
Monocytes (%)	24	0–1
Eosinophils ($10^3/\mu$L)	0	—
Eosinophils (%)	0	—
Basophils ($10^3/\mu$L)	0	—
Basophils (%)	0	—
Plasma protein (g/dL)	3.0	—
RBC ($10^6/\mu$L)	—	1.4–1.6
Hb (g/dL)	—	8.7–9.5
PCV (%)	20	25–27
Thrombocytes	Adequate	

[a]Lewbart (2005).

monocyte. The normal heterophils of goldfish have eccentric partially lobed nuclei with a colorless cytoplasm that contains distinct, rod-shaped, slightly acidophilic cytoplasmic granules. The heterophils in this image have nonlobed to partially lobed nuclei and deeply basophilic vacuolated cytoplasm with indistinct eosinophilic gran-

ules. A thrombocyte is also present. The image also indicates numerous smudge cells (likely to be free nuclei from erythrocytes), relatively few erythrocytes, and no polychromasia. The latter indicates a poor or no response to the anemia. Figure 81.3b shows a lymphocyte (top leukocyte), toxic metamyelocyte, and monocyte (center right leukocytes) among the erythrocytes and smudge cells. The morphological findings of toxic heterophils place the inflammatory response in the severe category.

The fluid was yellow and hazy with a clear supernatant. The refractometric protein was 2.1 g/dL. Figure 81.4a shows the predominant cells in the fluid, which are heterophils with round to slightly indented nuclei and resemble those found in the peripheral blood. Figure 81.4b reveals large mononuclear cells with basophilic cytoplasm and numerous discrete, small, clear vacuoles. It was unclear whether these represented activated macrophages or some other cell type. The cell count (using both the Natt–Herrick's and phloxine dye methods) was 3,300 cells/μL with a neutrophil (heterophil) count of 2,640/μL (80% of the cells), a large mononuclear cell count of 495/μL (15% of the cells), and a lymphocyte count of 165/μL (5% of the cells). The erythrocyte count was 673 RBCs/μL. No organisms were seen.

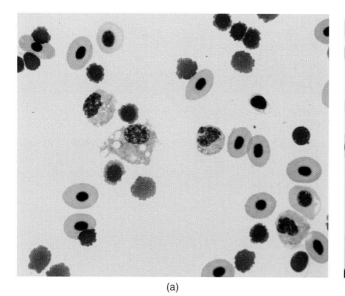
(a)

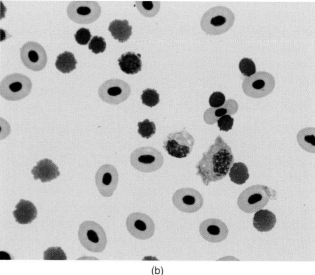
(b)

Fig. 81.3. (a and b) Images of the blood film (Wright–Giemsa stain, 100×).

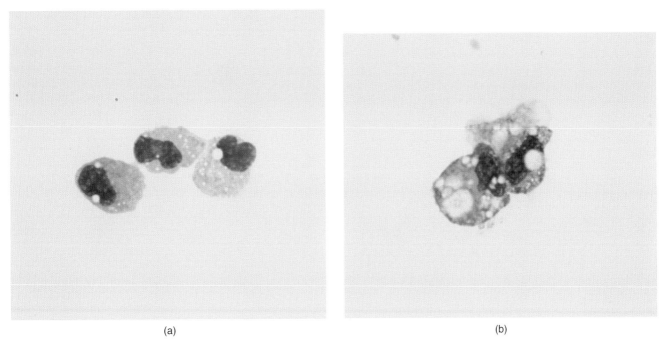

(a)

Fig. 81.4. (a and b) The image of coelomic fluid (Wright–Giemsa stain, 100×).

Summary

The leukogram and fluid analysis support a suppurative coelomitis. Causes for this condition include a septic bacterial infection, hepatobiliary disease, reproductive disease, or neoplasia. A coelomic ultrasound was offered as a means to further evaluate the coelomic cavity; however, this was declined by the client. The fish was given a poor prognosis for survival based on the diagnostic findings. Enrofloxacin (1 mL of a 22.7 mg/mL solution given intramuscularly using muscles near dorsal fin) was to be given daily for 10 days. The client was instructed to return in 2 weeks, if not sooner, for reevaluation.

The goldfish died 3 days later. On external examination at necropsy, there was marked generalized edema of the skin and scales. Additionally, the coelom was markedly distended. Present within the coelomic cavity, there was approximately 2 mL of purulent exudate. Disseminated throughout the kidneys bilaterally, there were multifocal, tan, firm lesions that were well-demarcated, compressive, and off-white on cut surface. Similar foci were present throughout the hepatic parenchyma. Ventral to the right pectoral fin, there was a focal cutaneous ulcer with minimal associated hemorrhage. Following histological review of the tissues, a diagnosis of a severe diffuse subacute granulomatous interstitial nephritis with necrosis, severe subacute multifocal to coalescing granulomatous hepatitis with necrosis, severe subacute generalized pyogranulomatous coelomitis, and a focal acute hemorrhagic and ulcerative dermatitis with cutaneous edema was made. No etiologic agent was found.

A 6-Year-Old Fish with a Red Mass Protruding from the Vent

82

Signalment

A 6-year-old Oscar (*Astronotus ocellatus*) was presented with a red mass protruding from the vent (Fig. 82.1).

History

The fish developed a red mass that protruded from the vent 2 days prior to presentation. The fish was housed in a 55-gallon freshwater aquarium with two Plecostomus fish (*Hypostomus* sp.) that had been housed with the Oscar for 4 years. The water temperature was kept at 80°F, and the water quality parameters were normal. The fish was fed a diet of shrimp, earthworms, and commercial cichlid pellets. There had been no additions or changes to the aquarium in 4 years.

Physical Examination Findings

The fish behaved normally and appeared to be in good body condition. It weighed 540 g. A 2 cm red tubular mass protruded from the vent (Fig. 82.1). The mass appeared to be a prolapsed rectum. The fish was placed under a general anesthetic using 100 ppm tricaine methanesulfonate with an equal amount of sodium bicarbonate for induction and maintained with 75 ppm for better evaluation. A 5 mm diameter spherical mass expanding from the rectum was found on closer inspection. The mass was removed using a CO_2 laser, using an 0.8 mm ceramic tip at a 4 W, continuous setting. The cut surface of the mass revealed an irregular, firm, and mottled red to tan tissue. An impression of the mass was made for cytologic evaluation (Figs. 82.2 and 82.3). The mass was placed in 10% neutral buffered formalin for histological examination. Reduction of the prolapsed rectum was attempted using 4-0 nylon suture to anchor the tissue to the vent using seven interrupted sutures. As soon as the prolapse was reduced, the fish was quickly

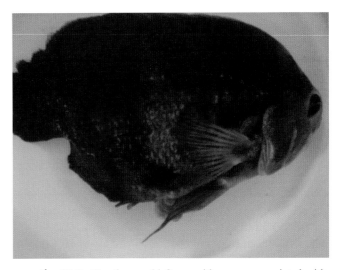

Fig. 82.1. The 6-year-old Oscar with a mass associated with the vent.

moved into a container with freshwater for anesthetic recovery. The fish recovered within 5 minutes of placement into the recovery water.

Interpretive Discussion

Figures 82.2 and 82.3 reveal a population of large cells with eccentric nuclei that tend to exfoliate as single cells and several erythrocytes. The cells have large, round to oval nuclei with coarsely clumped chromatin and large, round to oval nucleoli. The cells are pleomorphic and often have ill-defined borders in places. The cytoplasm is abundant, stains deeply basophilic, and appears foamy. The cytological features are those of malignancy and the cell type is more mesenchymal than epithelial, suggestive of a sarcoma. The features are not specific to the type of sarcoma, but the appearances of the cells suggest an aggressive malignancy.

333

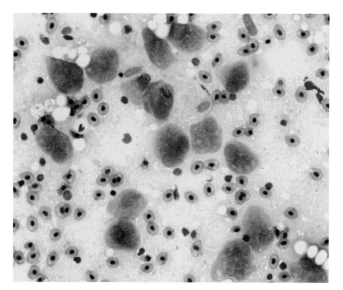

Fig. 82.2. An image from an imprint of the mass (Wright–Giemsa stain, 50×).

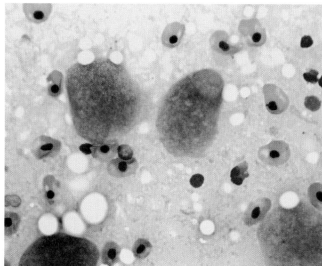

Fig. 82.3. An image from an imprint of the mass (Wright–Giemsa stain, 100×).

Summary

Histology of the biopsy of the mass was characterized by an outer layer composed of rectal mucosa, which was extensively eroded with multifocal areas of necrosis admixed with viable and degenerative neutrophils. Within the lumen of this outer layer, there was a segment of histologically normal intestine (colon). Between the eroded intestine and normal intestine, there was an infiltrate of a loose network of neoplastic endothelial cells, which arranged into clefts. These cells had indistinct cell borders with variable amounts of eosinophilic cytoplasm. Nuclei were pleomorphic, large, and round with finely stippled chromatin and one to two prominent round basophilic nucleoli. Nucleated erythrocytes were found within these clefts created by the endothelial cells. The neoplastic cells often rested on an amorphous eosinophilic scaffold. Mitoses were rare. Neovascularization was multifocally found throughout the tissue. These findings supported the histodiagnosis of a hemangiosarcoma.

The fish did well according to the owner for 1 week following surgery; however, after that period, the rectal prolapse recurred. Sutures remained intact around the vent, indicating the rectal tissue failed to hold the sutures. When this happened, the fish became lethargic and stopped eating and defecating. The fish was euthanized with an overdose of tricaine methanesulfonate 1 week later because of the recurrence of the prolapsed rectum and the cytologic and histologic findings of a malignant neoplasm. A necropsy revealed that the rectal mass and all other anatomical structures appeared normal.

An Adult Stingray with Skin Masses

83

Signalment

An adult female Southern stingray (*Dasyatis americana*) was presented for multiple skin masses on the underside of her wings of 2-month duration (Fig. 83.1).

History

This stingray is one of 24 stingrays housed in a 12,000-gallon touch pool exhibit in a public aquarium. Ten pounds of shrimp, squid, and cut fish, such as pollack, smelt, capelin, and mackerel, are fed to the stingrays in the exhibit each day and fish-fed by the public. The diet was supplemented weekly with a commercial elasmobranch vitamin. An aquarist at the aquarium had concerns about raised, red lesions on the ventral side of the stingray. The lesions had been slowly growing larger in a 2-month period.

Physical Examination Findings

The stingray was removed from the exhibit for evaluation. The ray had one large (2.5 cm diameter) and an adjacent small (1 cm diameter) raised reddened lesion on the ventral aspect of her right wing. An ultrasound examination revealed no abnormal findings. A blood sample was obtained via caudal venipuncture for a blood profile, and a fine-needle aspiration biopsy of one of the largest masses was obtained for cytologic examination. No bleeding was observed following the aspiration biopsy (Tables 83.1 and 83.2 and Figs. 83.2 and 83.3).

Interpretive Discussion

The hemogram indicates a normal packed cell volume and total leukocyte count; however, there is a heterophilia (increase in G_1 granulocytes) and lymphope-nia. This finding could be associated with a stress leukogram or a mild inflammatory response.

Figure 83.2a reveals a clump of seven heterophils (G_1 granulocytes) with normal morphology, a lymphocyte, three thrombocytes, and erythrocytes. Figure 83.2b reveals three heterophils, four lymphocytes, a monocyte, and erythrocytes. The cells in Fig. 83.2c include five thrombocytes, a lymphocyte (round cell with scant blue cytoplasm), and erythrocytes (the erythrocyte in the center appears hypochromatic).

In general, plasma chemistry values, except for blood urea nitrogen (BUN), of elasmobranchs are loosely interpreted in the same manner as those of other animals. Osmoregulation of marine elasmobranchs is maintained by a high concentration of urea nitrogen

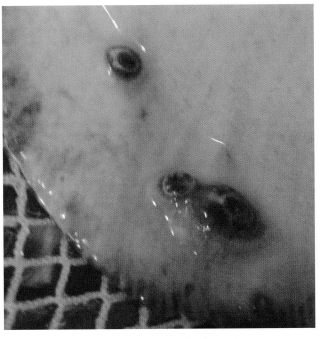

Fig. 83.1. The skin lesion on the Southern stingray.

Table 83.1. Hematology results.

		Reference[a]
PCV (%)	27	23–24
Leukocytes		
WBC ($10^3/\mu$L)	13.7	6.2–13.6
Heterophils (G$_1$) ($10^3/\mu$L)	12.5	2.9–5.7
Heterophils (G$_1$) (%)	91	42–47
Neutrophils (G$_2$) ($10^3/\mu$L)	0	0.1
Neutrophils (G$_2$) (%)	0	0–1
Lymphocytes ($10^3/\mu$L)	1.0	3.2–7.3
Lymphocytes (%)	7	52–54
Monocytes ($10^3/\mu$L)	0	0–0.3
Monocytes (%)	0	0–2
Eosinophils ($10^3/\mu$L)	0	0.1–0.2
Eosinophils (%)	0	1–3
Basophils ($10^3/\mu$L)	0.3	0–0.1
Basophils (%)	2	0–1
Thrombocytes		
Estimated number	Adequate	1–5/1,000× field
Morphology	Normal	
Plasma protein (refractometry) (g/dL)	6.7	5.7–7.8

[a]Range from previous two blood profiles during wellness examinations.

Table 83.2. Plasma biochemical results.

		Reference[a]	Reference[b]
Glucose (mg/dL)	40	26–32	36.5 (12–58)
BUN (mg/dL)	710	1,056–1,090	1,052.5 (609–1,330)
Creatinine (mg/dL)	<0.1	<0.1	0.35 (0–0.7)
Total protein (biuret) (g/dL)	3.8	2.8–4.8	2.7 (2.1–4.9)
Albumin (g/dL)	0.6	0–0.5	—
Globulin (g/dL)	3.2	2.3–3.8	1.6 (1.1–3.9)
A/G ratio	0.2	0.2–0.3	—
Alkaline phosphatase (IU/L)	7	8	21 (1–54)[c]
Aspartate aminotransferase (IU/L)	33	7–15	11 (1–55)[c]
Alanine aminotransferase (IU/L)	7	5	—
γ-Glutamyltransferase (IU/L)	1	1	7 (0–15)
Creatine kinase (IU/L)	680	124–336	312 (69–1,409)
Calcium (mg/dL)	16.6	16.1–17.1	16.3 (14–18.3)
Phosphorus (mg/dL)	4.3	5–5.9	4.35 (3.1–7.1)
Sodium (mEq/L)	280	273–274	273.5 (180–292)
Potassium (mEq/L)	2.7	1.7–3.7	3.5 (1.7–5.8)
Chloride (mEq/L)	283	229–280	265.5 (140–313)
Bicarbonate (mEq/L)	5.4	3–5.6	4.4 (3.1–5.7)
Anion gap (calculated)	−6	−6 to 41	—
Cholesterol (mg/dL)	116	157–175	143 (90–291)
Calculated osmolality	782	890–905	—
Amylase (IU/L)	8	—	—
Iron (μg/dL)	43	—	—
Lipemia (mg/dL)	1	—	—
Hemolysis (mg/dL)	61	—	—
Icterus (mg/dL)	0	—	—

[a]From previous blood profile during wellness examination.
[b]Median (min/max) from 20 Southern stingrays during routine physical examination.
[c]Collected from 11 stingrays.

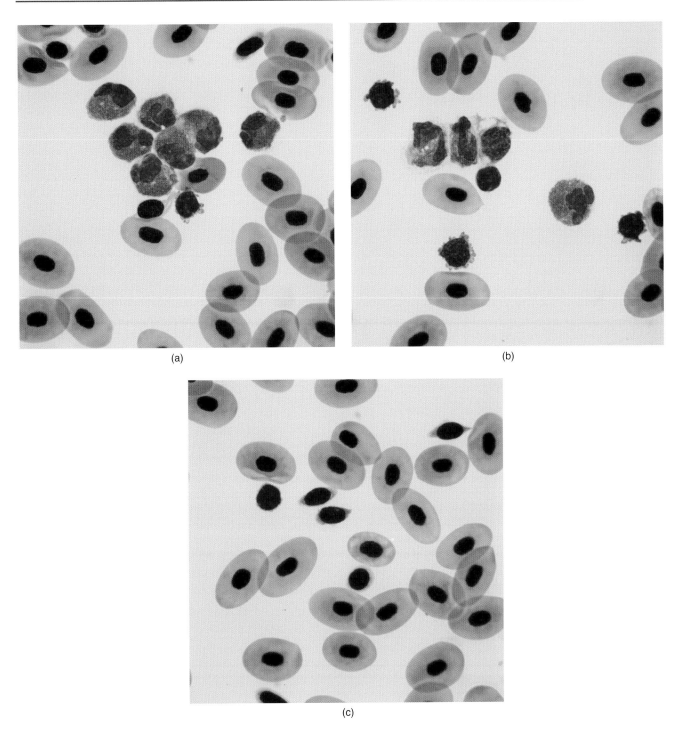

(a)

(b)

(c)

Fig. 83.2. (a–c) Blood films (Wright–Giemsa stain, 100×).

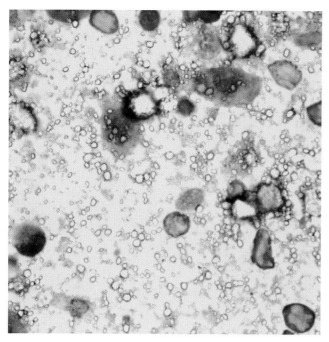

Fig. 83.3. An aspirate of skin mass (Wright–Giemsa stain, 100×).

and to some extent sodium and chloride in the blood and involves the kidneys, rectal glands, gills, and diet (Olson, 1999). A high level of urea is maintained by renal tubular reabsorption. The rectal gland of marine elasmobranchs is a salt-secreting organ; however, two-thirds of the total sodium and chloride excreted by elasmobranchs occur in the gills, whereas their gills have low permeability to urea. Finally, metabolic urea is directly related to food availability. Therefore, the low BUN in this ray is likely associated with either a decreased dietary intake or renal tubular reabsorption of urea.

The increased plasma creatine kinase activity is likely associated with muscle exertion or trauma associ-

ated with capture and restraint. Likewise, the increased plasma aspartate aminotransferase activity may also be associated with muscle activity; however, hepatocellular injury cannot be completely ruled out.

Figure 83.3 reveals refractile crystals of varying sizes. These crystals were seen throughout the specimen with few cells present. A cytodiagnosis of calcinosis circumscripta was made based on this finding.

Summary

One week later, a punch biopsy was obtained to further evaluate the lesions for histopathologic evaluation. A section of the tissue consisted of areas of mineralization. The mineralization was characterized by clumps of mineralized debris surrounded by large epithelioid macrophages and fibroblasts. There was fibrosis that dissects throughout the section, and the overlying epithelium was thickened, acanthotic, focally ulcerated, and covered by debris. This finding was indicative of calcinosis circumscripta, a typically benign lesion often seen in dogs and considered to be due to mineralization of necrotic tissues secondary to tissue trauma or inflammation (Marcos et al., 2006). The same pathogenesis was likely to be occurring within this Southern ray.

Complete surgical removal of the lesions is the recommended treatment for this disorder. Owing to the location and full-thickness nature of the lesions on the stingray, complete removal of the lesion would have resulted in the creation of large holes in the wing of the stingray. Instead, the ray was anesthetized using 100 ppm tricaine methanesulfonate (MS-222) with equal parts sodium bicarbonate, and the lesions were partially removed and ablated using a CO_2 laser (0.8 mm ceramic tip, 6 W, continuous superpulse settings). Four months postoperatively, the lesions were shrinking in size and barely noticeable.

84

An Adult Fish with a Mass Projecting from the Gills

Signalment

An adult Clown knife (*Chitala chitala*) of unknown gender was presented for a mass projecting from the gills (Fig. 84.1).

History

According to the aquarist at the public aquarium, a slow-growing mass had been developing on the right gill of the adult Clown knife during the past several months. The fish was housed in an 11,000-gallon freshwater aquarium with other Clown knife fish, Asian arowana (*Scleropages formosus*), Tiger fish (*Datnioides microlepsis*), Giant gourami (*Osphronemus gorami*), and Barramundi (*Lates calcarifer*).

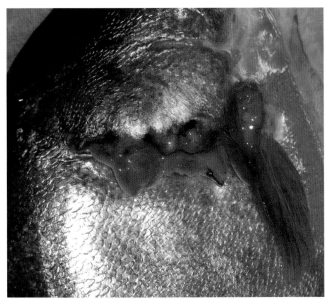

Fig. 84.1. The lesion on the Clown knife fish.

Physical Examination Findings

The physical examination was made following application of a general anesthetic using 100 ppm tricaine methanesulfonate (MS-222) with an equal concentration of sodium bicarbonate. The mass was determined to be growing from the trailing edge of the operculum, covering the right gill and not involving gill tissue. A biopsy was obtained using a CO_2 laser for cytologic and histopathologic examination.

Interpretive Discussion

Figure 84.2a reveals numerous erythrocytes and an aggregate of epithelial cells with abundant blue–gray cytoplasm and large nuclei with coarse nuclear chromatin. Figure 84.2b reveals squamous epithelial cells, resembling those in Fig. 84.2a. These cells appear more mature than those in the previous image. Figure 84.2c reveals numerous erythrocytes, three mesenchymal cells with darker blue cytoplasm, and oval nuclei with coarse chromatin. There is no evidence of inflammation and the cells do not have prominent features of malignant neoplasia; therefore, the cells in these images likely represent epithelial cell and mesenchymal cell hyperplasia.

Summary

A section of tissues obtained from the mass on the operculum revealed a proliferative mass on histopathology. The mass consisted of a central area of loose fibrous tissue that formed numerous papillary folds and fronds covered by thickened but normal-appearing epithelium. The histopathologic diagnosis was a fibropapilloma.

The fibropapilloma was removed in its entirety along its broad-based attachment to the operculum

339

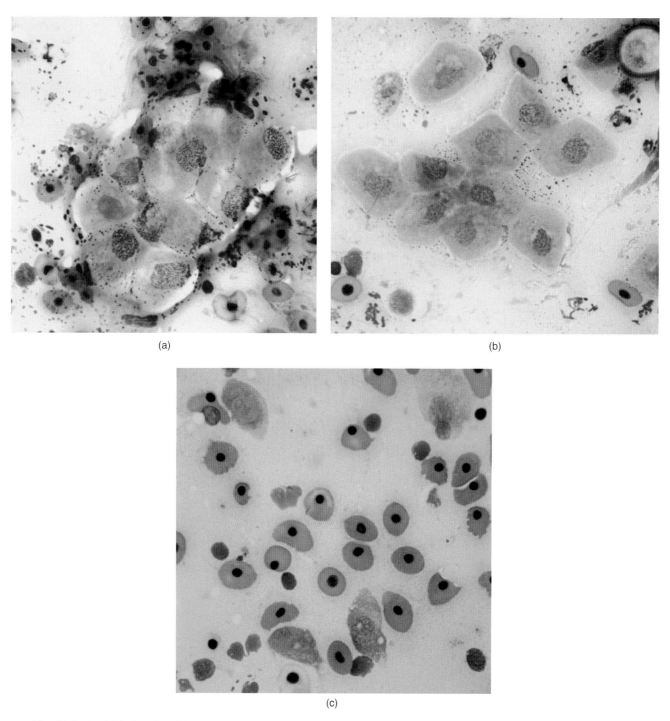

(a)

(b)

(c)

Fig. 84.2. (a–c) The imprint of the mass (Wright–Giemsa stain, 100 ×).

using the same anesthetic protocol and a CO_2 laser. Ablation of the base of the mass using the laser provided temporary resolution of the lesion, and recurrence was seen 1 year later. At that time, the procedure was repeated, except the base of the fibropapilloma was treated with cryosurgery. No recurrence has been noted after 12 months.

Papillomas have been reported in several species of freshwater and marine fish. The suspected etiologic agents for these growths include a virus (i.e., herpesvirus, retrovirus, or birnavirus), parasite, or toxin (i.e., okadaic acid from the dinoflagellates, *Prorocentrum*) (Noga, 2000). The benign papilloma form can progress to a locally invasive squamous cell carcinoma.

A 5-Year-Old Fish with Bloating and Constipation

85

Signalment

A 5-year-old Oscar (*Astronotus ocellatus*) was presented with a complaint of bloating and constipation.

History

The fish was housed in a 125-gallon freshwater aquarium with another cichlid, a Severum (*Hero severum*). The fish were usually fed a commercial cichlid pelleted diet; however, recently they had been fed peas as the owner thought the fish was constipated. The pea diet had not helped with the constipation. The fish were overfed 3 weeks earlier and a second Oscar died shortly afterward. Since then, this patient had not defecated. The other fish remained healthy. The water temperature was kept at 81°F and the water quality parameters had been normal. The aquarium was equipped with a bead filter and ultraviolet sterilizer. There had been no recent additions or changes to the aquarium.

Physical Examination Findings

On presentation, the 26-cm long fish behaved normally and appeared to be in good body condition. The skin on the head and lateral line revealed moderate ulcerations associated with lateral line disease. Bulging of the coelomic cavity was noted bilaterally just caudal to the pectoral fins in the area of the stomach (Fig. 85.1).

The fish was placed under a general anesthetic using 100 ppm tricaine methanesulfonate with an equal amount of sodium bicarbonate for induction and maintained with 75 ppm for a radiographic examination. The lateral radiographic image had poor coelomic detail and revealed only a lobed swim bladder; however, no radiodense foreign object or dilated loops of bowel could be found (Fig. 85.2).

An ultrasound examination of the coelomic cavity was also performed at that time. This examination

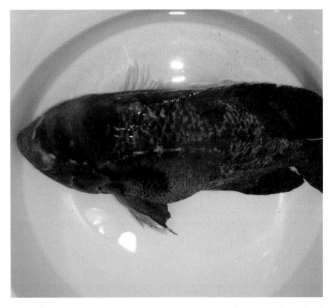

Fig. 85.1. The 5-year-old Oscar with possible gastrointestinal obstruction and lateral bulge seen here.

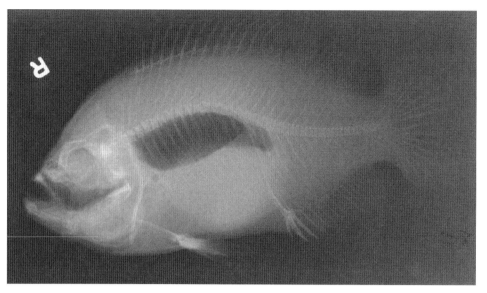

Fig. 85.2. The lateral radiograph of the fish.

revealed an enlarged fluid-filled stomach with roe-like (fish egg-like) material adhering to the stomach wall.

Interpretive Discussion

Figure 85.3a reveals erythrocytes and a cluster of five nondegenerate heterophils. Figure 85.3b shows erythrocytes and a macrophage exhibiting erythrophagocytosis. Figure 85.3c shows a large foamy macrophage, exhibiting erythrophagocytosis, numerous erythrocytes, and two nondegenerate heterophils. These images reveal a mixed cell inflammatory response associated with hemorrhage in the stomach and support the cytodiagnosis of a hemorrhagic gastritis.

Summary

An exploratory celiotomy was performed based on the cytodiagnosis of gastritis and the ultrasound findings, suggesting either gastric foreign bodies or impaction. The fish was again placed under a general anesthetic using 100 ppm tricaine methanesulfonate with an equal amount of sodium bicarbonate for induction and maintained with 75 ppm for an exploratory celiotomy.

The fish was placed in dorsal recumbency in a 75 ppm tricaine bath used for anesthesia. A number 5.5 endotracheal tube was placed in the mouth for delivery of the anesthetic solution across the gills. A number 10 blade was used to make a 4 cm incision on the ventral midline. The stomach was identified and two stay sutures were placed in the stomach using a 3-0 suture material (monofilament glycomer 631). A number 15 blade was used to make a 1 cm incision into the stomach, and 20 mL of a blood-like fluid was aspirated from the stomach using a syringe and suction. The mucosal surface of the stomach was lined with hemorrhagic bead-like mucus. The majority of the material was removed from the stomach (Fig. 85.4).

A number 5 French feeding tube was inserted into the stomach and passed through the intestines, causing a small amount of feces to exit from the vent indicating no obstruction distal to the stomach. A small biopsy of the stomach was collected for histopathologic examination. The stomach was closed with a 4-0 monofilament glycomer 631 using a simple continuous pattern. Enrofloxacin (0.3 mL of 2.27% solution) was deposited into the coelomic cavity before closure. The skin and body wall were closed with 3-0 nylon in a simple continuous pattern.

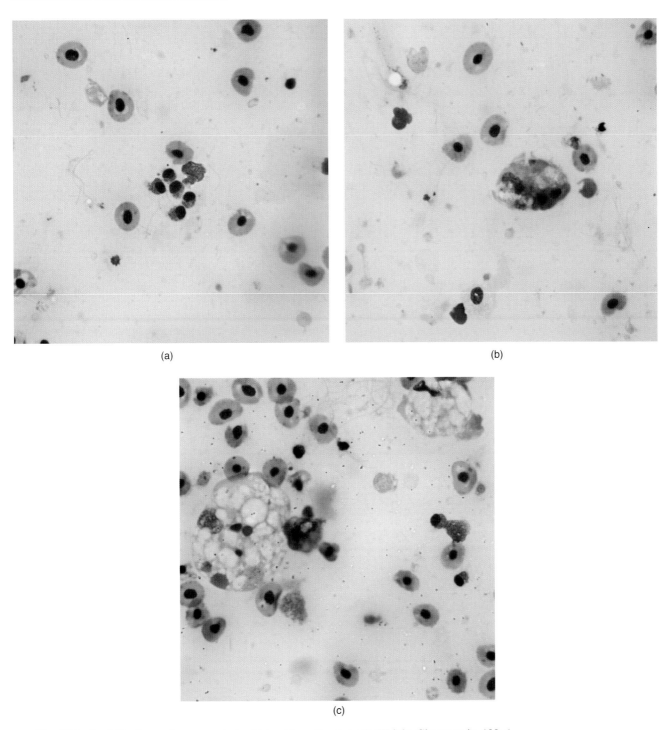

(a)

(b)

(c)

Fig. 85.3. (a–c) The image from an aspirate obtained from the stomach (Wright–Giemsa stain, 100×).

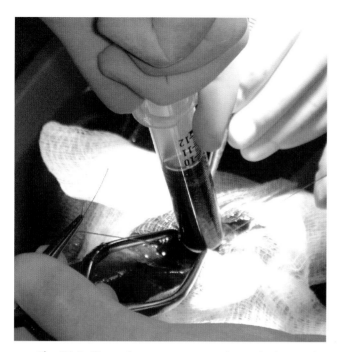

Fig. 85.4. The exploratory gastrotomy, hemorrhagic material removed.

Immediately following the closure of the body wall incision, the fish was moved into a container with freshwater for anesthetic recovery. The fish recovered within 5 minutes of placement into the recovery water.

A portion of the fluid obtained from the stomach was submitted for microbial culture. The fish was given a poor prognosis for survival because of the extent of the hemorrhagic gastritis. The client was instructed to give 0.3 mL of 2.27% enrofloxacin as an intracoelomic injection every other day for two treatments beginning in 2 days. Trimethoprim-sulfa (960 mg per 10 gallons of water) was also given as a prolonged immersion treatment for 5 days.

The histopathologic report of the stomach revealed many heterophils, lymphocytes, plasma cells, and chromatophores. There were areas of mineralization, but no evidence of neoplasia. The histopathologic diagnosis was heterophilic gastritis.

Bacterial culture of the stomach fluid failed to grow an organism. It is likely that the gastritis was associated with overfeeding that resulted in trauma to the stomach or the fish consumed an unknown toxin that severely irritated the lining of the stomach.

An Adult Fish with Lesions Around Its Mouth

86

Signalment

A banded rainbow fish (*Melanotaenia trifasciata*) was presented with lesions around its mouth.

History

This fish was one of many rainbow fish housed in a 1,200-gallon freshwater aquarium. Four rainbow fish were isolated into a separate aquarium because they had developed white, cotton-like lesions around the mouth. The lesions did not interfere with their ability to eat, and the fish displayed normal activity in the tank.

Physical Examination Findings

The four fish in quarantine were observed and appeared to have normal activity and swim function. The only abnormality noted on all fish was small, white, cotton-like lesions around the mouth (Fig. 86.1).

A scraping of the lesion for cytological evaluation was obtained from one fish after it was netted (Fig. 86.2).

Interpretive Discussion

Figures 86.3a and 86.3b reveal a highly cellular sample populated by round cells and erythrocytes. The majority of the round cells are large lymphocytes with scant amount of blue cytoplasm and nuclei with smooth nuclear chromatin. The nuclei frequently reveal prominent nucleoli, and mitotic figures are frequently seen. Figure 86.3b also reveals two macrophages. The cytologic examination indicates lymphoid neoplasia, lymphoma.

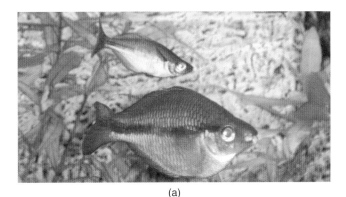

(a)

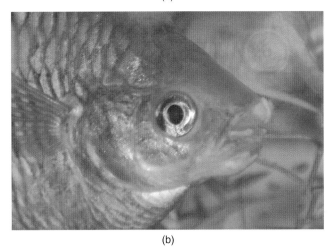

(b)

Fig. 86.1. (a) A gross image of lesion around the fish mouth. (b) A close-up of similar lesion from another fish in the same tank.

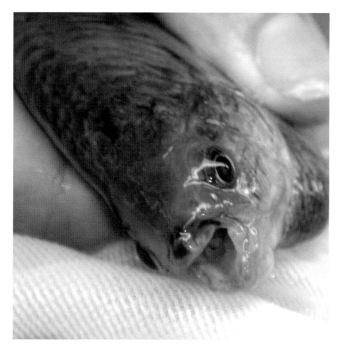

Fig. 86.2. The gross appearance of the mouth after the scraping.

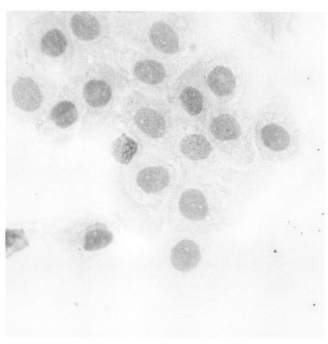

Fig. 86.4. The cytology of a second rainbow fish skin lesion (Wright–Giemsa stain, 100×).

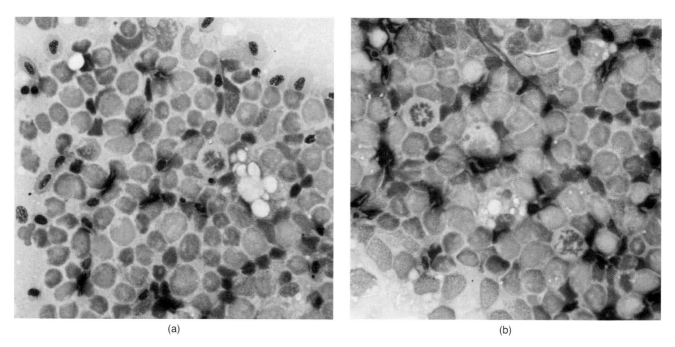

(a)   (b)

Fig. 86.3. (a and b) The cytology of the mouth lesion (Wright–Giemsa stain, 100×).

Summary

It is likely that the fish with lymphoma is not representative of the disease affecting the population of rainbow fish. The fish that was initially sampled died the following day; however, a necropsy was not performed. Subsequent samples were collected from other fish with similar lesions on two different occasions. Some of the fish exhibited similar lesions along the sides of their body as well. The cytology results from scrapings of the lesions on these fish revealed only sheets of a uniform population of epithelial cells indicative of epithelial hyperplasia, indicating chronic stimulation of the epithelium (Fig. 86.4). Several months later, as the problem continued, the Tiger prawn (*Panaeus monodon*) that shares the tank with the rainbow fish was observed eating one of the rainbow fish (Fig. 86.5). The lesions are possibly the result of trauma associated with encounters with the prawn.

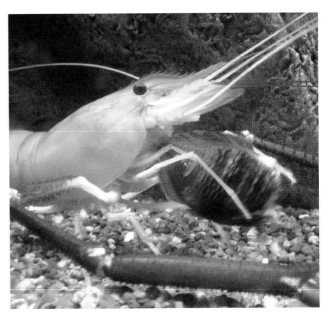

Fig. 86.5. A Tiger prawn eating a rainbow fish.

An Adult Fish with a Large Red Mass on Its Belly

87

Signalment

An adult Red-tailed catfish (*Phractocephalus hemioliopterus*) of unknown gender was presented for a large red mass on its belly (Fig. 87.1).

History

According to the aquarist at the public aquarium, a slow-growing mass had been developing on the abdomen of the grossly overweight Red-tailed catfish during the past several months. The fish was housed in a 9,482-gallon freshwater aquarium with Pacu (*Piaractus* sp.), Arapaima (*Arapaima gigas*), an Ocellated stingray (*Potamotrygon motoro*), and a Reticulated stingray (*Potamotrygon reticulata*).

Physical Examination Findings

The physical examination was made following application of a general anesthetic using 100 ppm tricaine methanesulfonate with an equal concentration of sodium bicarbonate. The mass was determined to be growing in the belly skin only. It appeared cystic and collapsed once the fluid (4 mL) was removed using a 22-gauge needle and 3 mL syringe. The fluid was poorly cellular and had a specific gravity of 1.002. The overlying tissue covering the cystic mass was surgically removed using a scalpel blade. An imprint for cytology was made and the tissue was submitted for histopathologic examination.

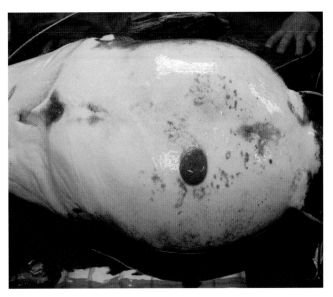

Fig. 87.1. An image of the Red-tailed catfish with a lesion on its belly.

Interpretive Discussion

Figure 87.2a shows a poorly cellular sample with a few erythrocytes and two lymphocytes. Figure 87.2b shows a few erythrocytes, a thrombocyte, and a single fibroblast. The appearance of the thrombocyte indicates peripheral blood contamination of the sample. The cytologic examination indicates a transudative effusion with mild peripheral blood contamination.

349

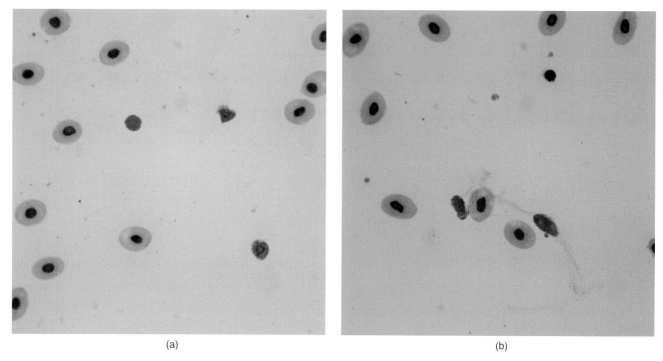

(a)   (b)

Fig. 87.2. (a and b) The imprint of the mass (Wright–Giemsa stain, 100×).

Summary

The tissue was lined by epidermis and was composed of varyingly maturing granulation tissue, according to the histopathology. Along the margins, this granulation tissue was moderately collagenous and contained numerous blood vessels. The blood vessels were perpendicular to the collagen deposition. Most of the center of this mass contained large sinus-like structures filled with moderately proteinaceous fluid, containing numerous vascular channels and wispy strands of fibroblastic tissues. The histopathologic diagnosis was an organizing seroma.

It is likely that this large blister was created by the skin rubbing along objects in the aquarium. This is likely related to the fish's obesity.

A 3-Year-Old Fish with a Growth below the Eye

88

Signalment

A 3-year-old plecostomus (*Hypostomus plecostomus*) was presented with a growth below the left eye.

History

The mass was first noticed by the owner approximately 5 days prior to presentation and had been increasing in size. The owner also noted the fish had a cloudy left eye. There were no other problems noted and the fish was eating and swimming normally. The fish lived in a large tank with catfish, Clown loaches (*Botia macracanthus*), and cichlids.

Physical Examination Findings

On physical examination, the fish was bright, alert, and responsive. He measured 12 cm in length. A 5 mm elliptical, pedunculated, subcutaneous, firm mass was noticed on the left side of the fish just cranial to the pectoral fin and ventral to the eye (Fig. 88.1). There was also corneal opacity associated with the left eye.

A fine-needle aspirate of the mass was performed. A radiograph was taken to evaluate for bony involvement (Figs. 88.2–88.4).

Interpretive Discussion

The radiograph (Fig. 88.2) showed a mild focal soft-tissue swelling laterally over the caudal aspect of the left side of the head. In this plane, the focal soft-tissue swelling occurs just caudal to the level of the operculum and at the same level of the base of the left pectoral fin. There were no underlying bony abnormalities.

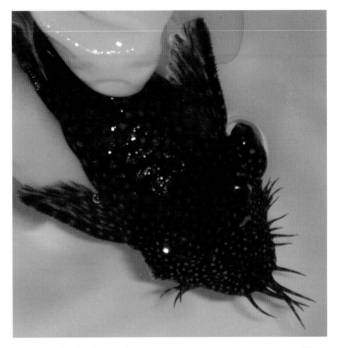

Fig. 88.1. A gross image of the mass on the plecostomus. Note the large mass just cranial to the left pectoral fin on the right side of the image of the fish. The corneal opacity in the left eye is also seen.

Figure 88.3 shows a highly cellular sample with a predominance of macrophages with foamy cytoplasm. Numerous erythrocytes and a heterophil (upper right corner of image) are also present. This indicates a macrophagic inflammation.

Figure 88.4a shows multinucleated macrophages. Figure 88.4b reveals crystals in the background that resemble cholesterol crystals. The cytologic result resembles that found in a xanthomatous lesion in avian and mammalian skin; however, the gross appearance of the

351

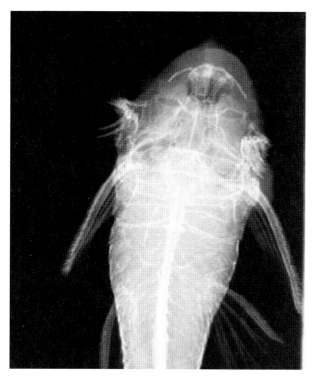

Fig. 88.2. The radiograph of dorsoventral view of the fish.

lesion lacks the yellow color of a xanthoma. The cytologic examination indicates a cholesterol granuloma.

Summary

The fish was placed under general anesthesia using 100 ppm tricaine methanesulfonate in the water (Fig. 88.5).

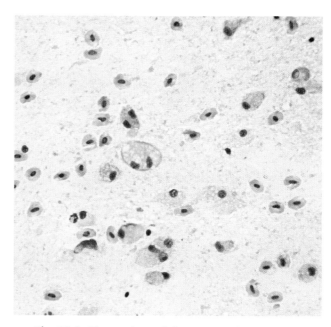

Fig. 88.3. The cytology of the mass (Wright–Giemsa stain, 50×).

A skin incision was made over the mass and an attempt to remove the entire mass was made; however, owing to a portion of the mass being adhered to the underlying bone and surrounding soft tissue, only part could be removed. The portion removed was submitted for histopathologic examination. The skin incision was closed using a simple interrupted 4-0 polytrimethylene carbonate suture.

The fish was treated postoperatively with an 18 ppm trimethoprim-sulfa solution as a 12-hour bath for

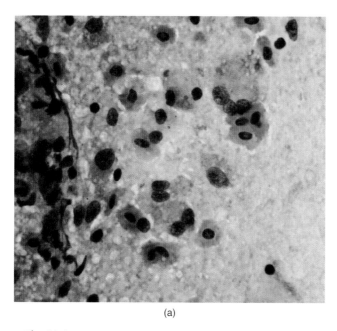

(a)

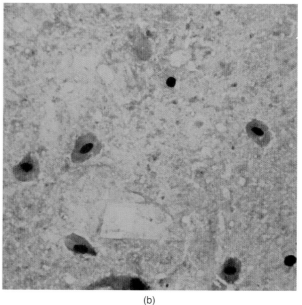

(b)

Fig. 88.4. (a and b) The cytology of the mass (Wright–Giemsa stain, 100×).

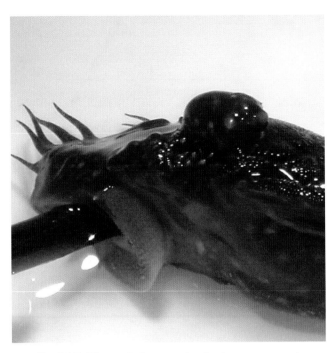

Fig. 88.5. The surgical preparation for the mass removal.

5–7 days. Fifty percent water changes were recommended daily between medications.

Histopathologic examination of the excised lesion revealed numerous cholesterol crystals associated with areas of previous hemorrhage or tissue necrosis, and a diagnosis of a cholesterol granuloma was made. It was not known how this fish developed this granuloma; however, traumatic injury resulting in hemorrhage into the tissue was a possible explanation. This condition is not often reported in fish. A cholesterol granuloma was reported in the heart of Piper gurnard (*Trigla lyra*), but the pathophysiology was unknown (Magi et al., 2009).

An Adult Fish with Increased Gilling and Eye Lesions

89

Signalment

An adult Lumpfish (*Cyclopterus lumpus*) was presented with increased gilling and eye lesions.

History

The Lumpfish was a recent arrival for exhibit at a public aquarium. It arrived with small, white spots above the eyes and exhibited rapid gilling behavior. It was shipped along with two other Lumpfish that also exhibited rapid gilling behavior. The fish were housed in a cold water (50°F) marine quarantine tank for observation.

Physical Examination Findings

On physical examination, the fish was gilling rapidly. There were small, white spots along the periorbital region of the left eye (Fig. 89.1).

A scraping of the lesion was conducted for cytological evaluation. The wet mount revealed numerous active organisms that moved around in a jerky manner. The organism in Figs. 89.2a and 89.2b repetitively stretched and recoiled when viewed under the microscope.

Interpretive Discussion

The parasites seen in this wet mount preparation (Figs. 89.2a and 89.2b) have a sucker-like appendage at one end that is surrounded with hooks. This structure resembles the opisthohaptor of a monogenean parasite (skin fluke). The organism appears to contain an embryo (the large vacuole-like structure inside the

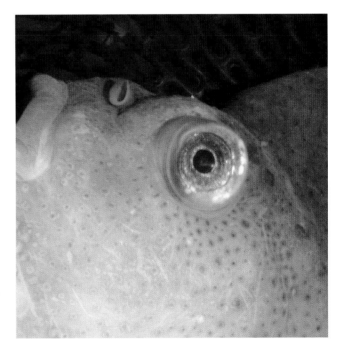

Fig. 89.1. A gross image of the white spots near the left eye of the Lumpfish.

parasite), suggesting that this monogenean is of the genus *Gyrodactylus*.

Summary

The quarantine tank was treated with 2 ppm praziquantel for 3 days. Following the treatment, the lesion above the eye disappeared and no monogeneans were seen on mucus scrapings. All three Lumpfish, however, continued their rapid gilling behavior.

355

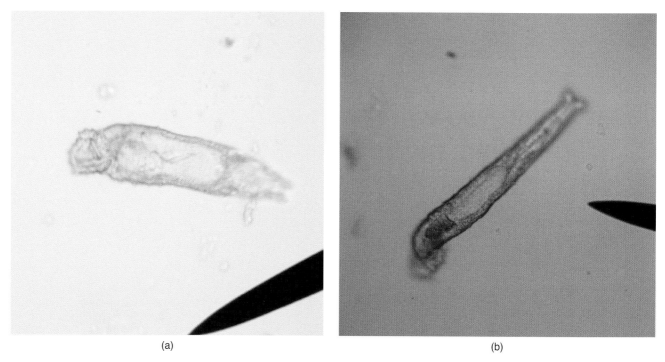

(a)   (b)

Fig. 89.2. (a and b) The wet mount of skin scraping (the organism measured 580 μm, 10×).

90

A Fish That Is a Sole Survivor of a Massive Fish Die-Off

Signalment

A Miniatus grouper (*Cephalopholis miniata*) was presented as a sole survivor of a saltwater aquarium that had experienced massive fish mortalities.

History

This grouper was kept in a 1,000-gallon aquarium with a variety of other fish, plants, and live coral and other invertebrates. According to the owner, the salinity of the aquarium varied from 30 ppt to 35 ppt owing to evaporation. The temperature was maintained at 80°F. The fish were fed either live feeder fish (goldfish, primarily) or frozen thawed fish cut into pieces. A new fish (Damselfish) was introduced into the aquarium 4 weeks earlier, but that fish died within a few days. The aquarium had experienced sporadic deaths during the past few weeks; however, all but one fish had died during the night. The grouper presented in grave condition and was not expected to survive.

Physical Examination Findings

The fish had been removed from the aquarium and presented in a 5-gallon bucket where it was floating on its side. The fish exhibited rapid gilling and had a marked buildup of the mucus covering on its skin. There were multifocal white patches or depigmented erosions on the skin. A mucus scraping was prepared for a wet mount examination. The wet mount preparation was teaming with motile protozoa (Figs. 90.1 and 90.2).

Interpretive Discussion

Figure 90.1 reveals the trophont of the holotrich ciliate protozoan, *Cryptocaryon irritans*. Cilia are evenly distributed over the spherical shaped body. The trophont

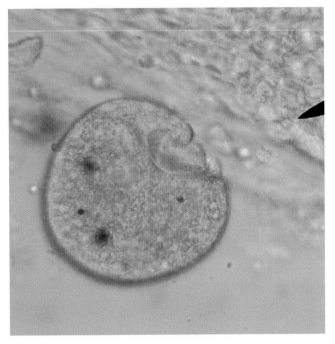

Fig. 90.1. A wet mount of mucus scraping (the round object at the end of the pointer measures 350 μm in diameter and moved in a slow rolling manner, 10×).

is identified by its round shape and slow tumbling movement on the wet mount. It is similar to *Ichthyophthirius multifiliis*, its freshwater counterpart. Unlike *I. multifiliis*, the macronucleus of *C. irritans* is concealed by the granular cytoplasm and is not seen on a wet mount preparation.

Figure 90.2 shows another holotrich ciliate protozoan, *Uronema marinum*. This active protozoan is identified by its pear shape and spiral movement. The one represented in the images appears more elongated than usual and thus has a greater long-axis measurement compared to others in the wet mount. *Uronema* is similar to *Tetrahymena* species, believed to be its counterpart found on freshwater fish.

357

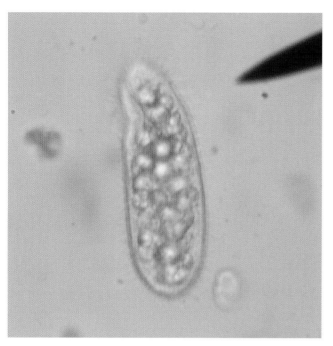

Fig. 90.2. A wet mount of mucus scraping (the ellipsoid object in the image measured 28 μm × 77 μm and rapidly moved around in a spiraling football-like motion, 40×).

Summary

Shortly following the mucus scraping, the grouper died. Treatment for ectoparasites in marine fish often involves the use of prolonged immersion with copper sulfate where free copper ions are maintained between 0.15 and 0.20 ppm or chelated copper. Formalin can also be used as a bath or prolonged immersion treatment for ectoparasites. The presence of live coral, plants, and invertebrates in the aquarium creates a challenge in effectively treating this aquarium for ectoparasites as copper and formalin treatments are likely to be lethal to those organisms. Treatment for *Cryptocaryon* involves lysis of the tomonts using hyposalinity (such as lowering the salinity to 18 ppt or less), which was suggested in the treatment of the aquarium. In this case, leaving the aquarium free of fish for 3 months was recommended as it may take a long time for emergence of the theronts left in the aquarium after the fish have gone. It is likely that the systemic or deep infestation with *Uronema* was the significant cause of the disease outbreak and high mortality in this case. The mixed infestation with two ectoparasites was likely a complicating factor as well.

91

An Adult Stingray Presented for Examination for Coccidia

Signalment

An adult male Yellow stingray (*Urobatis jamaicensis*) was presented for evaluation for coccidia.

History

One adult male and one adult female Yellow stingrays were recent arrivals to a local public aquarium. Prior to shipment, the rays were diagnosed with coccidia based on finding of oocysts in aspirates obtained from the spiral intestine. The stingrays were treated once with praziquantel before being shipped. On arrival to the aquarium, the stingrays were placed in a quarantine tank. Following 3 weeks since their arrival, the rays were presented for reevaluation of the coccidiosis. The rays were adjusting well and had no medical concerns.

Physical Examination Findings

On physical examination, both stingrays exhibited normal behavior and activity. They were captured with a small nylon net for closer observation and to collect samples (Fig. 91.1).

An ultrasound-guided aspirate of the spiral intestine of the male stingray was performed. The sample failed to show coccidian parasites or other significant findings. A cloacal wash was performed using a 5-French feeding tube and a 6 cc syringe. Approximately 1 mL of saltwater was administered into the cloaca of the male stingray and aspirated back into the syringe (Fig. 91.2).

Other Diagnostic Information

An ultrasound was also used to locate the spiral intestine of the female stingray in an attempt to aspirate the contents for detection of coccidian oocysts. An ultrasound image of the female stingray's uterus revealed an abundance of trophonemata (finger-like projections

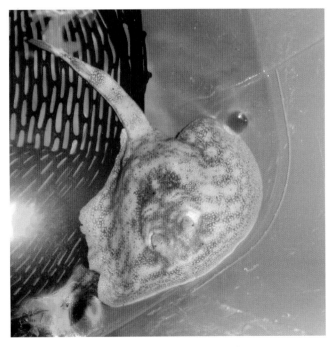

Fig. 91.1. The Yellow stingray at presentation.

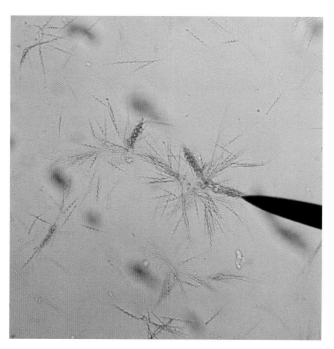

Fig. 91.2. The cloacal wash of the male Yellow-spotted stingray (wet mount, 10×).

of the uterine mucosa) among two fetuses. Trophone-mata are present during pregnancy to increase the surface area of the uterine mucosa. They deliver the histotroph (uterine milk) to the fetus during gestation (Hamlett and Koob, 1999).

Interpretive Discussion

The cloacal wash of the male stingray revealed many spiral-shaped spermatozoa. They were very active on the wet mount preparation and had a tendency to clump together as seen in Fig. 91.2.

Summary

An attempt to aspirate the contents of the spiral intestine of the female stingray was not performed because of her pregnancy. The female remained in quarantine throughout gestation.

92

An Adult Fish with a Large Mass on Its Operculum

Signalment

An adult Tinfoil barb (*Barbus schwanenfeldi*) was presented with a large mass caudal to the left operculum.

History

The Tinfoil barb was part of a large freshwater exhibit in a public aquarium. The fish lived in a 12,600-gallon aquarium inhabited by a variety of freshwater fish that was part of a water feature in an exhibit for Sumatran tigers (*Panthera tigris sumatrae*).

The mass was originally noted approximately 1 year prior to presentation and had recently demonstrated extensive growth. The fish was removed from the exhibit and placed in a quarantine facility for further examination.

Physical Examination Findings

On physical examination, the fish appeared to be in good body condition and was swimming in a normal fashion. The mass was located caudal to the left operculum and dorsal to the left pectoral fin. The mass measured 4 cm in diameter and protruded 1.5 cm from the body (Fig. 92.1a). It was ulcerated and felt firm on palpation (Fig. 92.1b). A fine-needle aspiration biopsy

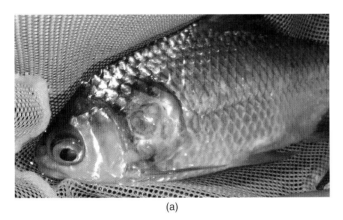

(a)

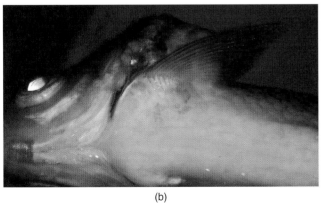

(b)

Fig. 92.1. The gross lesion on the Tinfoil barb: (a) lateral view of the lesion and (b) ventral view of the lesion.

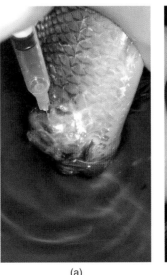

(a)

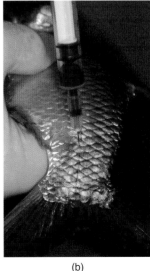

(b)

Fig. 92.2. (a) A fine-needle aspirate of the mass and (b) caudal venipuncture, lateral tail.

361

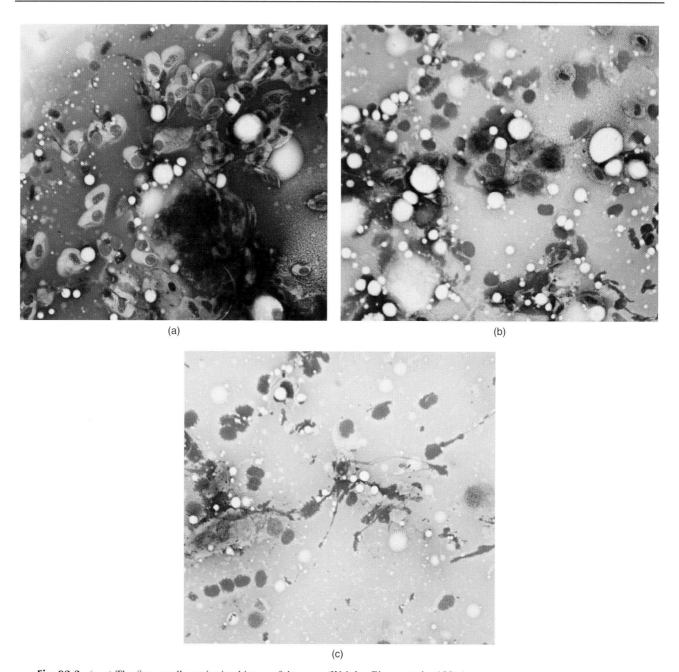

Fig. 92.3. (a–c) The fine-needle aspiration biopsy of the mass (Wright–Giemsa stain, 100×).

of the mass was performed for cytology, and a small blood sample was obtained via caudal venipuncture for preparation of a blood film (Figs. 92.2a and 92.2b). During the aspirate, the tumor felt "gritty." The packed cell volume of the blood was 32%, and the leukocyte differential revealed 31% neutrophils, 67% lymphocytes, and 2% monocytes (Figs. 92.3 and 92.4).

Interpretive Discussion

The images of the fine-needle aspiration biopsy of the mass reveal a poorly cellular sample that contains many erythrocytes. Cells other than erythrocytes appear to be embedded in a heavy eosinophilic background substance. These pleomorphic cells tend to be elongated to spindle-shaped with a basophilic cytoplasm and an

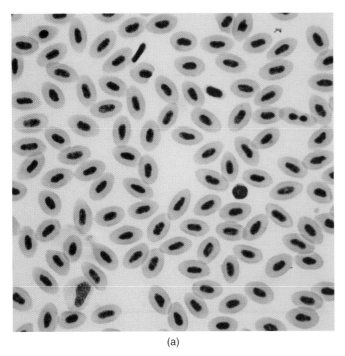

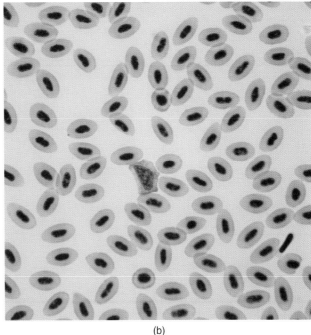

(a)

(b)

Fig. 92.4. (a and b) Blood films (Wright–Giemsa stain, 100×).

eccentrically positioned nucleus that contains coarsely granular nuclear chromatin and large prominent nucleoli. Figure 92.3a shows numerous erythrocytes with cells embedded in a heavy eosinophilic background, making it difficult to evaluate the cells. Figure 92.3b shows a thinner area that reveals cells with indistinct cytoplasmic margins, a high nucleus–cytoplasm ratio, basophilic cytoplasm, and nuclear pleomorphism. Figure 92.3c shows a thinner area with scattered mesenchymal cells with eccentrically positioned oval nuclei that contain coarsely granular chromatin and prominent large nucleoli. The cytoplasm is light blue and more abundant than cells observed in other fields. The oval to spindled cell on the right of the image has an abundant blue foamy cytoplasm with a distinct Golgi and an eccentrically positioned nucleus, features of an osteoblast. This poorly cellular sample that contains mesenchymal cells with features of malignancy embedded in a heavy eosinophilic background substance is indicative of either a chondrosarcoma or an osteosarcoma.

Figure 92.4a shows a neutrophil with a nonlobed nucleus, a lymphocyte, and two thrombocytes. Figure 92.4b shows a monocyte, a thrombocyte, and two polychromatic erythrocytes. The packed cell volume and leukocyte differential are presumed to be normal for a freshwater bony fish. The cells in the image reveal normal hemic cell morphology; therefore, the hematology appears to be within normal expectations for a healthy fish and not affected by the mass.

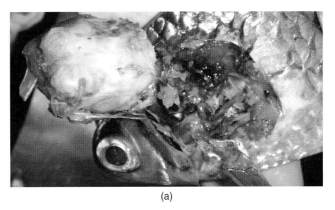

(a)

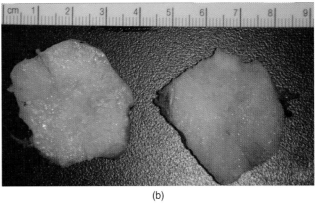

(b)

Fig. 92.5. (a) The mass removed during necropsy and (b) the cut surface of the mass.

Summary

Because of the location and apparent bony involvement of the lesion, the fish was euthanized with an overdose of tricaine methanesulfonate in the water. The necropsy revealed a well-circumscribed mass that extended deep into the operculum tissue. The tissue was very firm, difficult to remove, and the solid and white cut surface had a chalk-like texture (Figs. 92.5a and 92.5b).

Histopathologic results revealed the mass consisted of cartilage; however, the cartilage proliferated in a somewhat haphazard fashion. Cells were embedded within lacunae within a cartilaginous matrix. Nuclei were mildly pleomorphic, round, and had small nucleoli. Mitoses were not observed. Centrally, there were areas of ossification of the cartilage in the formation of bone. The histopathologic diagnosis was a chondrosarcoma.

93

An Adult Fish with a Mass on Its Side

Signalment

An adult Red-eye tetra (*Moenkhausia sanctaefilomenae*) was presented with a mass on its left side just behind the operculum.

History

The fish was presented with a 2-month history of having the mass on its left side. The owner reported that the fish exhibited normal behavior and activity but was concerned about the mass that had been growing in size.

Physical Examination Findings

On physical examination, the fish appeared to be in good body condition. There were no other abnormalities noted other than the raised lesion on the left side. The mass was 7 mm in diameter and not ulcerated although it was not covered by normal scaled skin (Fig. 93.1).

An impression of the mass was taken for cytological evaluation.

Interpretive Discussion

Figure 93.2a shows a macrophagic inflammation. Figure 93.2b also shows macrophagic inflammation along with the presence of numerous large rod-shaped organisms that stain negative with the Wright–Giemsa stain. This is supportive of a *Mycobacterium* sp. infection.

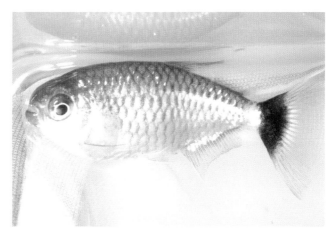

Fig. 93.1. The Red-eye tetra on presentation.

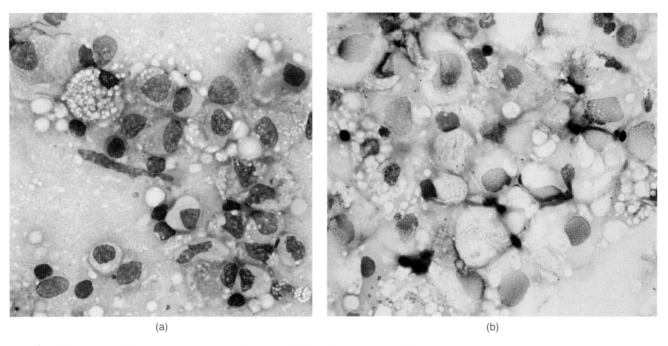

(a)   (b)

Fig. 93.2. (a and b) The impression smear of the mass (Wright–Giemsa stain, 100×).

Summary

An acid-fast stain was applied to a sample obtained from the lesion to help confirm the presence of *Mycobacterium*; however, that sample stained negatively for acid-fast. Although no acid-fast positive organisms were seen, a strong presumptive diagnosis of mycobacteriosis was made. An offer for microbial culture was made but declined by the owner owing to the zoonotic potential of an infection with *Mycobacterium* and the associated poor prognosis for treatment and survival. The client elected euthanasia. An offer for a postmortem examination was made, but declined by the client.

94

An Adult Fish with Ulcerative Skin Lesions

Signalment

An adult Koi (*Cyprinus carpio*) was presented for ulcerative skin lesions.

History

The client obtained the Koi from a farm in Hawaii approximately 1 year prior to presentation. The Koi was housed with 20 other Koi in a 17,000-gallon pond. During the previous summer, the pond experienced an increase in nitrite concentration. This was followed by this Koi along with three others in the pond developing ulcerative skin lesions in the fall. The other three Koi died within a few weeks of onset of the ulcerative skin lesions. Necropsies performed on those fish revealed a diagnosis of *Aeromonas salmonicida* infection (furunculosis), according to the owner. No treatment was given to any of the fish and no other fish became ill. This Koi survived the winter. It was presented now (spring) owing to continued ulcerative cutaneous lesions on its body and head.

Physical Examination Findings

On physical examination, the Koi appeared to be in good body condition and exhibited normal behavior and activity. The fish measured 12 inches in length. The only abnormalities found on examination were three ulcerative skin lesions, two on the body and one on the head (Fig. 94.1). The two lesions on the body were located on the right side near the dorsal fin and on the left side toward the tail. The lesion on the head was just caudal to the left eye.

A mucus scraping was performed after sedation of the fish using a 50 ppm concentration of tricaine methanesulfonate (MS-222). A wet mount preparation was made for immediate analysis (Figs. 94.2a–94.2d).

Interpretive Discussion

Figures 94.2a–94.2c show a monogenean parasite, *Gyrodactlylus*. This parasite may be found on freshwater or marine fish during stressful situations. This organism moves along the surface of the fish by extending its body and attaching its haptor to the skin, gills, or fins (Campbell and Ellis, 2007). The haptors are located on the caudal end of the parasite where 2 hooks and up to 16 hooklets are located (Gratzek, 1993; Noga, 2000). The cranial portion exhibits the V-shaped head. The circular area seen in the body is the embryo.

Figure 94.2d shows a protozoan, *Trichodina*. These parasites may also be found on freshwater and marine fish. This is a round ciliate protozoan with a ring of internal denticles (Campbell and Ellis, 2007). It is not uncommon for compromised fish to exhibit different parasitic infestations such as in this case.

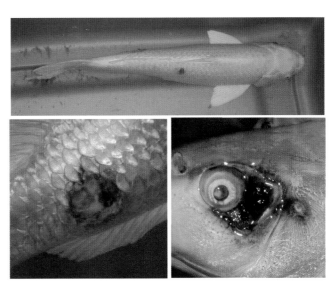

Fig. 94.1. The Koi on presentation and during physical examination.

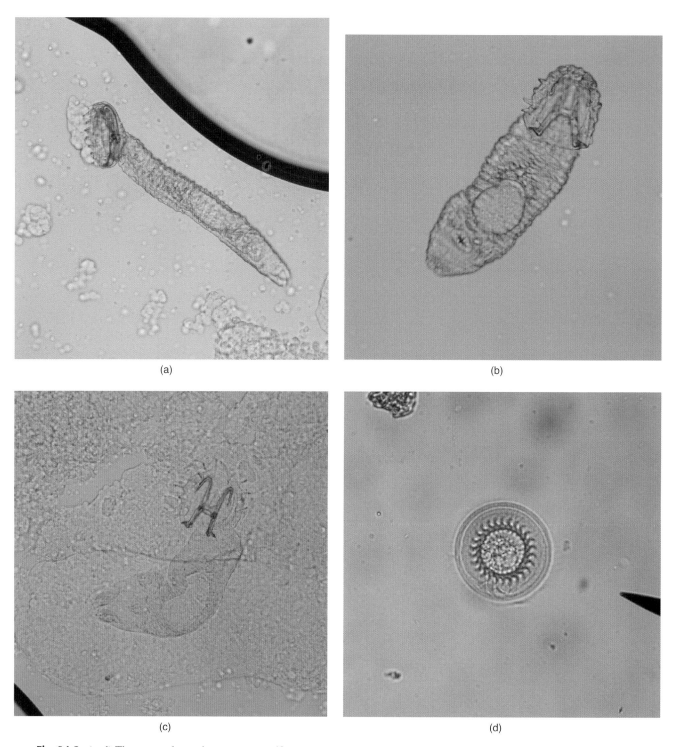

(a)

(b)

(c)

(d)

Fig. 94.2. (a–d) The mucosal scraping wet mount, 40×.

Summary

Ulcer disease associated with *Aeromonas* species and/or ectoparasitism is common among Koi (Wildgoose, 1998). These pathogens may rapidly reproduce during stressful situations, such as poor water quality, thus threatening the health of the fish. It is difficult to determine if the initial condition of the fish in this case was primarily caused from the presumed bacterial infection or an ectoparasite, such as *Gyrodactylus*, that may act as a vector in spreading bacterial pathogens (Cusack and Cone, 1985, 1986). Regardless, it is important to treat both the bacterial infection and the parasitic infestation. This fish was treated with enrofloxacin (0.1 mL/6 inches of fish or 14 mg/kg IM daily for 3 days, then every other day for two treatments) for the *Aeromonas* infection. It was also treated with praziquantel for the monogenean infestation.

The owner reported that this fish recovered after treatment; however, other fish suffered from similar clinical signs approximately 6 months later. These conditions can be difficult to control as shown in other reports (Wildgoose, 1998). The owner was prescribed ciprofloxacin, which was to be given in the following gel diet recipe:

Add together and blend:
- Two and one-fourth cups pellet diet ground into powder
- Two and half cups water
- Twenty-five milliliters cod liver oil (optional)
- Twenty-five milliliters vegetable oil (optional)
- One can sardine, tuna, or spinach baby food
- Add powdered ciprofloxacin (250 mg tablet)

Prepare gelatin:
- Two and half cups boiling water
- Add ten packets (1/4 oz) of unflavored gelatin
- Allow to begin to set up before adding all together
- Place in a large ice cube tray
- Cut up when feeding; feed for 10–14 days

The owner prepared the medicated diet to give to the entire pond population in an effort to control the disease.

REFERENCES

Barker G. 2001. Bacterial diseases. In *BSAVA Manual of Ornamental Fish*, 2nd ed., edited by Wildgoose WH. Quedgeley, UK: British Small Animal Veterinary Association, pp. 185–193.

Bavelaar FJ, Beynen AC. 2003. Severity of atherosclerosis in parrots in relation to the intake of α-linolenic acid. *Avian Diseases* 47:566–577.

Briggs L, Burgin S. 2003. A rapid technique to detect chytrid infection in adult frogs. *Herpetological Review* 34:124–126.

Bryden SL, Burrows AK, O'Hara AJ. 2004. *Mycobacterium goodii* infection in a dog with concurrent hyperadrenocorticism. *Veterinary Dermatology* 15:331–338.

Cain DK, Harms CA, Segars A. 2004. Plasma biochemistry reference values of wild-caught Southern Stingrays (*Dasyatis Americana*). *Journal of Wildlife and Zoo Medicine* 35(4): 471–476.

Campbell TW. 2000. Normal hematology of waterfowl. In *Schalm's Veterinary Hematology* 5th ed., edited by Feldman BF, Zinkl JG, Jain NC. Philadelphia, PA: Lippencott Williams & Wilkins, pp. 1161–1163.

Campbell TW, Ellis CS. 2007. *Avian and Exotic Animal Hematology and Cytology*, 3rd ed. Ames, IA: Blackwell Publishing.

Carpenter JW. 2005. *Exotic Animal Formulary*, 3rd ed. St. Louis, MO: Elsevier Saunders.

Coles EH. 1986. Erythrocytes. In *Veterinary Clinical Pathology*, 4th ed., edited by Coles EH. Philadelphia, PA: WB Saunders, p. 32.

Cray C. 2000. Blood and chemistry tables. In *Manual of Avian Medicine*, edited by Olsen G, Orosz S. St. Louis, MO: Mosby.

Cusack R, Cone DK. 1985. A report of bacterial microcolonies on the surface of *Gyrodactylus* (Monogenea). *Journal of Fish Diseases* 8:125–127.

Cusack R, Cone DK. 1986. A review of parasites as vectors of viral and bacterial diseases of fish. *Journal of Fish Diseases* 9:169–171.

Depaolo LV, Masoro EJ. 1989. Endocrine hormones in laboratory animals. In *The Clinical Chemistry of Laboratory Animals*, edited by Loeb WF, Quimby FW. NY: Pergamon Press, pp. 279–308.

Diethelm G. 2005. Reptiles. In *Exotic Animal Formulary*, 3rd ed., edited by Carpenter JW. St. Louis, MO: Elsevier Saunders, pp. 100–101.

Diethelm G, Stein G. 2006. Hematologic and blood chemistry values in reptiles. In *Reptile Medicine and Surgery*, 2nd ed., edited by Mader D. St. Louis, MO: Saunders Elsevier.

Fernandez-Beneitez MJ, Ortiz-Santaliestra ME, Lizana M, Dieguez-Uribeondo J. 2008. Saprolegnia diclina: Another species responsible for the emergent disease "*Saprolegnia* infections" in amphibians. *FEMS Microbiology Letters* 279:23–29.

Fettman MJ. 2004. Fluid and electrolyte metabolism. In *Veterinary Hematology and Clinical Chemistry*, edited by Thrall MA. Philadelphia, PA: Lippincott Williams & Wilkins, pp. 329–353.

Fox JG. 1988. Normal clinical and biological parameters. In *Biology and Diseases of the Ferret*, edited by Fox JG. Philadelphia, PA: Lea and Febiger, pp. 159–173.

Graesser D, Spraker TR, Dressen P, Garner MM, Raymond JT, Terwilliger G, Kim J, Madri JA. 2006. Wobbly hedgehog syndrome in African pygmy hedgehogs (*Atelerix* spp). *Journal of Exotic Pet Medicine* 15:59–65.

Gratzek JB. 1993. Parasites associated with freshwater and tropical fishes. In *Fish Medicine*, edited by Stoskopf MK. Philadelphia, PA: W.B. Saunders Company, pp. 573–593.

Hamlett WC, Koob TJ. 1999. Female reproductive system. In *Sharks, Skates, and Rays the Biology of Elasmobranch Fishes*, edited by Hamlett WC. Baltimore, MD: The Johns Hopkins University Press, pp. 417–420.

Hawkey CM, Samour JH. 1988. The value of clinical hematology in exotic birds. In *Exotic Animals: Contemporary Issues in Small Animal Practice*, edited by Jacobson ER, Kollias GV Jr. London: Churchill Livingstone.

Hess L. 2005. Ferret lymphoma: The old and the new. *Seminars in Avian and Exotic Pet Medicine* 14 (3):199–204.

Jackson CA, deLahunta A, Dykes NL, Divers TJ. 1994. Neurological manifestation of cholesterinic granulomas in three horses. *Veterinary Record* 135:228–230.

Johnston-Delaney CA, Harrison LR (eds.). 1996. *Exotic Companion Medicine Handbook for Veterinarians*. Lake Worth, FL: Wingers Publishing.

Lassen ED. 2004a. Laboratory evaluation of the exocrine pancreas. In *Veterinary Hematology and Clinical Chemistry*, edited by Thrall MA. Phladelphia, PA: Lippincott Williams & Wilkins, pp. 377–385.

Lassen ED. 2004b. Laboratory evaluation of the liver. In *Veterinary Hematology and Clinical Chemistry*, edited by Thrall MA. Phladelphia, PA: Lippincott Williams & Wilkins, pp. 355–375.

371

Lewbart GA. 2005. Fish. In *Exotic Animal Formulary*, 3rd ed., edited by Carpenter J. St. Louis, MO: Elsevier Saunders, p. 24.

Magi GE, Iannacconne M, Gili C, Rossi C. 2009. Cardiac cholesterol granuloma in a piper gurnard, *Trigla lyra* (L.). *Journal of Fish Disease* 32:473–475.

Marcos R, Santos M, Oliveira J, Vieira MJ, Vierira AL, Rocha E. 2006. Cytochemical detection of calcium in a case of calcinosis circumscripta in a dog. *Veterinary Clinical Pathology* 35:239–242.

Mulley RC. 1979. Haematology and blood chemistry of the black duck (*Anas superciliosa*). *Journal of Wildlife Diseases* 15:437–441.

Mulley RC. 1980. Haematology of the wood duck (*Chenoneta jubata*). *Journal of Wildlife Diseases* 16:271–273.

Mylniczenko N. 2009. Amphibians. In *Manual of Exotic Pet Practice*, edited by Mitchell MA, Tully TN. St. Louis, MO: Saunders Elsevier, pp. 73–111.

Nevarez J. 2009. Lizards. In *Manual of Exotic Pet Practice*, edited by Mitchell MA, Tully TN. St. Louis, MO: Saunders Elsevier, pp. 164–206.

Noga EJ. 2000. *Fish Disease Diagnosis and Treatment*. Ames, IA: Blackwell Publishing.

Olson KR. 1999. Rectal gland and volume homeostasis. In *Sharks, Skates, and Rays the Biology of Elasmobranch Fishes*, edited by Hamlett WC. Baltimore, MD: The Johns Hopkins University Press, pp. 329–352.

Pessier AP, Nichols DK, Longcore JE, Fuller MS. 1999. Cutaneous chytridiomycosis in poison dart frogs (*Dendrobates* spp) and white's tree frogs (*Litoria caerulea*). *Journal of Veterinary Diagnostic Investigation* 11:194–199.

Pollack C, Carpenter JW, Antinoff, N. 2005. Birds. In *Exotic Animal Formulary*, 3rd ed., edited by Carpenter J. St. Louis, MO: Elsevier Saunders, p. 268.

Quesenberry KE, Donnelly TM, Hillyer EV. 2006. Biology, husbandry, and clinical techniques of guinea pigs and chinchillas. In *Ferrets, Rabbits, and Rodents Clinical Medicine and Surgery*, 2nd ed., edited by Quesenberry KE, Carpenter JW. Philadelphia, PA: WB Saunders.

Saunders DC. 1958. The occurrence of *Haemogregarina bigemina*, Laverna and Mesnil, and *H. dasyatus* N. sp. in marine fish from Bimini, Bahams, B.W.I. *Transactions of the American Microscopical Society* 77(4):404–412.

Schmidt RE, Reavill DR, Phalen DN. 2003. *Pathology of Pet and Aviary Birds*. Ames, IA: Wiley-Blackwell.

Schultze AE. 2000. Interpretation of canine leukocyte responses. In *Schalm's Veterinary Hematology*, 5th ed., edited by Feldman BF, Zinkl JG, Jain NC. Philadelphia, PA: Lippincott Williams & Wilkins, pp. 366–381.

Sedacca CD, Campbell TW, Bright JM, Webb BT, Aboellail TA. 2009. Chronic cor pulmonale secondary to pulmonary atheroscerlosis in an African Grey parrot. *Journal of the American Veterinary Medical Association* 234:1055–1059.

Straub J, Pees M, Krautwald-Junghanns M-E. 2002. Measurement of the cardiac silhouette in psittacines. *Journal of the American Veterinary Medical Association* 221:76–79.

Sykes JM, Garner MM, Greer LL, Lung NP, Coke RL, Ridgley F, Bush M, Montali RJ, Okimoto B, Schmidt R, Allen JL, Rideout BA, Pesavento PA, Ramsay EC. 2007. Oral eosinophilic granulomas in tigers (*Panthera tigris*)—a collection of 16 cases. *Journal of Zoo and Wildlife Medicine* 38(2):300–308.

Thrall MA. 2004. Erythrocyte morphology. In *Veterinary Hematology and Clinical Chemistry*, edited by Thrall MA. Philadelphia, PA: Lippincott Williams & Wilkins, pp. 69–82.

Walker D. 1999. Peripheral blood smears. In *Diagnostic Cytology and Hematology of the Dog and Cat*, edited by Cowell RL, Tyler RD, Meinkoth JH. St. Louis, MO: Mosby, Inc., pp. 254–283.

Wildgoose WH. 1998. Twelv-month study of ulcer disease in a pond of koi carp (*Cyrinus carpio*). *Fish Veterinary Journal* 2:13–28.

Williams BH, Weiss CA. 2004. Neoplasia. In *Ferrets, Rabbits and Rodents*, 2nd ed., edited by Quesenberry KE, Carpenter JW. Philadelphia, PA: WB Sauders, pp. 91–106.

Zinkl JG. Avian hematology. 1986. In *Shalm's Veterinary Hematology*, 4th ed., edited by Jain NC. Philadelphia, PA: Lea & Febiger, pp. 256–273.

INDEX